CONTENTS

Special Issue: Plasticity in Spatial Neglect – Recovery and Rehabilitation
Guest Editors: Georg Kerkhoff and Yves Rosetti

Editorial
   G. Kerkhoff and Y. Rossetti — 201

Basic mechanisms

Impact of neglect on functional outcome after stroke – a review of methodological issues and recent research findings
   M. Jehkonen, M. Laihosalo and J.E. Kettunen — 209

Neglect and extinction: Within and between sensory modalities
   C. Brozzoli, M.L. Dematté, F. Pavani, F. Frassinetti and A. Farnè — 217

Stimulus- and goal-driven biases of selective attention following unilateral brain damage: Implications for rehabilitation of spatial neglect and extinction
   J.C. Snow and J.B. Mattingley — 233

Anosognosia for motor and sensory deficits after unilateral brain damage: A review
   G. Vallar and R. Ronchi — 247

Diagnostic issues

What do eye-fixation patterns tell us about unilateral spatial neglect?
   S. Ishiai — 261

A battery of tests for the quantitative assessment of unilateral neglect
   P. Azouvi, P. Bartolomeo, J.-M. Beis, D. Perennou, P. Pradat-Diehl and M. Rousseaux — 273

Spatial and non-spatial attention deficits in neurodegenerative diseases: Assessment based on Bundesen's theory of visual attention (TVA)
   P. Bublak, P. Redel and K. Finke — 287

Construction and psychometric properties of a novel test for body representational neglect (Vest Test)
   D. Glocker, P. Bittl and G. Kerkhoff — 303

Postural disorders and spatial neglect in stroke patients: A strong association
   D. Pérennou — 319

Treatment techniques

Development of a rehabilitative program for unilateral neglect
   L. Pizzamiglio, C. Guariglia, G. Antonucci and P. Zoccolotti — 337

Neglect and prism adaptation: A new therapeutic tool for spatial cognition disorders
   G. Rode, T. Klos, S. Courtois-Jacquin, Y. Rossetti and L. Pisella — 347

Repetitive optokinetic stimulation induces lasting recovery from visual neglect
   G. Kerkhoff, I. Keller, V. Ritter and C. Marquardt — 357

Alertness-training in neglect: Behavioral and imaging results
   W. Sturm, M. Thimm, J. Küst, H. Karbe and G.R. Fink — 371

Using limb movements to improve spatial neglect: The role of functional electrical stimulation
   G.A. Eskes and B. Butler   385

Future directions for research and treatment

The need for randomised treatment studies in neglect research
   N.B. Lincoln and A. Bowen   401

Prism adaptation first among equals in alleviating left neglect: A review
   J. Luauté, P. Halligan, G. Rode, S. Jacquin-Courtois and D. Boisson   409

Simulating unilateral neglect in normals: Myth or reality?
   C. Michel   419

Virtual reality applications for the remapping of space in neglect patients
   C. Ansuini, A.C. Pierno, D. Lusher and U. Castiello   431

Author Index Volume 24 (2006)   443

Editorial

Plasticity in Spatial Neglect – Recovery and rehabilitation

G. Kerkhoff[a,*] and Y. Rossetti[b]

[a]Clinical Neuropsychology Unit, Department of Psychology, Saarland University, Postbox 151150, 66041 Saarbrucken, Germany
[b]Espace et Action, UMR-S 534 INSERM et Université Claude Bernard, 16 avenue Lepine, 69676 Bron, France
Tel.: Lab: +33 4 72 91 34 16; Hospital: +33 4 78 86 50 23; Fax: +33 4 72 91 34 01;
E-mail: rossetti@lyon.inserm.fr/yves.rossetti@chu-lyon.fr

1. Scientific perspective

Hemineglect (synonymous: unilateral spatial neglect) denotes the impaired or lost ability to react to or process sensory stimuli (visual, auditory, tactile, olfactory, imaginal) presented in the hemispace contralateral to a lesioned cerebral hemisphere or to act upon such stimuli motorically (motor neglect). Despite recovery of the most obvious signs of hemineglect in the first 2–3 months after stroke a considerable portion of neglect patients – especially those with *large* right-hemispheric lesions – remains severely impaired in cognitive and motor tasks, as well as in functional activities of daily living (ADL). Apart from its clinical significance, neglect has attracted many researchers from different faculties because of its multifaceted nature, the associated breakdown of conscious awareness found in victims with this disease, as well as the multimodal nature of the syndrome which provides fascinating opportunities to study crossmodal integration and attention as well as spatial orientation and representation.

Although much progress has been made in the understanding of the basic impairments in spatial neglect in the past two decades, which is documented by many conferences held, numerous conference proceedings and text books, only recently significant progress has been made in the development and evaluation of novel treatment approaches for patients with neglect. This lag is partially explained by the fact that theory-based treatment-approaches can only be developed when new theories for the explanation of the basic mechanisms have been formulated and tested experimentally. Another reason may be the fact that controlled and randomized large-scale treatment studies require tremendous efforts and resources, both with respect to the availability of clinics, patients, treatments, potential financial incomes and researchers designing and coordinating such studies.

Clinically, spatial neglect and associated disorders are a major neurological handicap in many societies. The incidence of stroke in man is relatively high in all societies and will probably rise with increasing age, at least in most societies. Spatial neglect occurs in some 25–30% of all stroke patients, which means that 3–5 million *new* victims will suffer from neglect every year worldwide. Despite recovery of the most obvious signs of the disease in a portion of these, chronic impairments will persist in the remaining persons for years or even the rest of their life. While motor system plasticity as well as language recovery following stroke have been repeatedly a scientific topic the recovery of spatial

---

*Corresponding author: Clinical Neuropsychology Unit, Department of Psychology, Saarland University, Postbox 151150, 66041 Saarbrucken, Germany. Tel.: +49 681 302 57380; Fax: +49 681 302 57382; E-mail: kerkhoff@mx.uni-saarland.de.

0922-6028/06/$17.00 © 2006 – IOS Press and the authors. All rights reserved

neglect – both naturally and by treatment interventions – has only recently moved into the focus of researchers.

Therefore, as guest editors of this special issue of RNN we thought that time is mature to focus especially on those topics of neglect which are related to plasticity (both behavioural and neural), recovery, improved diagnostics, novel treatment techniques and their outcome. We therefore invited many of the leading researchers in this field from Australia, Canada, Finland, France, Germany, Great Britain, Italy and Japan, to collate lab reviews or broader topical reviews that might guide the reader to novel, influential ideas, improved diagnostic and treatment techniques as well as to fruitful concepts for future research and applications in this field. While a complete coverage of all relevant research was definitely beyond the scope of this special issue we selected 18 different contributions dealing with basic mechanisms of neglect, extinction and unawareness, diagnostic issues, treatment techniques, and perspectives for future research. We trust that this broad collection of papers will be stimulating both for researchers interested in basic mechanisms of spatial neglect as well as clinicians involved in the clinical management of patients with neglect. Furthermore, this broad focus may facilitate the scientific cross-talk between specialists in basic science and others primarily interested in clinical applications and treatment.

2. Basic mechanisms of neglect and associated disorders

The review by Jehkonen, Laihosalo and Kettunen from Tampere/Finland [9] addresses major aspects regarding the impact of neglect on functional outcome after stroke. While the negative impact of neglect on the patient's outcome is common knowledge, few is known about the long-term outcome. The available studies with respect to the long-term outcome of neglect have often relied on test scores instead of measuring functional activities, motor or cognitive functions related to daily life. In the light of the international classification of diseases (ICF) it is essential for future studies not only to collect test scores, but also to include motor, cognitive and social activity measures when studying the effects of neglect and neglect therapy. This will provide a more accurate figure of the limits but also of the resources of the patients suffering from spatial neglect, as well as their families caring for them. By the same logic, treatment studies should in the future also include measures of activities and participation to measure outcome in order to show whether these can be improved by a specific intervention. This could – in the long run – improve the management of neglect patients. Furthermore, homogenous patient groups should be used, and the knowledge about right-sided neglect after left-hemisphere lesions is very limited.

In the second article Brozzoli, Dematté, Pavani, Frassinetti and Farné (Lyon/France, Trento/Italy, Bologna/Italy) [4] deal with the complex interplay of neglect and extinction within and between sensory modalities. While formerly extinction has been considered as a minor form of neglect during its recovery stage this view is no longer tenable. Neglect occurs without extinction and vice versa. These double dissociations and the interplay of different modalities show that both disorders have different mechanisms (both behavioural and neural), but share similar principles of multimodal and crossmodal integration. Thus, most patients with visual neglect will also have auditory or somatosensory neglect. Furthermore, the authors highlight novel findings about neglect and extinction in the so-called "lower senses", olfaction and taste. The final message of this review is that a deeper understanding of the multisensory nature of the deficits in neglect and extinction will eventually lead to more powerful, multisensory-based rehabilitation approaches.

In the following review Snow (Birmingham/UK) and Mattingley (Melbourne/Australia) [16] point to the need to distinguish between stimulus-driven and goal-driven aspects of patients' selective attention deficits. They discuss the interaction between bottom-up factors, such as stimulus salience, and top-down factors, such as task goals, in the manifestations of spatial neglect and extinction. They argue that these conditions are characterised by a failure to integrate bottom-up and top-down neural signals, with specific reference to impairments of stimulus selection that affect the ipsilesional side of space.

A special issue about neglect would be incomplete without dealing with one of the most conspicuous features of neglect patients: their unawareness (anosognosia) of the(ir) disease. Vallar and Ronchi (both at Milano/Italy) [18] summarize all relevant published studies on unawareness of hemiplegia and hemianopia after brain damage including a recent neuroanatomic analysis of the lesions in patients showing neglect with and without anosognosia. In summary, these data show that although neglect and unawareness are indeed often combined, the may dissociate in single cases. Analysis of the lesions shows that anosognosia for hemiplegia most often is found after lesions to the motor cortex, hence lesions causing the hemiplegia. The authors frame their review with a theory of unawareness according to which awareness of motor functions (i.e. intactness of one's own limbs) is generated within the same cortical regions that are involved in motor control. Put differently, motor functions and motor awareness are coded in neighbouring or even identical cortical regions.

3. Diagnostic issues

While the bedside-assessment of neglect phenomena in acute stroke patients does not require very sophisticated instruments such tests have only limited value in detecting nonvisual neglect, and are often useless in detecting chronic or more subtle neglect phenomena. Therefore, other techniques are required. A more sophisticated analysis of visual neglect phenomena is dealt with in the review by Ishiai (Tokio/Japan) [8]. His results indicate that in patients with neglect, the representational image of a horizontal line may be formed on the basis of the attended segment between the right endpoint and the favored point of fixation. As the favored point of fixation is nearly always shifted to the ipsilesional side, the resulting bisection is mostly shifted to this side. Furthermore, these eye movement analyses show clearly that neglect patients do not explore the contralesional part of a line during line bisection tasks. Thus, the combination of eye tracking devices with line bisection tasks may further elucidate the mechanisms underlying neglect. This elegant combination of behavioural and oculomotor techniques might eventually be used for other domains of neglect as well.

The comparison of neglect in different studies is often difficult due to the use of different screening tests for the diagnosis of neglect. The lack of standardized, internationally adapted measures that all researchers agree on often lead in the past to largely diverging results between different studies. We therefore believe that it is necessary in the future – as in other areas of medicine or psychology – to use standardized, internationally available test instruments. One such new instrument is the test battery developed and normed by the French group on neglect including Azouvi (Garches/France), Bartolomeo (Paris/France), Beis (Nancy/France), Pérennou (Dijon/France), Pradat-Diehl (Paris/France) and Rousseau (Lille/France) [2]. They collected normative values on a large patient sample ($n = 456$–472) in a test battery including paper-and-pencil-tests, an assessment of personal neglect, extinction, anosognosia and a behavioural rating of neglect by staff. Their results show that a multifaceted diagnostic approach is more sensitive to neglect and that paper-and-pencil-tests may miss neglect phenomena that are readily detected by behavioural ratings or behavioural tests of neglect. Another important finding is that age, education and acting hand may influence the performance already in normal subjects and therefore these factors have to be controlled for.

The complex interplay between lateralized and non-lateralized attentional capabilities in neurodegenerative diseases is highlighted in the contribution by Bublak (Jena/Germany) and Finke (München/Germany) [5]. While spatially non-lateralized impairments of attention and working memory have been reported in a number of recent studies in neglect patients suffering from stroke, there exist only few methods to delineate these deficits in greater detail. Furthermore, subtle disturbances – as seen frequently in slowly progressive degenerative disease – can not be precisely mapped with these methods. Bublak and Finke suggest the assessment of nonlateralized and lateralized attentional capacities by techniques based on Bundesen's theory of visual attention. This is a parameter-based estimation of visual perceptual processing speed, visual working memory storage, and spatial attentional weighting. Their lab-review shows that this method is highly sensitive to detect subtle pathological impairments in neurodegenerative disease, and to delineate different profiles of impairments in different diseases (i.e. Alzheimer's versus Huntington's disease).

In the next article Glocker, Bittl (both from Eichstätt/Germany) and Kerkhoff (Saarbrücken/Germany) [7] describe the development, psychometric validation and clinical results of a novel test designed to assess body representational neglect. Little is known about body neglect and its relationship to other forms of neglect. One reason is the lack of standardized tests to detect it. The authors show that the novel test is highly reliable and sensitive and that nearly 80% of right-brain and 47% of left-brain damaged patients are impaired in this apparently simply test. Apart from this clinical significance, preliminary data show that body neglect and other neuropsychological disorders that also involve knowledge of the own body (apraxia) can be dissociated. This result may be taken as an indication of multiple cortical mechanisms devoted to different aspects of body knowledge (i.e. pantomiming hand gestures versus searching the own body surface).

In the last chapter of the diagnostic section Pérennou (Dijon/France) [13] provides a comprehensive review examining the association between postural disorders and neglect. While it is long known that patients with right-brain-damage have a poor motor outcome after stroke the reasons for this finding have been less clear. Unawareness, neglect and spatial disorders have been identified as influential factors. This review provides also a description of the most useful tasks and devices suitable for the measurement of postural deficits in stroke patients with neglect. Pérennou theorizes that postural disorders are so prominent in neglect because of disturbed graviceptive and visuospatial informations both subserving postural control. This review should encourage neglect researchers to incorporate postural measurements into their research as well as clinical assessment routines.

4. Treatment techniques

The treatment section covers five different types of treatment approaches for spatial neglect. In the first contribution, Pizzamiglio, Guariglia, Antonucci and Zoccolotti (all from Rome/Italy) [14] give a topical as well as historical review about the development of a rehabilitative program for unilateral neglect. This review, covering a period of the past 30 years, summarizes the major milestones in the development of the so-called visual scanning training, the first systematic and effective treatment for patients with neglect. Furthermore, typical problems in neglect rehabilitation are addressed (i.e. limited transfer to daily life). Rode (Lyon/France), Klos (Erlangen/Germany), Courtois-Jacquin (Lyon/France) and Rossetti (Lyon/France) [15] report novel findings of the prism-adaptation technique for the rehabilitation of spatial cognition disorders, i.e. spatial dysgraphia. Spatial dysgraphia and constructional apraxia are known for many decades but have been largely neglected by researchers. This contribution shows that prism adaptation improves spatial-cognitive abilities relevant for spatial writing number processing and constructional abilities.

In the subsequent contribution by Kerkhoff (Saarbrücken/Germany), Keller (Bad Aibling/Germany), Ritter and Marquardt (both Munich/Germany) [10] it is shown that optokinetic stimulation with active tracking of the moving targets by the patient yields significantly greater and lasting improvements as compared to the conventional scanning training procedure. While this does not necessarily imply to abandon scanning training it shows that this form of optokinetic training may be particularly useful in acute neglect patients because it does not require a consciuous, top-down-directed strategy for compensation. Sturm (Aachen/Germany), Thimm and Fink (both Aachen and Jülich/Germany) [17] summarize ongoing studies of alertness training in neglect patient and its effect on behavioural and neural measures of neglect. They show that alertness training leads to a reduction of neglect by recruitment of frontal cortical areas in both cerebral hemispheres, whereas optokinetic stimulation of the type designed by Kerkhoff et al. [10]. These results suggest the complementary use of attentional and optokinetic training procedures, which in turn might produce a combined and possibly greater behavioural recovery in neglect patients. Finally, in the last contribution of the treatment section Eskes and Butler (both Halifax/Canada) [6] show that the use of functional electrical stimulation may yield promising results in activating contralateral limb movements in those neglect patients with severely impaired motor functions due to hemiplegia. This novel combination approach might be an interesting avenue for future research and shows the potential when combining behavioural treatments with prosthetic or technical devices in neglect rehabiliation. Though space was too limited to deal with all currently available techniques in the treatment section, it summarizes novel ideas, provides updates of currently used techniques and suggests novel treatment combinations. Furthermore, the treatment potential when *combining* such single treatments – a common strategy in other areas of medicine and psychology – is not at all exhausted at the moment. The partially divergent profiles of action of the different treatments strongly suggest that an intelligent combination (not necessarily at the same time) could produce more, quicker and more stable treatment-induced recovery. This is not only clinically relevant, but poses also central basic science questions of how such integrative effects are enabled on the neuroanatomic and neurophysiological level.

5. Future directions for research and treatment

In this section Bowen and Lincoln (Nottingham/UK) [3] give a meta-analysis of the overall effects of neglect therapy. Their critical conclusion is also formulated in their title: there is a need for randomized treatment studies in neglect research because few studies so far used a randomized allocation to treatments. The most likely explanation for this is that the collection of large, homogenous patient groups takes years to complete – when one centre performs the study alone. This problem probably could be solved by conducting multicentre studies. Furthermore, the stability of the treatment effects is often evaluated only in short time intervals after the cessation of treatment. Finally, as already pointed out in the first contribution by Jehkonen et al. [9] functional tasks documenting treatment-induced recovery after a specific intervention have been used only very rarely. Hence, the best we can say at the moment is that neglect rehabilitation reduces neglect in neglect tasks – whether or not functional gains follow from such improvements is an open research question for the next years.

In the subsequent contribution Luauté (Lyon/France), Halligan (Cardiff, UK), Rode, Jacquin-Courtois and Boisson (Lyon/France) [11] give a comprehensive review of prism-adaptation studies in neglect rehabilitation. This therapeutic intervention is probably the best evaluated technique among the other novel treatment approaches, although no randomized control trial is available yet. Prism adaptation has been shown to affect patients with spatial neglect as well as normal subjects. C. Michel (Dijon/France) [12] studied neglect-like behaviour in healthy individuals and in particular the use of prism adaptation as a procedure for simulating various symptoms of clinical neglect in normals. Such neglect-like symptoms offer insights as to the mechanisms of spatial neglect and provides an understanding of the interaction between low level sensorimotor processes and spatial cognition. Implications for the functional mechanisms and the anatomical substrates of prism adaptation are discussed in terms of inter-sensory plasticity and sensorimotor coordination.

In the final contribution by Ansuini (Padova/Italy), Pierno (Padova/Italy), Lusher (Melbourne/Australia) and Castiello (London/UK and Padova/Italy) [1] the authors describe the effect of virtual reality applications for the remapping of contralesional (neglected) space in patients. The authors show that patients with lesions sparing the parietal cortex benefit from this novel technique. Their results also highlight the pivotal role of the parietal cortex for this induced remapping of neglected space.

6. Concluding remarks and further perspectives

Brain repair, adaptive reorganisation, compensatory strategies, prostheses and medications all can contribute to functional recovery from spatial neglect and associated disorders after brain damage. Animal experiments, functional imaging studies and longitudinal outcome studies suggest that injured brains can change their function and connectivity, both on the behavioural and neural level, and both spontaneously (i.e. without intervention) as well in response to specific treatments. However, many questions in this context remain still open. Some of these are: Is spontaneous recovery similar to treatment-induced-recovery? Which treatments are best in which type of neglect, and when after stroke? How often and how long should a treatment be applied? Could an enriched environment improve the outcome additionally, as suggested by animal experiments? Another interesting question is whether top-down-compensatory strategies and bottom-up stimulation maneuvers can be combined to yield a better outcome? Despite significant progress in the development of novel and more effective treatments in the past 10 years little is known about the long-term-stability of such treatment-related improvements (over a timescale of years after treatment). How can transfer to daily life be improved? What is the relative role of the anatomically intact and of the lesioned hemisphere in recovery? Furthermore, patients differ considerably in their individual response to the same type of treatment. Although lesion size, location, diffuse lesions and related factors are without doubt relevant here, individual psychological factors like motivation, intelligence and affective style have not been considered until now. As they all influence cognitive functioning and the underlying neural circuitry in the healthy brain these parameters might be relevant prognostic factors when researchers try to tailor individually optimized treatments. Finally, how can the unawareness issue be successfully addressed?

In conclusion, the study of these questions in spatial neglect provides excellent opportunities for an interdisciplinary exchange of research ideas between basic neuroscience, applied clinical neuropsychology, neurorehabilitation and neuro-technology.

Acknowledgements

This issue would have not been possible without the help of others. We are grateful to all authors for their dedicated contributions. We also gratefully acknowledge the reviewers work, the continuous help of St. Matzke from the editorial office of RNN, as well as the support of IOS press.

References

[1] C. Ansuini, A.C. Pierno, D. Lusher and U. Castiello, Virtual reality applications for the remapping of space in neglect patients, *Restor. Neurol. Neurosci.* **24**(4–6) (2006), 431–441.

[2] P. Azouvi, P. Bartolomeo, J.-M. Beis, D. Perennou, P. Pradat-Diehl and M. Rousseaux, A battery of tests for the quantitative assessment of unilateral neglect, *Restor. Neurol. Neurosci.* **24**(4–6) (2006), 273–285.

[3] A. Bowen and N.B. Lincoln, The need for randomized treatment studies in neglect research, *Restor. Neurol. Neurosci.* **24**(4–6) (2006), 401–408.

[4] C. Brozzoli, L. Demattè, F. Pavani, F. Frassinetti and A. Farne, Neglect and extinction: within and between sensory modalities, *Restor. Neurol. Neurosci.* **24**(4–6) (2006), 217–232.

[5] P. Bublak and K. Finke, Spatial and nonspatial attentional deficits in neurodegenerative diseases: Assessment based on Bundesen's theory of visual attention, *Restor. Neurol. Neurosci.* **24**(4–6) (2006), 287–301.

[6] G.A. Eskes and B. Butler, Using limb movements to improve neglect: the role of functional electrical stimulation, *Restor. Neurol. Neurosci.* **24**(4–6) (2006), 385–398.

[7] D. Glocker, P. Bittl and G. Kerkhoff, The Vest test: construction and psychometric validation of a novel test for the measurement of body representational neglect, *Restor. Neurol. Neurosci.* **24**(4–6) (2006), 303–317.

[8] S. Ishiai, Eye movement measurement in the diagnosis of visual neglect, *Restor. Neurol. Neurosci* **24**(4–6) (2006), 261–271.

[9] M. Jehkonen, M. Laihosalo and J.E. Kettunnen, Impact of neglect on functional outcome after stroke – a review of methodological issues and recent research findings, *Restor. Neurol. Neurosci.* **24**(4–6) (2006), 209–215.

[10] G. Kerkhoff, I. Keller, V. Ritter and C. Marquardt, Repetitive optokinetic stimulation with active tracking induces lasting recovery from visual neglect, *Restorative Neurology and Neuroscience* **24**(4–6) (2006), 357–369.

[11] J. Luauté, C. Michel, G. Rode, D. Boisson, P. Halligan and Y. Rossetti, Prism adaptation: first among equals in alleviating neglect – a review, *Restor. Neurol. Neurosci.* **24**(4–6) (2006), 409–418.

[12] C. Michel, Simulating unilateral neglect in normals: myth or reality? *Restor. Neurol. Neurosci.* **24**(4–6) (2006), 419–430.

[13] D. Perennou, Postural disorders and spatial neglect in stroke patients: a strong association, *Restor. Neurol. Neurosci.* **24**(4–6) (2006), 319–334.

[14] L. Pizzamiglio, C. Guariglia, G. Antonucci and P. Zoccolotti, Development of a rehabilitative program for unilateral neglect, *Restor. Neurol. Neurosci.* **24**(4–6) (2006), 337–345.

[15] G. Rode, T. Klos, S. Courtois-Jacquin, Y. Rossetti and L. Pisella, Neglect and prism adaptation: A new tool for spatial cognition disorders, *Restor. Neurol. Neurosci.* **24**(4–6) (2006), 347–356.

[16] J.C. Snow and J.B. Mattingley, Competition, salience and selection: interactions between bottom-up and top-down signals in spatial neglect and extinction, *Restor. Neurol. Neurosci.* **24**(4–6) (2006), 233–245.

[17] W. Sturm, M. Thimm and G.R. Fink, Alertness-Training in Neglect – Behavioural and Imaging Results, *Restor. Neurol. Neurosci.* **24**(4–6) (2006), 371–384.

[18] G. Vallar and R. Ronchi, Anosognosia for motor and sensory deficits after unilateral brain damage: A review, *Restor. Neurol. Neurosci.* **24**(4–6) (2006), 247–257.

Basic mechanisms

Impact of neglect on functional outcome after stroke – a review of methodological issues and recent research findings

M. Jehkonen*, M. Laihosalo and J.E. Kettunen
Tampere University Hospital, Department of Neurology and Rehabilitation, P.O. Box 2000, 33521 Tampere, Finland

Received 27 September 2005
Revised 4 January 2006
Accepted 3 February 2006

Abstract. *Purpose*: This study provides an update on recent research findings concerning neglect and its impact on functional outcome. The review covers studies published during the past ten years.
Methods: A systematic review was carried out on reports drawn from electronic databases (MEDLINE and PSYCHLIT, January 1996–August 2005) and identified from the lists of references in these reports. Unpublished reports, articles in other than the English language, and studies with non-human and non-adult subjects were excluded. The selection criteria were met by 26 articles.
Results: 15 of the 26 studies recruited heterogeneous patient groups (patients with right and left and/or unspecified lesions). The results from homogeneous groups (right hemisphere patients) were more consistent, emphasizing neglect as an independent predictor of functional outcome. Studies with homogeneous patient groups used consecutive series of patients, standardized measures of neglect, and a broader concept of functional outcome (both motor and cognitive items) than those with heterogeneous patient groups. Follow-ups longer than one year were very rare.
Conclusions: Neglect has a significant negative impact on functional outcome, either as an independent predictive factor or in connection with other variables. The results, however, are inevitably affected by differences in patient samples and in the methods used in assessing neglect and functional outcome. Research focusing on homogeneous patient groups and especially on left hemisphere patients is needed. Neglect should be assessed with a standardized test battery rather than a single test, and functional outcome should be measured with scales consisting of cognitive, social and motor items. Also longer follow-ups are needed to verify the long-term functional outcome of neglect patients.

Keywords: Stroke, neglect, perceptual disorders, daily living

1. Introduction

Neglect is characterised by failure to orient, report, or respond to stimuli located predominantly on the side opposite to the site of the brain lesion. The condition cannot be explained by either primary sensory or motor deficits [20]. In everyday life, patients with neglect often fail to shave or dress the left side of their body, fail to attend to events and people situated on the left, and collide with objects to their left. Several authors have found that presence of neglect predicts poor functional recovery and inability to manage activities of daily living (ADL) after stroke [8,24,25,28]. However, there are also conflicting findings which emphasize the impact of anosognosia instead of neglect on poor recovery and functional outcome [14,39]. These apparent discrepancies may be due to differences in patient se-

---

*Corresponding author: Mervi Jehkonen, PhD, Tampere University Hospital, P.O. Box 2000, 33521 Tampere, Finland. Tel.: +358 3 3116 6498; Fax: +358 3 3116 5314; E-mail: mervi.jehkonen@pshp.fi.

lection, the methods used in assessing neglect and outcome, and the amount of time elapsed between stroke onset and assessment.

Neglect is a heterogeneous syndrome and several different subtypes have been reported (e.g. motor neglect, personal neglect, visual neglect, representational neglect) [44]. Neglect can also be classified according to spatial domains, such as peripersonal (reaching space), personal (body space), extrapersonal (far space), and representational space [44]. Most tests are designed to evaluate neglect in the peripersonal space (e.g. line bisection, visual scanning and cancellation, copying and drawing). In addition, there are some tests measuring other than peripersonal space, e.g. the Fluff test [10] or Comb and Razor/compact task evaluating the personal domain [48]. It is unlikely then that any single test can provide a sufficient evaluation of all forms of neglect. The sensitivity of different neglect tests varies widely according to their ability to measure the underlying deficits [18]. One of the most frequently used test batteries in clinical practice and neglect research is the Behavioural Inattention Test (BIT) [46]. Another widely used standardized test battery for screening neglect has been developed by Pizzamiglio et al. [42].

Wade [45] says that the term ADL refers to the basic, physical functions that underlie normal living, such as going to the toilet, dressing, and walking. This definition stresses the purely motor aspects of recovery, but there are also several comprehensive measures that additionally take into account the cognitive and social domains when evaluating overall disability after stroke. The most widely used ADL scales are those that emphasize motor functions, e.g. the Barthel Index (BI) [31], the Katz ADL Index (KADLI) [27], and the Rivermead Mobility Index (RMI) [11]. Well-known extended ADL scales include the Functional Independence Measure (FIM) [17], which comprises both motor and cognitive subscales, and the Frenchay Activities Index (FAI) [21], which considers social activities as well as motor and cognitive domains.

The presence of neglect and its impact on recovery has received extensive attention in the literature, which has been reviewed among others by Ferro and collaborators [13]. The first author of this paper also provided an overview in her dissertation [23]. However, we were unable to find any recent systematic reviews.

Our review here gives a systematic update on research findings concerning the influence of neglect on functional outcome after stroke during the past ten years (from January 1996 to August 2005). It covers the following aspects of neglect and patients' functional recovery: patient selection, evaluation methods, timing of the assessment(s) after stroke, and variables affecting functional outcome.

2. Materials and methods

2.1. Definition of the main terms used in the search

Because there are so many different subtypes, neglect is described in the literature by a variety of different concepts. The terms that appear most frequently are *neglect* and *perceptual disorders*. Some of the studies we reviewed were concentrated on specific subtypes of the clinical syndrome of neglect. Since we wanted to include all these studies in our review, we started our search with the general terms of *neglect* or *perceptual disorders*. In data analysis it was not possible to distinguish between the subtypes of neglect since most of the studies were concerned with visual neglect.

Functional abilities were also described with a wide range of definitions and at different levels of accuracy. In our search we used the general term of *daily living* in order not to exclude any study that might have been focused on a specific functional ability. Studies selected for inclusion in our review were to have used some commonly known ADL scale.

2.2. Selection of articles

We used the same method that has been used in earlier reviews [5,9,41] to identify the relevant literature. The first step was to search the Cochrane Library database in order to see whether there were any recent or ongoing reviews on this subject, but we found none.

All published studies reporting data on the impact of neglect on functional outcome after stroke were included in this review. Those studies were also included that were primarily concerned to determine the effect of neglect on daily living. Likewise, we chose to include studies that were interested in general recovery from stroke, provided that the data on the recovery of neglect patients in activities of daily living could be examined independently.

We searched MEDLINE and PSYCHLIT for articles published between January 1996 and August 2005. The search was carried out using terms *stroke, neglect, perceptual disorders,* and *daily living*. The exclusion criteria were as follows: 1) non-English articles, 2) studies on non-human and 3) non-adult subjects (< 19 years) and 4) articles published before January 1996.

We found 337 articles and read the abstracts of all of them. Next, studies that were concerned exclusively with the effects of a specific intervention method, case reports, studies failing to specify any functional outcome measure after stroke, theoretical articles or reviews, and experimental studies were excluded. Neither book chapters nor published letters were included. These criteria were met by 22 of the 337 abstracts. The full articles of these 22 studies were reviewed and their lists of references searched; this yielded four additional articles. The total number of articles reviewed for this study was thus 26.

For our review we collected data on the selection of patients, the methods used to assess neglect and outcome, the timing of assessment(s) and variables affecting the functional outcome. All the studies were checked by three independent reviewers.

3. Results

3.1. Demographic and clinical data

The sample sizes and patients' characteristics are described in Table 1. The number of patients in the 26 studies included in our review ranged from 32 to 602 (median 146), and their mean age from 57 to 76 years (not specified in three studies) [22,26,38] (median 68 years). Eleven (42%) [3,6–8,12,16,24,25,28,30,34] of the 26 studies, recruited only right hemisphere damaged patients (RH). Seven (27%) [32,33,35–37,40,43] studies had both right and left hemisphere patients (RH and LH) and five (19%) [1,2,15,22,47] studies included RH and LH patient groups and also patients whose lesion laterality was not classified (NUD). In three (12%) [26,29,38] studies the patients' lesion laterality was not clearly stated (NUD). The etiology of stroke (infarction, hemorrhage, or other) is given in Table 1.

3.2. Patient selection

In 13 (50%) studies [7,8,12,15,24,26,28,29,33–37] the patient sample was drawn from consecutive cases of stroke, either at admission to general hospitals ($n = 3$) or to rehabilitation facilities ($n = 9$). The setting of the consecutive cases was not specified in one [12] of these studies. Five (19%) studies [3,25,30,32,43] recruited selected groups of patients and four (15%) studies [1,2,40,47] were community-based. Three (12%) studies [6,16,22] were retrospective and one (4%) was a population-based study [38]. Table 2 provides a detailed summary of patient selection in each subgroup.

Table 1
Sample sizes and characteristics of the subgroups in the 26 studies reviewed

	No. of studies
I Studies with only RH patients	11
of which:	
only infarct patients	3
only hemorrhage patients	1
infarct and hemorrhage patients	3
infarct and hemorrhage and other patients	0
not specified	4
No. of patients	32–178 (Md 52)
II Studies with RH and LH patients	7
of which:	
only infarct patients	0
infarct and hemorrhage patients	4
infarct and hemorrhage and other patients	1
not specified	2
No. of patients	100–602 (Md 157)
III Studies with RH, LH, and NUD patients	5
of which:	
only infarct patients	0
infarct and hemorrhage patients	0
infarct and hemorrhage and other patients	1
not specified	4
No. of patients	119–279 (Md 248)
IV Studies with NUD patients	3
of which:	
only infarct patients	1
infarct and hemorrhage patients	0
infarct and hemorrhage and other patients	1
not specified	1
No. of patients	100–179 (Md 146)

RH = Right hemisphere, LH = Left hemisphere,
NUD = Lesion laterality not classified,
Md = median.

3.3. Assessment methods and timing

3.3.1. Evaluation of neglect

Most of the studies concentrated on evaluating neglect at a general level rather than classifying it into subtypes. Neglect was assessed with a large variety of different tests, most of which assessed visual or peripersonal forms of neglect (e.g. copying/drawing, line bisection, cancellation tasks). In a few studies [1, 3,6,12] subtypes of neglect were specified at different levels of accuracy, with evaluations presented for example of personal and motor neglect. In 16 (62%) studies [1–3,6–8,12,24,25,28,33–37,43] a standardized test battery of neglect (the BIT or the four-test battery of Pizzamiglio et al.) was conducted, whereas four (15%) studies [22,26,30,40] applied two or more separate tests (e.g. cancellation tasks, line bisection, copying and drawing). Five (19%) studies [15,16,29,32,47] used only a single test to define neglect (e.g. cancellation tasks, line bisection). One study [38] did not specify its method of assessing neglect.

Table 2
Patient selection

	No. of studies
I Studies with only RH patients	
of which:	
consecutive series	6
selected groups	3
retrospective study	2
II Studies with RH and LH patients	
of which:	
consecutive series	4
selected groups	2
community based	1
III Studies with RH, LH and NUD patients	
of which:	
consecutive series	1
community based	3
retrospective study	1
IV Studies with NUD patients	
of which:	
consecutive series	2
population based	1

RH = Right hemisphere, LH = Left hemisphere, NUD = Lesion laterality not classified.

Table 3
Occurrence of the six most frequently used functional outcome measures

Measure of outcome	No. of studies using this measure*
Barthel Index	11
Functional Independence Measure	8
Length of Stay	4
Rivermead Mobility Index	4
Katz ADL Index	3
Frenchay Activities Index	3

*Note: Several studies used more than one measure.

3.3.2. Functional outcome measures

In 13 studies [1,2,7,12,26,29,30,33–37,40] functional outcome was measured with scales designed to assess motor abilities only (e.g. BI or KADLI); in nine studies [3,6,8,15,16,22,28,32,43] it was measured with scales assessing motor and cognitive abilities (e.g. FIM; the Functional Autonomy Measurement System, SMAF) [19]; and in three studies [24,38,47] with scales assessing motor, cognitive and social abilities (e.g. FAI). Another commonly used outcome measure was length of stay, e.g. the time from stroke to discharge to home. Table 3 lists the six most commonly used functional outcome measures.

3.3.3. Timing of the first evaluation and the follow-up studies

The timings of the first assessment (assessment of neglect and related neurological and neuropsychological disorders) and the follow-up measurements of func-

Table 4
Timing of assessments

	No. of studies
1st evaluation (range: 1–378 days)	
Interval between onset and 1st evaluation:	
less than 1 week	6
1–4 weeks	8
more than 4 weeks	11
not specified	1
Follow-up times (range: 8 weeks to 3 years)	
Interval between 1st evaluation and follow-up time:	
up to 3 months	8
over 3 months, up to 6 months	4
over 6 months, up to 12 months	8
over 12 months	3
no follow-up	3

tional outcome are shown in Table 4. The first assessment was made between 1 and 378 days after stroke. Most typically, the first assessment took place more than four weeks after onset (11 out of 26 studies). The timing of the follow-ups varied from two months to three years. The majority of the follow-up studies (16 out of 26) were performed either before three months [7,8,12,16,26,29,34,40] or between 6 to 12 months [2,3,15,22,24,25,28,47] after onset. Longer follow-ups than 12 months were rare [36–38]. In three studies [1,6,32] no follow-up was conducted. One of these was a cross-sectional study [6].

3.4. Main findings concerning outcome

With just one exception [40], all the 26 studies reviewed provided consistent results of the impact of neglect on functional outcome. In most studies neglect was addressed in general terms, without classifying it into different subtypes. Only four studies [1,3,6,12] made a distinction between subtypes of neglect, but none of them specified the possible impact of these subtypes on outcome.

In 11 studies [3,6–8,12,16,26,28,34,35,43] that used multivariate analyses, neglect was reported to have an independent predictive value on poor functional outcome, while in six studies [1,22,24,33,36,37] neglect had a predictive value together with one additional variable (age, hemiparesis, severity of stroke, anosognosia, other cognitive impairment). In eight studies [2,15,25,29,30,32,38,47] neglect predicted poor functional outcome in combination with more than one additional variable.

The independent negative effect of neglect on functional outcome was emphasized [3,6–8,12,16,28,34] most particularly in studies with homogeneous RH groups. These samples consisted mainly of consecutive series of patients [7,8,12,24,28,34], and they typically used a standardized battery for assessing neglect [3,6–8,12,24,25,28,34]. The most common functional outcome scales used in these homogeneous RH groups were the FIM [3,6,8,16,28] and the BI [7,30,34].

In heterogeneous patient groups (RH and LH; RH, LH and NUD; NUD) neglect was most frequently mentioned as one of the variables affecting the outcome; it was reported as having an independent predictive value in only three studies [26,35,43]. There was greater variation in patient selection in these studies than in the homogeneous RH groups, even though the samples were mainly based on consecutive series [15,26,29,33,35–37]. For purposes of assessing neglect, a standardized test battery was used in seven studies [1,2,33,35–37,43]. In most of these studies [1,2,26,29,33,35–37,40] the outcome was measured in terms of motor abilities only, and the most common functional outcome measure was the BI. Six studies [15,22,32,38,43,47] used functional scales measuring both motor and cognitive abilities.

As was mentioned earlier, one study [40] concluded that hemineglect per se has no negative prognostic value on functional outcome. Pedersen et al. [40] studied 602 consecutive stroke patients on admission. Visual neglect was assessed with a single cancellation task and anosognosia for hemiparesis and/or for hemianopia was evaluated using the procedure of Bisiach et al. [4]. Functional outcome was assessed by the BI, which emphasizes motor recovery after stroke. The assessments were made during the first week after admission, every week during the hospital stay, and at discharge. The authors suggested that anosognosia had an independent value in the prediction of the BI at discharge from hospital. However, the two forms of anosognosia were treated together in the analyses, making it impossible to determine which form of anosognosia was related to outcome.

Two studies [29,32] included neglect in a broad category of perceptual disorders, but offered no definition of the concept of neglect. In both these studies neglect was measured with a single test and the authors reported that perceptual factors contributed significantly to the outcome. Nevertheless, the independent value of neglect was not specifically analysed in either of these studies.

4. Discussion

The studies included in our review showed differences both in patient selection, in the accuracy of the methods used to assess neglect and functional outcome, and in the timing of the baseline and follow-up assessments. Differences were also seen in the results concerning the impact of neglect on functional outcome. Some of the studies indicated that neglect is an independent predictor of poor functional outcome, others reported that neglect has an impact on functional outcome only in connection with other factors. The reported incidence of neglect and the definition of functional outcome (purely motor versus motor, cognitive and social) are probably influenced by the range of different methods used, which therefore undermines the generalizability of the results.

The methods and criteria used in sampling the patients also varied. The samples included patients referred to rehabilitation centres as well as consecutive series of patients from a certain district. Moreover, the time intervals from stroke to the first assessments and follow-up assessments differed markedly between the studies. The last follow-up usually took place during the first year after onset, but there were also studies with very short follow-ups or no follow-up at all. The functional outcome of neglect patients after stroke was frequently evaluated in mixed or heterogeneous groups of patients with left and right hemisphere hemorrhagic or ischaemic stroke. Some studies even recruited patients whose type of stroke remained unclear. A minority of the studies reviewed concentrated on examining patients who only had hemorrhage [30] or patients who only had brain infarction [24–26,28]. This means that the outcome may be affected by a large number of confounding factors. Longer follow-ups are therefore needed to confirm the effect of neglect on long-term outcome.

The studies reviewed also had different definitions of the concepts of neglect and functional outcome and used different methods of assessment. Most of the studies addressed neglect as a general disorder, without specifying its subtypes. The few studies that did categorize neglect into subtypes failed to specify whether those subtypes had an effect on functional outcome. Although most studies used a standardized test battery of neglect, some were content to use a single task to define neglect. As Halligan et al. [18] have pointed out, however, neglect should not be assessed on the strength of just one single task, because several tests are more likely to uncover evidence of neglect than a single test. The effect of mild residual neglect on functional outcome was not evaluated in the studies reviewed, probably because of the lack of adequate tools available. In addition, many functional outcome measures emphasize motor functioning instead of social and cognitive abilities. There is a shortage of outcome measures that take into account the specific features of cognitive disorders and their impact on everyday functioning after stroke. The variety in definitions and methods used in assessing neglect and outcome therefore greatly complicates the task of comparing the results.

A few comments are also in order on the limitations of our review. The articles reviewed included five studies by Paolucci and collaborators [33–37], and the patient samples in some of their studies maybe be overlapping. The subjects in these studies were drawn from a consecutive series of patients referred to a rehabilitation institution, thus representing a selected sample of stroke patients, which should be taken into account when generalizing our results. The rehabilitation setting also affects the timing of first evaluation (usually more than one month after onset), which may be an additional confounding factor affecting the evaluation of outcome. In addition, three studies by Appelros and collaborators [1–3] were included. Two of these studies [1,2] included the same patients. The first study [1] was confined to the acute phase of stroke, while the second study [2] completed the results with a one-year follow-up. There were also two other studies [6,32] that involved no follow-up, but that evaluated neglect and functional outcome at the same point of time. These studies were included in the review because they met the inclusion criteria of our study and because we wanted to illustrate the wide range of studies from which the conclusions concerning the poor prognostic value of neglect have been drawn.

To conclude, the role of neglect in predicting functional outcome after stroke depends on how and when the variables are measured, what other predictors are included in the multivariate analyses and how the patients are selected. The terminology used in the studies reviewed lacked consistency, and very few of the studies provided detailed definitions of the concept of neglect. This needs to be borne in mind when interpreting the results of the studies reviewed.

Our review suggests several recommendations for future research. First, it would be important to focus on homogeneous patient groups so that generalizations can be made on at least those patient groups. Secondly, more research is needed that focuses on LH patient groups with right-sided neglect and their functional outcome. The third recommendation for future research is that it should assess various forms of neglect with a standardized test battery rather than a single test, and functional outcome with measures that consist of motor, cognitive and social items. This would provide a more coherent and broader foundation for assessing the neglect syndrome and the relationship of its different subtypes to the outcome, and thus increase the reliability and comparability of studies.

Acknowledgements

We wish to thank Professor Juhani Vilkki from the University of Helsinki for his helpful comments on this paper.

References

[1] P. Appelros, G.M. Karlsson, Å. Seiger and I. Nydevik, Neglect and anosognosia after first-ever stroke: incidence and relationship to impairment and disability, *J Rehabil Med* **32** (2002), 215–220.

[2] P. Appelros, G.M. Karlsson, Å. Seiger and I. Nydevik, Prognosis for patients with neglect and anosognosia with special reference to cognitive impairment, *J Rehabil Med* **35** (2003), 254–258.

[3] P. Appelros, I. Nydevik, G.M. Karlsson, A. Thorwalls and Å. Seiger, Recovery from unilateral neglect after right-hemisphere stroke, *Disabil Rehabil* **26** (2004), 471–477.

[4] E. Bisiach, G. Vallar, D. Perani, C. Papagno and A. Berti, Unawareness of disease following lesions of the right hemisphere: anosognosia for hemiplegia and anosognosia for hemianopia, *Neuropsychologia* **24** (1986), 471–482.

[5] A. Bowen, K. McKenna and C.T. Tallis, Reasons for variability in the reported rate of occurrence of unilateral spatial neglect after stroke, *Stroke* **30** (1999), 1196–1202.

[6] L.J. Buxbaum, M.K. Ferraro, T. Veramonti, A. Farné, J. Whyte, E. Lavadas, F. Frassinetti and H.B. Coslett, Hemispatial neglect: subtypes, neuroanatomy, and disability, *Neurology* **62** (2004), 749–756.

[7] T.P. Cassidy, S. Lewis and C.S. Gray, Recovery from visuospatial neglect in stroke patients, *J Neurol Neurosurg Psychiatry* **64** (1998), 555–557.

[8] L.R. Cherney, A.S. Halper, C.M. Kwasnica, R.L. Harvey and M. Zhang, Recovery of functional status after right hemisphere stroke: relationship with unilateral neglect, *Arch Phys Med Rehabil* **82** (2001), 322–328.

[9] K.D. Cicerone, C. Dahlberg, J.F. Malec, D.M. Langenbahn, T. Felicetti, S. Kneipp, W. Ellmo, K. Kalmar, J.T. Giancino, J.P. Harley, L. Laatsch, P.A. Morse and J. Catanese, Evidence-based cognitive rehabilitation: updated review of the literature from 1998 through 2002, *Arch Phys Med Rehabil* **86** (2005), 1681–1698.

[10] G. Cocchini, N. Beschin and M. Jehkonen, The Fluff test: a simple task to assess body representation neglect, *Neuropsychol Rehabil* **11** (2001), 17–31.

[11] C. Collen, D.T. Wade, D.T. Robb and C.M. Bradshaw, The Rivermead Mobility Index: a further development of the Rivermead Mobility Assessment, *Int Disabil Stud* **13** (1991), 50–54.

[12] A. Farné, L.J. Buxbaum, M. Ferraro, F. Frassinetti, J. Whyte, T. Veramonti, V. Angeli and H.B. Coslett, Patterns of spontaneous recovery of neglect and associated disorders in acute right brain-damaged patients, *J Neurol Neurosurg Psychiatry* **75** (2004), 1401–1410.

[13] J.M. Ferro, G. Mariano and S. Madureira, Recovery from aphasia and neglect, *Cerebrovasc Dis* **9** (1999), 6–22.

[14] B. Gialanella and F. Mattioli, Anosognosia and extrapersonal neglect as predictors of functional recovery following right hemisphere stroke, *Neuropsychol Rehabil* **2** (1992), 169–178.

[15] S. Giaquinto, S. Buzzelli, L. Di Francesco, A. Lottarini, P. Montenero, P. Tonin and G. Nolfte, On the prognosis of outcome after stroke, *Acta Neurol Scand* **100** (1999), 202–208.

[16] R. Gillen, H. Tennen and T. McKee, Unilateral spatial neglect: relation to rehabilitation outcomes in patients with right hemisphere stroke, *Arch Phys Med Rehabil* **86** (2005), 763–767.

[17] C.V. Granger, A.C. Cotter, B.B. Hamilton and R.C. Fiedler, Functional Assessment Scales: a study of persons after stroke, *Arch Phys Med Rehabil* **74** (1993), 133–138.

[18] P. Halligan, J.C. Marshall and D.T. Wade, Visuospatial neglect: underlying factors and test sensitivity, *The Lancet* **ii** (1989), 908–911.

[19] R. Hébert, R. Carrier and A. Bilodeau, The functional autonomy measurement system (SMAF): description and validation of an instrument for the measurement of handicaps, *Age Ageing* **17** (1988), 293–302.

[20] K.M. Heilman, E. Valenstein and R.T. Watson, The neglect syndrome, in: *Handbook of clinical neurology 45*, P.J. Vinken, G.W. Bruyn and H.L. Klawans, eds, Elseviere Science Publishers, Amsterdam, 1985, pp. 152–183.

[21] M. Holbrook and C.E. Skilbeck, An activities index for use with stroke patients, *Age Ageing* **12** (1983), 166–170.

[22] D. Jackson, H. Thornton and L. Turner-Stokes, Can severely disabled stroke patients regain the ability to walk independently more than three months poststroke, *Clin Rehabil* **14** (2000), 538–547.

[23] M. Jehkonen, *The role of visual neglect and anosognosias in functional recovery after right hemisphere stroke*, Tampere, Tampere University Press, 2002.

[24] M. Jehkonen, J.P. Ahonen, P. Dastidar, A.M. Koivisto, P. Laippala, J. Vilkki and G. Molnár, Visual neglect as a predictor of functional outcome one year after stroke, *Acta Neurol Scand* **101** (2000), 195–201.

[25] M. Jehkonen, J.P. Ahonen, P. Dastidar, A.M. Koivisto, P. Laippala, J. Vilkki and G. Molnár, Predictors of disharge to home during the first year after right hemisphere stroke, *Acta Neurol Scand* **104** (2001), 136–141.

[26] L. Kalra, I. Perez, S. Gupta and M. Wittink, The influence of visual neglect on stroke rehabilitation, *Stroke* **28** (1997), 1386–1391.

[27] S. Katz, A.B. Ford, R.W. Moskowitz, B.A. Jackson and M.W. Jaffe, Studies of illness in the aged. The index of ADL: a standardized measure of biological and psychosocial function, *JAMA* **185** (1963), 914–919.

[28] N. Katz, A. Hartman-Maier, H. Ring and N. Soroker, Functional disability and rehabilitation outcome in right hemisphere damaged patients with and without unilateral spatial neglect, *Arch Phys Med Rehabil* **80** (1999), 379–384.

[29] B. Lofgren, L. Nyberg, P.O. Osterlind, M. Mattson and Y. Gustafson, Stroke rehabilitation – discharge predictors, *Cerebrovasc Dis* **7** (1997), 168–174.

[30] S. Maeshima, A. Ueyoshi, T. Matsumoto, S. Boh-oka, M. Yoshida, T. Itakura and N. Dohi, Unilateral spatial neglect in patients with cerebral hemorrhage: the relationship between hematoma volume and prognosis, *J Clin Neurosci* **9** (2002), 544–548.

[31] F.I. Mahoney and D.W. Barthel, Functional evaluation: The Barthel Index, *Md State Med J* **14** (1965), 61–65.

[32] L. Mercier, T. Audet, R. Hébert, A. Rochette and M.F. Dubois, Impact of motor, cognitive, and perceptual disorders on ability to perform activities of daily living after stroke, *Stroke* **32** (2001), 2602–2608.

[33] S. Paolucci, G. Antonucci, L.E. Gialloreti, M. Traballesi, S. Lubich, L. Pratesi and L. Palombi, Predicting stroke inpatient rehabilitation outcome: the prominent role of neuropsychological disorders, *Eur Neurol* **36** (1996), 385–390.

[34] S. Paolucci, G. Antonucci, M.G. Grasso and L. Pizzamiglio, The role of unilateral spatial neglect in rehabilitation of right brain-damaged ischemic stroke patients, *Arch Phys Med Rehabil* **82** (2001), 743–749.

[35] S. Paolucci, G. Antonucci, L. Pratesi, M. Traballesi, S. Lubich and M.G. Grasso, Functional outcome in stroke inpatient rehabilitation: Predicting No, Low and High Response Patients, *Cerebrovasc Dis* **8** (1998), 228–234.

[36] S. Paolucci, M.G. Grasso, G. Antonucci, M. Bragoni, E. Troisi, D. Morelli, P. Coiro, D. De Angelis and F. Rizzi, Mobility status after inpatient stroke rehabilitation: 1 year-follow-up and prognostic factors, *Arch Phys Med Rehabil* **82** (2001), 2–8.

[37] S. Paolucci, M.G. Grasso, G. Antonucci, E. Troisi, D. Morelli, P. Coiro and M. Bragoni, One-year follow-up in stroke patients discharged from rehabilitation hospital, *Cerebrovasc Dis* **10** (2000), 25–32.

[38] M. Patel, C. Coshall, A.G. Rudd and C.D.A. Wolfe, Natural history of cognitive impairment after stroke and factors associated with its recovery, *Clin Rehabil* **17** (2003), 158–166.

[39] P.M. Pedersen, H.S. Jorgensen, H. Nakayama, H.O. Raaschou and T.S. Olsen, Frequency, determinants, and consequences of anosognosia in acute stroke, *J Neurol Rehabil* **10** (1996), 243–250.

[40] P.M. Pedersen, H.S. Jorgensen, H. Nakayama, H.O. Raaschou and T.S. Olsen, Hemineglect in acute stroke – incidence and prognostic implications: the Copenhagen stroke study, *Am J Phys Med Rehab* **76** (1997), 122–127.

[41] S.R. Pierce and L.J. Buxbaum, Treatments of unilateral neglect: a review, *Arch Phys Med Rehabil* **83** (2002), 256–268.

[42] L. Pizzamiglio, A. Judica, C. Razzano and P. Zoccolotti, Toward a comprehensive diagnosis of visuospatial disorders in unilateral brain-damaged patients, *Psychol Assess* **5** (1989), 199–218.

[43] H. Ring, M. Feder, J. Schwartz and G. Samuels, Functional measures of first-stroke rehabilitation inpatients: usefulness of the functional independence measure total score with a clinical rationale, *Arch Phys Med Rehabil* **78** (1997), 630–635.

[44] I.H. Robertson and P.W. Halligan, *Spatial neglect: A clinical handbook for diagnosis and treatment*, Hove, Psychology Press, 1999.

[45] D.T. Wade, *Measurement in neurological rehabilitation*, New York, Oxford University Press, 1992.

[46] B. Wilson, J. Cockburn and P.W. Halligan, *Behavioural Inattention Test, Manual*, Titchfield, Hampshire: Thames Valley Test Company, 1987.

[47] J. Young, S. Bogle and A. Forster, Determinants of social outcome measured by the Frenchay Activities Index at one year after stroke onset, *Cerebrovasc Dis* **12** (2001), 114–120.

[48] P. Zoccolotti and A. Judica, Functional evaluation of hemineglect by means of a semistructured scale: Personal extrapersonal differentation, *Neuropsychol Rehabil* **1** (1999), 33–44.

Neglect and extinction: Within and between sensory modalities

Claudio Brozzoli[a,b], M. Luisa Dematté[c], Francesco Pavani[c], Francesca Frassinetti[d] and Alessandro Farnè[a,b,]*

[a]INSERM, UMR-S 534, Espace et Action, Bron, F-69500, France
[b]Université Claude Bernard Lyon I, Lyon, F-69000, France
[c]Center for Mind/Brain Sciences, University of Trento, Rovereto, 38068, Italy
[d]Dipartimento di Psicologia, Università degli Studi di Bologna, Bologna, 40100, Italy

Received 2 February 2006
Revised 12 April 2006
Accepted 22 June 2006

Abstract. *Purpose:* The interest in human conscious awareness has increasingly propelled the study of neglect, the most striking occurrence of an acquired lack of conscious experience of space. Neglect syndromes commonly arise after unilateral brain damage that spares primary sensory areas nonetheless leading to a lack of conscious stimulus perception. Because of the central role of vision in our everyday life and motor behaviour, most research on neglect has been carried out in the visual domain. Here, we suggest that a comprehensive perspective on neglect should examine in parallel evidence from all sensory modalities.
Methods: We critically reviewed relevant literature on neglect within and between sensory modalities.
Results: A number of studies have investigated manifestations of neglect in the tactile and auditory modalities, as well as in the chemical senses, supporting the idea that neglect can arise in various sensory modalities, either separately or concurrently. Moreover, studies on extinction (i.e., failure to report the contralesional stimulus only when this is delivered together with a concurrent one in the ipsilesional side), a deficit to some extent related to neglect, showed strong interactions between sensory modality for the conscious perception of stimuli and representation of space.
Conclusions: Examining neglect and extinction by taking into account evidence from all sensory modalities in parallel can provide deeper comprehension of the neglect syndrome mechanisms and possibly more effective multi-sensory based rehabilitation approaches.

1. Introduction

Unilateral spatial neglect is a relatively common deficit that most frequently arises after right brain damage (RBD). Its main characteristic is a lack of awareness for sensory events located in the contralesional side of space (towards the left side space following a right lesion) and a loss of exploratory search and other actions normally directed toward that side. Most readers would be familiar with some of the classic presentation (and descriptions) of neglect patients: they typically behave as if the left half of their world no longer existed, so that in daily life they may only eat from one side of their plate, shave or make-up only one side of their face [50,89], draw or verbally describe only the right side of a remembered image or place [22,136]. This shortened version of a commonly used description of what neglect is, already conveys the equally common (though often implicit) assumption that neglect is mainly a visual disturbance. This probably relies on the well-funded argument that visually-guided behaviour entails most of our daily living activities. As such, visual neglect certainly gained most of the scholars' at-

*Corresponding author: A. Farnè, Espace et Action, UMR-S 534, INSERM-UCBL, AVENIR Team "Multisensory space & action" 16 av. Doyen Lépine, 69500 Bron, France. Tel.: +33 0 4 72913412; Fax: +33 0 4 72913401; E-mail: farne@lyon.inserm.fr.

tention over the expression of this syndrome in other modalities and, accordingly, the main visually-centred aspects of neglect will be first briefly reviewed here.

However, there is now large consensus that neglect and extinction[1] can virtually affect all of the other sensory modalities (separately or jointly), as well as the motor domain. We will address such a diversity of the neglect symptomathology to provide an up-to-date multisensory-motor framework. In addition, we will argue that the multisensory nature of neglect is most likely to have profound implications for rehabilitation of this cognitive deficit. Accordingly, we will conclude by reviewing some recent multisensory-based approaches to neglect rehabilitation.

2. Visual neglect and extinction

The last "decade of the brain" studies have brought convergent and definite evidence that neglect is a protean disorder, whose definition escapes from the boundaries of any theoretical unifying attempt [75]. Despite its heterogeneity, several core aspects of visual spatial neglect have been identified and, although they might be present at different levels in different patients, they are quite widely acknowledged to represent main aspects of this multifaceted syndrome. It is beyond the scope of this work to provide a comprehensive review of visual neglect and its theoretical accounts (see [107]). What follows is instead a brief list of examples with two purposes. First, to show how deeply the study of visual neglect has contributed to the understanding of the anatomo-functional structure of human conscious experience. Second, to recall the core aspects of the syndrome that should be taken into account when examining the literature on non-visual manifestations of neglect and extinction.

The diagnosis of visual neglect typically requires a comparison of performance on the left-side of a display with that on the right-side in tasks such as line bisection, cancellation, drawing (from model or memory). These tasks commonly reveal the presence of a spatial bias towards the ipsilesional side, in terms of rightward deviation and/or omissions of left-sided items. The presence of abnormal biases across hemispaces, in absence of contralateral primary sensorimotor loss, highlights neglect as a higher-order deficit of spatial cognition. This defective behaviour has been alternatively taken as evidence of patients' defective spatial attention and/or representation, or altered computation of an egocentric reference frame (for review, see [149]).

Indeed, neglect patients suffer from reduced visual spatial attention [49], especially in its exogenous component ([95] for review, see [6]). Not only simple reaction time (RT), but also search times for contralesional target are lengthened, increasing with the number of ipsilesional distractors, thereby indicating a difficulty in disengaging attention from ipsilesional stimuli [11,127]. Despite the presence of attentional deficits, preattentive processing has been shown to be relatively preserved in visual neglect and extinction, proceeding up to the level of the extraction of the meaning of contralesional "neglected" items [19,50,97], thus confirming that implicit visual processing can influence explicit visuo-motor performance.

Problems of attentional orienting towards the left side of space are compelling when observing neglect patients' behaviour. An interesting debate in the recent past has concerned what should be intended as "left" in left visual neglect and extinction. When asked to copy, for example, neglect patients typically draw the right side of a perceptual scene, omitting several details, or even leaving incomplete the left part of centrally located, single element of the scene. This behaviour is most likely responsible for the word "hemispatial" neglect, as implicitly referring to a corporeal midline that should represent the vertical cleavage line with respect to which conscious perception is preserved (to the right), or more or less absent (to the left). Although the trunk is one of the most important egocentric reference frames' origin [85], visual neglect and extinction can also be manifest according to other reference frames. For example, neglect patients have been reported to miss out the respective left part of two objects present in a scene (object-based neglect), instead of missing the leftmost one (space-based neglect), and vice-versa [48, 74]. Moreover, visual neglect can be selectively present for the vertical, not the horizontal dimension [123,128].

Dissociations of this kind have largely contributed to thinking of visual neglect as an increasingly fractionating entity [73,107]. Along the same line, patients may show left visual neglect for a limited sector of space around their body, the peripersonal/reaching space [20, 72]. On the contrary, neglect can affect selectively a farther sector of the extrapersonal space [5,157]. Neglect for near space can also be "transferred" into far

---

[1] The issue of whether (and to what extent) neglect and extinction should be conceived of as separate deficits is outside the scope of this work (for review, see [106]; see also [64]). Nonetheless, throughout this review we will clearly specify whether the reported studies concerned extinction or neglect patients.

space when using tools as physical extensions of the body for bisecting lines of constant visual angle [20]. Visual neglect can even be confined to either internally generated representations of visual images or perceptually presented scenes [70].

The role potentially played by non lateralised deficits of sustained attention and arousal on the genesis of visual neglect has been recently stressed [83,135]. By studying sustained attention through the use of an auditory target detection test, Hjaltason and colleagues [80] found a strong relationship between the presence of sustained attention deficits and visual neglect severity. Similarly, neglect patients may show a significantly longer "dwell time" for a secondary visual target being detected after presentation of a first target (attentional blink [82]). However, the degree of impairment on tasks for sustained attention does not always differentiate between RBD patients populations with and without visual neglect, although neglect patients are certainly affected by non lateralised attentional deficits when compared with age-matched healthy subjects [55]. Indeed, neglect seems to be mainly characterised by spatial deficits, though non lateralised attentional deficits are also present, without being specifically responsible for the major manifestations of the syndrome.

Another non-lateralised aspect of visual neglect that has recently raised great interest is the possible involvement of a spatial working memory deficit in the genesis of the syndrome. When invited to ocularly explore a scene to report targets amidst distractors, neglect patients do not only avoid exploring left-sided elements, but also produce a high number of rightwards saccades bringing their eyes to re-fixate items on their ipsilesional side that had already been "visited" [100]. Most important, many of these re-fixations were associated with a failure to keep track of spatial locations across saccades, the patients being unaware of revisiting previously visited locations. The presence of spatial working memory deficits should not be conceived of as an alternative account for visual neglect, but could certainly contribute to exacerbating omission of left sided items, especially in patients with lateral parietal involvement [100].

A different approach has been undertaken by Pisella and Mattingley [122], whose arguments propose that the origin of some re-visiting behavioural deficits in neglect might not be due to the proposed spatial working memory disorder. They suggest that the manifestations of visual neglect that are hardly grasped by more traditional accounts solely based upon deficits of spatial attention, representation, or working memory can actually be accounted for by an additional underlying disorder of spatial remapping due to parietal dysfunction (for another alternative account, see [139]).

One important issue that is currently the object of a very lively debate is the fine-grained anatomy of visual neglect. There is controversy as to whether lesions of the inferior posterior parietal cortex are still to be considered as the crucial anatomo-pathological counterpart of visual neglect [150], or whether and to what extent the mid-temporal gyrus may also play a role in the genesis of neglect [86,137]. Most of the recent studies, although employing different techniques, seem to confirm the crucial involvement of the inferior parietal lobule and the temporo-parietal junction [27,55, 75,109], as well as the crucial contribution of parieto-frontal connections [44,46]. It is out of the scope of this review to fully address this topic, but the interested reader can also refer to neurointerference studies using TMS in healthy participants [58,111], although it is worth noting that the criteria used for defining neglect are becoming important for comparing anatomical lesions studies [107].

As noted by Halligan and colleagues [75, p. 125], "Deficits of attention, intention, global-local processing, spatial memory and mental representation can all contribute to the clinical picture of neglect, which accordingly cannot be traced back to the disruption of a single supramodal process." More recently, the neglect literature has actually seen some attempts to provide a re-unifying interpretation, not by referring to a unique feature of the syndrome, as was the tendency in the past three decades, but by advocating the need of the joint presence of (some) deficits of lateralised and non-lateralised attention, eye movement, and manual exploratory behaviour, spatial working memory and remapping to fully account for the puzzling lack of awareness for contralesional events that is the hallmark of neglect (see [35,83,122]).

From this brief review, it is apparent how much the study of visual neglect has contributed to the refinement of our understanding of human conscious awareness. Although this supremacy of vision studies over the other sensory modalities can be explained, at least in part, by the fact that the appropriate technology has been made available for vision well before than for touch, audition or the chemical senses, it is quite surprising that relatively few(er) studies have addressed neglect and extinction in the other senses, or even in the motor domain [77,102]. In the following sections, we will review the current knowledge for non-visual manifestations of neglect and extinctions.

3. Tactile neglect & extinction

Generally, neglect is less evident and usually less strong in the tactile domain than for the visual modality. Many authors [30,62,79] failed to demonstrate tactile neglect in right brain damaged patients with visual neglect, when using tasks such as rod tactile bisection or haptic exploration. Fuji and colleagues asked visual neglect patients to bisect a tactually presented stick. The examiner placed the blindfolded patients' index finger on the centre of the stick and asked him to move the finger and stop it at the estimated midpoint of the stimulus. Although the patients showed rightward errors on a visual bisection task, they performed normally on the tactile test. Similar findings were described by Hjaltason and colleagues in an analogous study, where RBD patients were asked to perform the visual and tactile bisection, as well as a visuo-tactile variant of the same task. In the latter task, patients had to indicate the midpoint of a rod in the same way as in the tactile version, but in a free vision condition. Rightward bias was present only in the visual task and no difference was found between the tactile and the visuo-tactile rod bisection.

Evidence for tactile neglect comes from studies that employed spatial exploration tasks like in the maze test [41], whereby RBD patients were asked to move their forefinger along the alleys of a maze hidden behind a curtain, in order to search marbles placed at the end of one of its four lateral arms. Failure to find the targets in the contralesional part of the maze was taken as evidence of tactile neglect. Following this criterion, RBD patients with visual neglect showed more "tactile neglect" than control groups. Although these results have been replicated [21], Villardita [154] reported that patients with left visual neglect engaged at the same test preferred to explore the left part of the maze, thus suggesting an inconsistency between the phenomena described for vision and touch. Other studies have concentrated on the weak relationships between visual and tactile neglect, which seem to be double dissociable [21, 30,33]. One of the possible reasons for the paucity of tactile neglect studies may derive from its definition, most often diverging from the classical "omission" of left-sided targets that is so clearly and astonishingly present in the visual modality. Strictly speaking, one may ask the question of whether pure tactile neglect exists at all. Indeed, the difficulties in describing tactile neglect might be overcome if one admits that some cases of apparent hemisensory loss are, at least partially, mimicked by tactile neglect ([25], see also [108]).

Several studies have shown that vestibular stimulation (cold water in the left ear) may induce a transient remission of diverse neglect symptoms in RBD patients. However, a contralesional supposedly somatosensory deficit may also be ameliorated by vestibular stimulation [25,151], thus revealing a higher order problem and suggesting that tactile neglect may be mistaken for a mere sensory deficit. In this respect, it would be interesting to establish which proportion of RBD patients seemingly affected by hemisensory loss is, in fact, affected by unisensory tactile neglect.

While tactile neglect has been rarely documented, tactile extinction is much more frequently reported [113], even when assessed by simple confrontation methods. Extinction patients are able to detect a single stimulus presented alone either to the ipsi- or the contralesional side of space, but fail to report the same contralesional stimulus when this is delivered concurrently to a second one in the ipsilesional side of space (for review, see [103]). In the tactile domain, extinction has been reported to occur at the level of the hands, the face-neck, the arms-legs, both in case of symmetrical and asymmetrical stimulation [7,15,56], or between the two sides of a single body-part [110,147].

To some extent, both neglect and extinction show a similar lack of awareness for tactile inputs delivered in the side of the body opposite to the brain lesion, despite relatively intact primary sensory pathways, such that extinction has long been considered as a residual form of spatial neglect [50]. However, they also differ in some respects and double dissociations have been documented [31,64,134,153], suggesting that the underlying neural mechanism of extinction and neglect might differ [87].

Both "tactile neglect" and tactile extinction may manifest according to different reference frames. For example, they can be modulated by body posture and by the relative position of the stimulated body parts. Left tactile extinction is reduced when the left hand crosses the body midline and lies in the right hemispace, or even occupies a relative left location as compared to the right hand in the same hemispace [1,7,141]. Moreover, a single-case study of a RBD patient [148] illustrated that right hand touches may also be extinguished by a concurrent ipsilesional elbow stimulus (see [15,63]) when the right hand lies on the left and the elbow on the right of the patient's body midline. Similar effects of posture arise in neglect patients [109], whereby detection of single contralesional tactile stimuli increases when the stimulated hand lies in the ipsilesional hemispace, whereas touches delivered to the ipsilesional "good" hand are omitted to a variable degree when the right hand lies in the contralesional affected hemispace [1,7]. Similar to what has been reported for visual neglect [124], improvements in tactile neglect and extinction have been observed following a reduction of gravitational inputs, obtained by placing the subjects in a supine position [120].

Moreover, in the visual domain it is typically assumed that extinction is maximal under conditions in which competing stimuli occur simultaneously [95]. One may ask whether, in addition to posture, time (e.g., asynchronous stimulation) could also modulate tactile extinction in a similar fashion. The more a stimulus is temporally tied apart from another, the more reliably contralesional events should be perceived [26]. In this respect, Mattingley et al. [103] examined tactile detection in a RBD patient with tactile extinction, introducing a variable stimulus onset asynchrony (SOA) between bilateral stimulations. The occurrence of a right-sided competitor interfered with detection of left targets across a range of asynchrony from −400 to 1200 ms (minus means that left leads), showing an asymmetry in the effect. The point of subjective simultaneity appears thus to be biased in favour of ipsilesional stimuli. These results suggest that sensory timing problems might be present in both visual and somatosensory neglect [10].

In the case of tactile extinction considerable processing can still take place prior to the level at which loss of awareness arises. Although the extinguished tactile stimulus does not access consciousness, it may interfere with perception of the ipsilesional one [2]. More direct evidence comes from measures of patients' neural activity through functional imaging or event-related potentials. Some studies in the visual domain observed that the relatively early components of visual processing may be abnormal for contralesional stimuli in visual extinction [101]. Similarly, it is possible to examine the fate of extinguished tactile stimuli in those bilateral conditions where extinction arises, by comparing correct unilateral ERPs with incorrect ones in case of extinction [52]. In a single RBD patient study, bilateral trials with extinction still revealed residual early components (P60 & N110) over the right hemisphere in response to the extinguished left touches. These components were completely absent in the right hemisphere after a single right hand stimulation, although these kind of stimuli have the same conscious report of the other ones. However, the somatosensory neural activity in the right hemisphere was reduced in amplitude when compared to the one elicited by right hand stimulation on the left hemisphere. This suggests that, although tactile extinction is not a pure sensory deficit and is defined in conditions of bilateral stimulation, there may be an underlying pathology for the contralesional unilateral stimulation too, in agreement to what has been suggested for visual extinction [101]. Finally, these results demonstrate that somatosensory cortex activity is not sufficient for tactile inputs to reach awareness. In the same vein, a PET study [129] revealed that tactile extinction is associated with reduced activity in the secondary somatosensory cortex, but not in the primary one, suggesting that processing of bilateral tactile stimuli takes place at a "higher" stage and that extinction arises at a high level of tactile input processing.

4. Chemical neglect & extinction

To date, only a limited number of investigations concerning the suppression of (or competition among) spatial information processed through the so-called 'chemical senses' (i.e., olfaction and taste) have been reported [12,13,16,18,105]. A number of various different reasons may account for this lack of research. First, the distinction between pure chemical versus somatosensory information is often problematic (e.g. [18]). Second, it is widely assumed that olfaction and taste are senses that are not specialized for conveying spatial information (e.g. [92]). In olfaction, in particular, it is still unclear whether humans can localize at all the source of the olfactory stimulation by distinguishing between odours that are processed through the right versus the left nostril. This is particularly true when the stimulus is a pure odorant rather than trigeminal, that is when the odour does not cause any somatosensory stimulation that is known to be encoded by the trigeminal system (see [47]).

4.1. Olfaction

With respect to olfaction, Mesulam [105] first described a case of left-sided olfactory extinction revealed under double simultaneous stimulation of both nostrils in a patient with a brain lesion localized in the right parietal cortex. A few years later, Bellas and colleagues [12,13] assessed the ability of a group of fifteen RBD patients who were affected by left tactile extinction on the hand to identify and localize a series of bilaterally presented olfactory stimuli. On each trial, patients were presented with two stimuli (one in each nostril) using squeezing bottles and their task was to name each of the odours that were perceived. Participants could receive either the same pure odorant in both nostrils, or different odorants in each nostril, or else an odorant in one nostril and a trigeminal odour (vinegar) in the other. As the authors could not find another appropriate trigeminal odour, the vinegar odour was only presented singularly to one of the two nostrils while the other nostril was stimulated with a pure odorant. Bellas and colleagues [12] reported the presence of an extinction-like phenomenon in the patients' performance. Specifically, when two different stimuli (being either two pure odorants or an odorant and the trigeminal odour) were delivered to each nostril, RBD patients consistently failed to report the stimulus delivered to the left nostril. As the olfactory system would predominantly project its fibres ipsilaterally while the trigeminal system would be a contralaterally innervated system, the authors considered these results as evidence supporting the representational theory of neglect (see [22]). Indeed, if the sensory theory (see [37]) was responsible for the olfactory and trigeminal extinction, the pure odorants presented to the right nostril rather than those presented to the left nostril should have been extinguished. Bellas et al. [13] also reported that the patients affected by olfactory extinction showed a large number of displacements in that the correctly-identified stimuli presented to the left nostril were described as being in the right nostril.

The studies conducted by Bellas and colleagues represent a first step in the investigation of phenomena such as extinction and neglect in the olfactory modality. Nevertheless, it is not completely possible to determine the exact influence exerted by the nasal somatosensation in the olfactory extinction reported, since one of the odours considered as being pure odorants was later found to be processed probably also by the trigeminal system (i.e., a soap odour; see [13]). Finally, the possibility of highlighting deficits related to the localization of stimuli in the olfactory sensory modality should be interpreted within a much wider debate regarding whether the olfactory system could extract spatial information from pure odorants (i.e., without any interventions of the trigeminal system; e.g., see [47,92]; though see [126,155]).

Kobal and colleagues [92], for instance, claimed that the human olfactory system appears to be able to localize the source of the olfactory stimulation only when the odour elicits also a trigeminal response. This would appear to be in contradiction with the pioneering work of von Békésy [155] who showed that trained participants localized both trigeminal stimuli and pure odorants between the two nostrils. Moreover, Porter et al. [126] showed recently that naive participants were able to reliably localize pure odorants between the two nostrils in a setting in which olfactory stimuli were delivered by a computer-controlled air-dilution olfactometer that controlled for the exact timing in stimuli presentation. The stimuli were presented to the nose through a compartmentalized nasal mask that allowed for mono-rhinal odour presentation and the sniff flowrate was controlled in real-time. Clearly, if the ability of the olfactory system to extract spatial information from non-trigeminal stimuli turns out to be true, new light could be shed on the extinction phenomena described for odours. In fact, the relative contribution of pure odorant and somatonsensory information to olfactory localization could be disentangled using experimental methods similar to those described by Porter and colleagues.

4.2. Taste

The existence of neglect and/or extinction in taste has been even less explored than in olfaction, even though in humans the ability to localize taste stimuli presented on the tongue has been previously described (e.g. [140, 156]). Bender and Feldman [17] first reported a single case of a patient with a wide parietal-occipital tumor and tactile extinction on the upper limbs who also showed extinction of taste sensations on the left part of the tongue when two tastes were presented simultaneously on each hemi-tongue. Taste stimuli were applied on the tongue surface by means of cotton buds and they were all accurately identified and localized by the patient when presented singularly. The results of the assessment revealed that the patient was not only affected by unimodal taste extinction, but that he also displaced taste sensations under crossmodal taste-tactile stimulation. In particular, when a touch or a pinprick was delivered to the right hemi-tongue and a taste was applied on the left hemi-tongue, the patient repeatedly reported bilateral taste stimulation, thus surprisingly extinguishing the right touch and partially misplacing the left taste stimulus. Unfortunately, Bender and Feldman did not describe in detail the method that was used to generate the tactile sensations.

More recently, Berlucchi and colleagues [18] described a study carried on two groups of patients (i.e., having a right or left brain lesion) and a control group. The RBD patients were affected by tactile (on the hands), visual, and/or auditory extinction with different degrees. By using a highly controlled stimulus presentation (e.g., use of micro-pipettes and controlled water temperature), Berlucchi and colleagues could disentangle (contrary to [17]) between the presence of taste and/or tactile extinction on the tongue. A sub-group of the RBD patients showed tactile extinction under bilateral simultaneous stimulation of the tongue. However, the authors failed to find any significant presence of taste extinction even among these tactile extinguishing patients, thus highlighting for the first time the existence of dissociations between extinction phenomena occurring in somatonsensory or in purely chemical information processing. There also appeared not to be any consistent correlations between the presence of tactile extinction on the tongue and that of tactile (on the hands), visual, and auditory extinction. Berlucchi and colleagues suggested that a distributed taste representation could account for the existence of such dissociation. Namely, the processing of somatosensory information coming from the tongue would be predominantly contralateral, whereas the taste stimulation would activate the brain areas ipsilateral to the hemitongue being stimulated (e.g., see [3,114]). Moreover, according to Berlucchi and colleagues, the fact that a dissociation between gustatory and tactile extinction could be highlighted would suggest that gustatory extinction occurs consequently to a severe tactile extinction (see [17]). The patients involved in their study would have been affected by a mild tactile extinction, thus allowing the gustatory information to be processed by the preserved left hemisphere.

To date, thus, there is still no clear evidence of the existence of purely taste extinction and/or neglect, while few studies provided evidence about the presence of tactile extinction on the tongue or inside the mouth following a right brain lesion [4,18]. In the study of extinction and neglect, a wide number of questions related to the chemical senses are still waiting for answers. Today, it would appear to be possible to devise studies where information conveyed by the chemosensory modalities and by the collateral somatosensory modality could finally be investigated separately [18,126,140]. Therefore, future research will be in charge of furthering our understanding about odours and tastes and their links with spatial representations.

5. Auditory neglect & extinction

Patients with focal brain lesions can also suffer a number of disturbances in the auditory modality that can be characterised as auditory manifestations of the neglect syndrome. Patients with right hemispheric lesions might either fail to respond when addressed verbally from the left, or more commonly behave as if they heard the voice originating from their right (e.g. [16,38]). This suggested a deficit in detection and localisation of auditory stimuli, especially when they originate in contralesional space, which could emerge for hearing as well as for vision. Although this clinical observation has generally been confirmed, a number of recent evidence has now highlighted important differences between the manifestations of neglect in hearing and vision.

5.1. Deficits of sound localisation

The disturbance for sound localisation, originally described as 'alloacusis' [16], has been the topic of several experimental works in the last two decades (see [118] for review). A first aspect that emerged from these systematic investigations is that auditory spatial disturbances in neglect patients might reflect increased spatial uncertainty for sound position, especially for contralesional stimuli, instead of a strictly systematic shift in heard azimuth towards the ipsilesional side. For instance, when asked to discriminate verbally the relative position (same vs. different) of two sounds in close succession, neglect patients typically perform worse for pairs of sounds originating from the contralesional side (e.g. [117,146]; see also [40] for evidence of reduced mismatch negativity response in scalp recordings of event-related potentials for contralesional vs. ipsilesional free-field sounds). In addition, it has recently been shown that patients with neglect perform less efficiently than control right-hemisphere patients without neglect in a discrimination task that concerns the vertical position free-field sounds [116,119]. Thus, a disturbance in auditory space perception emerges even when localisation involved the vertical dimension, orthogonal to any potential horizontal shift.

Horizontal bias in sound localisation have instead been typically documented when neglect patients are asked to point to a sound presented in free-field (i.e., from an external source [115,121]; but see [138]), or over headphones (pointing to a location on their head; e.g. [23]). In addition, deficits have been observed when using 'auditory midline' tasks, in which patients adjust a continuous sound (or make judgments on a discrete sound) to locate it relatively to the centre of the head or body midline (e.g. [23,90,146,152]; but see [34]). For sounds presented over headphones (with either varied intensity at the two ears, or varied interaural timing cues to sound localisation), neglect patients typically report a sound to be central when it is actually lateralized towards the left (i.e. more intense or arriving earlier at the left ear), as if there were a rightward shift in perceived location (e.g. [23,146]). By contrast, for sounds presented free-field, neglect patients often reported that an external sound seemed aligned with their head/body midline when it was actually presented to the right (thus implying a leftward shift in sound localization if one assumes that perceived head/body midline is veridical, which it might not be in neglect patients [90, 152]). As proposed recently [115], some of these discrepancies concerning the direction of lateral shifts in sound localization for neglect patients might actually relate to non-auditory aspects of the task. Specifically, motor or visuo-motor biases in pointing tasks [115], or pathological distortions of perceived head/body midline in auditory-midline tasks [57] could in principle affect performance.

5.2. Detection and identification deficits

Although auditory spatial deficits have often been reported in neglect patients for single auditory stimuli, especially when they originate in contralesional space, the patients usually detect these single sounds with apparent ease in most localization studies (e.g. [23,115–119,121,146]). This might appear to contrast with characteristic clinical deficits affecting the visual modality in neglect patients, where complete failures to detect or respond to contralesional visual events are commonly noted, rather than merely failures in localization. Two critical differences between hearing and vision may account for this discrepancy. First, the anatomical organization of the auditory system, which is less crossed than for other senses, with some ipsilateral as well as major contralateral cortical projections of the input reaching each ear. Second, the typical reduced complexity of the auditory environment in experimental setups. Unlike experiments in vision, in which targets are often embedded among many distracters, the typical experiment in the auditory domain presents a single strong sound against silence [115]. Indeed, when even a minimal version of concurrent competing stimulation is produced, usually by presenting one sound on each side of the head, a consistent failure to detect and/or identify contralesional sounds emerged, for both free-field sounds [39,142] and headphone stimuli [14,42]. Strictly speaking, however, such effects with two concurrent competing sounds might be considered the auditory equivalent of visual or tactile extinction, rather than manifestations of neglect.

A long standing debate in relation to detection and/or identification deficits under double simultaneous auditory stimulation has been whether poor detection of sounds at the contralesional ear could be related to neglect of contralesional auditory space [81], or instead should be ascribed solely to poor processing (or suppression) of the auditory information entering the contralesional ear [8,9]. Indeed, free-field sounds presented from a contralesional location will tend to be more intense at the contralesional ear, and if presented monaurally over headphones, will only reach that ear. However, there is now mounting evidence suggesting a role for higher-level spatial factors (e.g., perceived external position, spatial attention, relation to visual neglect) in the contralesional detection/identification deficits for auditory stimuli observed for neglect patients (e.g. [14,29,142]). For instance, it has been shown that identification of left free-field sounds can sometimes improve in the presence of a fictitious visible sound source (a 'dummy' loudspeaker) on the right, which reportedly made it seem that the sounds originated from the right side [142]. In addition, a direct investigation of the role of apparent sound location with respect to which ear the information enters was recently conducted by Bellman and colleagues [14], presenting each auditory stimulus (heard words) either to one ear only ('dichotic' stimulation), or binaurally but with interaural time difference serving as the only lateralization cue ('diotic' stimulation). Under double simultaneous presentation, two out of four neglect patients tested in the study showed poorer performance for left than right words only with dichotic presentation (consistent with a deficit for sounds entering the contralesional ear), whereas the other two patients were impaired in reporting left words for both methods of lateralized presentation (consistent with an identification deficit for sounds perceived as originating from contralesional space).

5.3. Non spatial auditory deficits

A final aspect that merits attention is the description of non-spatially-lateralized auditory deficits in patients with visual neglect [34,80,135]. Robertson and colleagues, for instance, documented a non-spatial difficulty in sustaining attention and maintaining arousal in the auditory modality, in a task where neglect patients were required to count the number of occurrences of a particular auditory target among a stream of sounds, of variable length, all presented centrally. Non-spatial auditory deficits have also emerged when patients with visual neglect were asked to listen to a short rapid sequence of auditory stimuli over headphones, to detect which of the stimuli had a higher pitch [34]. Despite auditory stimuli were always presented centrally, and patients were able to detect subtle pitch modulation for single auditory objects, they were severely impaired at any comparison between two sounds in a rapid sequence, possibly as a result of pathologically limited attentional capacity.

6. Multisensory neglect and extinction

The previous sections on non-visual manifestations of neglect and extinction clearly showed that in many circumstances neglect and extinction can emerge for a single sensory modality, or for multiple sensory modalities in a given patient [43,153]. Note however that all the works reviewed so far were concerned with stimulation delivered within a single sensory modality at a time. We now turn to examine how neglect and extinction affecting a unimodal sensory system can be influenced (enhanced or degraded further) by the concurrent activation of another modality.

A number of evidence has now systematically shown that extinction in particular can emerge even when concurrent stimuli are presented in different sensory modalities, i.e., different sensory inputs delivered to the ipsi- and contra-lateral side of the patient's body [17, 45]. Tactile extinction, for example, can be modulated by visual events simultaneously presented in the space region near the tactile stimulation, increasing or reducing tactile perception, depending upon the spatial arrangement of the stimuli. In particular, the visual stimulation in the ipsilesional side exacerbates contralesional tactile extinction, whereby the presentation of visual and tactile stimuli on the same contralesional side can reduce the deficit [96]. Moreover, the modulation described is most consistently manifest when visual-tactile interaction occurs in the space close to the body than when the space far from the body is visually stimulated.

In a similar way, visual and tactile information are integrated in other peripersonal space regions, such as around the face [56,99]. In this case, extinction patients were presented with unilateral and bilateral tactile stimulation on both cheeks and, in addition, visual stimuli were concurrently presented in the contralesional or ipsilesional side. As for the hand, exacerbation of the deficit was found in the ipsilesional visual condition, whereby the visual stimulus enhanced tactile detection when delivered in the contralesional side. The modulation, again, is more evident when the visual stimulus is presented in a near-body region of space rather than in a farther region, thus implying that sensory integration arising from the same near-the-body location allows for the tactile input to reach awareness.

Similar modulations of tactile extinction have been reported following another kind of multisensory interaction, between audition and touch [98]. When sounds are concurrently presented with single touches delivered at the level of the neck in tactile extinction patients, their contralesional tactile detection is most likely to be hampered by proximal, as compared to far loudspeakers. Interestingly, such a multisensory effect observed in the front space with respect to the patients' head was even stronger when cross-modal auditory-tactile extinction was assessed in the patients' back space, thus suggesting that different degrees of multisensory integration may occur depending upon the functional relevance of a given modality for that particular sector of space [54].

These results support the existence of a peripersonal multisensory space in humans, akin to that described in animals studies [94]. Evidence from animal studies [51,68,69,131,132] revealed a dissociation between a space far from the body that can not be reached by a simple arm movement, and a near peripersonal space, a region of space extending only a few centimetres out from the body surface. Indeed, a strong multisensory integration takes place at single neuron level in this region of space: the same neurons activated by tactile stimuli delivered on a given body-part are also activated by visual or auditory stimuli delivered in the space near that body-part. In this respect, the selectivity of visual-tactile extinction for the proximal sector of space is reminding of the spatial bias observed in unimodal visual neglect, which may selectively arise in the near peripersonal space [32,72].

An interesting characteristic of the space region surrounding the body is its plasticity. Through tool-use, for example, it is possible to remap the space so that "far becomes near" [20]. When asked to use a long stick to bisect distant horizontal lines the neglect patients' selective bias, formerly present only in the near space, was transferred to the far space. Similar results have been described in extinction patients who, after tool-use, showed increased contralesional tactile extinction when a visual stimulus was presented far from the body at the extremity of a hand-held tool. Therefore, using a tool to retrieve distant objects increases the strength of visual-tactile integrative effects in a region of space far from the patients' body. Such a phenomenon has been ascribed to a tool-use dependent size-change of the peri-hand multisensory space [53].

Altogether, these results show that the expression of cross-modal interaction seems to be a rather frequent occurrence, which can be selectively modulated by several parameters relative to the relationship between the stimulus and the body: like distance, spatial location, auditory complexity, spatial and temporal coincidence. Therefore, these findings are in good agreement with a modular organization of space in which several neuronal structures are devoted to the processing of different space sectors, in different co-ordinates, across different modalities, most probably for different behavioral purposes [143]. Among these structures, the representation of near and far peripersonal space in humans parallels the functioning of the circuit of multisensory areas that has been well documented in monkeys, which is similarly sensitive to the same parameters listed above.

7. Multisensory-based rehabilitation approaches

The reported frequency of hemispatial neglect varies widely from 13% to 81% of patients who have had right hemisphere stroke [145]. The presence of neglect has been associated with poor outcome measures on functional activities following a stroke [55,65,67]. Patients with neglect[2] have been found to have longer lengths of stay in rehabilitation facilities and lower scores on the Functional Independence Measure (FIM) [71] and thus require more assistance at discharge than patients without neglect [36,88]. Neglect severity also predicts the degree of family burden more accurately than the extent of brain damage [27].

These are the main reasons why it is important to know whether or not neglect spontaneous pattern of evolution tends towards recovery, in which proportion of patients and to which degree. In this respect, a recent study [55] has shown that only 43% of neglect patients improved spontaneously during a two-week long assessment in the acute phase (up to six weeks post-stroke) and only 9% of patients showed complete recovery. When a subset of this patient population was re-assessed during the chronic phase, the proportion of patients who recovered increased up to 63%, although recovery was complete only in 25% of them. Since spontaneous recovery in the acute and chronic phase of the disease is not axiomatic and, when present, does not allow for complete remission of neglect symptoms in most patients, it is very important to individuate efficient treatment strategies to improve recovery of patients with chronic and persistent unilateral neglect.

Neglect rehabilitation approaches have been classically divided into two classes: rehabilitation procedures based on a voluntary reorientation of attention toward the contralesional space and rehabilitation procedures based on the sensory stimulation of the affected (contralesional) field, or sensory deprivation of the good (ipsilesional) field. The second class of rehabilitation procedures are based on an interpretation of neglect as an attentional-representational deficit due to the competition between left and right space representations. After a right brain damage, the contralateral space representation is weak and, as a consequence, the competition with intact ipsilesional space representation induces neglect in that sector of space. The antagonism between left and right space representation may be reduced by sensory stimulating the contralesional hemispace (i.e. vestibular, optokinetic, left-sided transcutaneous mechanical vibration, left-sided electrical nervous stimulation and left-limb proprioceptive stimulation), or by suppressing sensory inputs from the ipsilesional hemispace (i.e., hemiblinding technique). Needless to say, most of the studies focussed on the visual components of neglect, although several non-visual aspects of neglect and associated disorders may also benefit from some of these approaches [104,149].

More recently, many studies have outlined that space representation is based not only on input and output responses, that is on sensory and motor information, but on the integration of these information from multiple sensory modalities. As reviewed above, neuropsychological findings have shown the existence of multisensory systems devoted to the integrated coding of spatial information, e.g., a visuotactile system [96,99], an auditory – tactile system [54,98], and an auditory-visual system [59,61]. These integrated systems can offer a unique opportunity to improve the performance of patients with spatial representational deficit, such as patients with visual neglect. As a consequence, potential therapeutic implications could derive from the integration of visual and proprioceptive information, and visual and auditory information; for example, a multisensory based approach to neglect rehabilitation may

---

[2]To date, rehabilitation studies have focussed on neglect rather than extinction, most likely because extinction is not known to have such a negative impact on patients' everyday life as neglect, although some approaches have nonetheless proved to ameliorate extinction, for example in the tactile modality [76,112].

enable patients to detect "bimodal" stimuli for which unimodal components are below behavioural threshold. Concerning the integration of proprioceptive and visual information it has been shown that passive movements of the contralesional arm in the contralesional space may improve visual neglect. As far as the integration of visual and auditory integration, bimodal audiovisual stimulation of the affected field can improve perception of the visual events in the neglected hemispace [59]. This amelioration of visual detection was observed only when the two simultaneous stimuli were spatially coincident, or when they were located near one another in space (at a distance of 16°). In contrast, when the spatial disparity between the two sensory stimuli was larger than 16°, patients' visual performance remained unvaried. Moreover, multisensory enhancement was greater when visual stimuli were presented in the most peripheral positions of the affected visual field where the impairment was more severe. This is in keeping with the functional properties of multisensory neurons described in animal studies [144]: a greater enhancement of bimodal neurons' response is observed when visual and auditory stimuli originate at the same time (temporal rule) and from the same position and, as a consequence, fall within the excitatory receptive fields of a visual-auditory multisensory neuron (spatial rule), and when two weaker, rather than two strong stimuli are combined (inverse effectiveness rule). These functional integrative properties are well suited to explain the amelioration of visual neglect patients following multisensory stimulation, thus providing a potential neuronal substrate for a multisensory based treatment of neglect.

Beyond the existence of beneficial effects of audio-visual stimulation, showing that a sound can ameliorate visual detection in neglect patients, the characteristics of patients who can benefit from audio-visual integration effects would be important to establish. It is well known that sensory deficits, such as visual field deficit (e.g. hemianopia), are frequently associated with neglect and may represent a negative predictive factor for cross-modal audiovisual integration in neglect patients [61]. Moreover, since it has been shown that, not only the superior colliculus [144], but also "heteromodal" [66] and "sensory-specific" [28,66] cortices are involved in cross-modal integration, it is possible that the site of cerebral lesions may affect audio-visual integration. The presence of cross-modal audio-visual integration effects has been recently investigated in patients with either neglect or hemianopia and in patients with both hemianopia and neglect [61]. Patients were asked to detect visual stimuli presented alone or in combination with auditory stimuli that could be spatially aligned or not with the visual ones. As in the previously reported study, an enhancement of visual detection was found when a sound was presented in the same position of the visual one, but only in patients affected either by neglect or hemianopia; by contrast, enhancement dependent upon the multisensory integration did not occur when patients presented with both deficits. Moreover, a different influence of the site of the cortical lesion on multisensory integration has been found. When patients' lesion was mainly confined to fronto-temporo-parietal areas (neglect patients), or to the occipital areas (hemianopic patients), the visual and auditory stimuli were effectively integrated, whereas when the lesion involved all the previous lobes, although to different degrees in different patients, the effects of multisensory integration were no longer present (neglect patients with hemianopia).

The results of these studies underline the relevance of cross-modal integration in enhancing visual processing in neglect patients and in patients with visual field deficits. The possibility of a sound improving the detection of visual stimuli is very promising with respect to the possibility to take advantage of the brain's multisensory capabilities for a rehabilitation approach of visual attention deficit and visual field defects [24,61]. In this respect, one question which needs to be addressed in the future is whether a systematic bimodal stimulation, by affecting orientation towards the neglected/blind hemifield and modulating the processing of visual events, can improve visual exploration, perhaps with long-lasting effects. A cross-modal training might reinforce the innate ability of our brain to perceive multisensory events, hidden in the normal condition in which unimodal processes are usually at work on unisensory events that are sufficiently salient to be perceived. This possibility is particularly relevant in terms of rehabilitation perspectives because it is non-invasive, as compared with other rehabilitative procedures, and does not require the voluntary displacement of the patients' attention to the affected side, which can be particularly difficult for neglect patients.

8. Summary and conclusions

As it results from the experimental evidences reviewed above, some core aspects of neglect and extinction are observed across different modalities. Whatever explanation is proposed for the lack of perceptual awareness, the deficits can not be solely attributed to early sensory problems. For example, patients' performance in visual and tactile detection may strongly vary according to different reference frames and postural changes. In addition, Pavani and colleagues [119] recently showed that discrimination performance for auditory stimuli presented in the contralesional auditory hemifield of visual neglect patients can actually improve when patients gaze towards the left. A pure sensory deficit would imply a complete loss of perception irrespective of spatial relationship between bodyparts or gaze direction. However, the presence of subtle sensory dysfunctions has been recently consistently reported in visual, tactile, and auditory studies of neglect and extinction. Although still unclear, the role possibly played by early sensory deficits can no longer be excluded, as degradation or slowing of sensory inputs processing may concur to the difficulty in perceiving contralesional events.

Other features of neglect and extinction studies recently gained considerable interest, such as the presence of non lateralised deficits and their contribution to the syndrome. However, the latter have been mainly reported in vision and audition, whereas their potential role in the chemical and tactile modalities has not been systematically explored. In the same vein, clear evidence of processing without awareness is mainly available for the visual and tactile modality.

Although we did not intend to provide an exhaustive critical review of what the multisensory approach tells us about the current neurocognitive models of neglect and extinction, we believe the study of unisensory and multisensory neglect and extinction is both theoretically and clinically relevant. The within- and between-modality approach would hopefully proceed in parallel, the other senses possibly filling the gap with vision, which is still dominant. We undertook this direction as it may provide a wider framework within which multisensory-based rehabilitation approaches may be devised. An increasing attention devoted to non-visual manifestations of neglect may be of great interest for deepening our knowledge of human spatial awareness.

Acknowledgements

This work was supported by the European Mobility Fellowship (CB), the Università degli Studi di Trento (MLD), the MIUR and RFO (FF, AF, FP), the EC Marie Curie Fellowship #HPMF-CT-2000-00506 (FP), the Integrated Action Program "Galileo" (FP, AF) and the AVENIR project funding #R05265CS (AF, FP).

References

[1] S.M. Aglioti, N. Smania and A. Peru, Frames of reference for mapping tactile stimuli in brain-damaged patients, *Journal of Cognitive Neuroscience* **11** (1999), 67–79.

[2] S.M. Aglioti, N. Smania, V. Moro and A. Peru, Tactile salience influences extinction, *Neurology* **50** (1998), 1010–1014.

[3] S.M. Aglioti, G. Tassinari, M. Fabri, M. Del Pesce, A. Quattrini, T. Manzoni et al., Taste laterality in the split brain, *European Journal of Neuroscience* **13** (2001), 195–200.

[4] J.-M. André, J.-M. Beis, N. Morin and J. Paysant, Buccal hemineglect, *Archives of Neurology* **57** (2000), 1734–1741.

[5] A.M. Barrett, R.L. Schwartz, G.P. Crucian, M. Kim and K.M. Heilman, Attentional grasp in far extrapersonal space after thalamic infarction, *Neuropsychologia* **38** (2000), 778–784.

[6] P. Bartolomeo and S. Chokron, Orienting of attention in left unilateral neglect, *Neuroscience And Biobehavioral Reviews* **26** (2002), 217–234.

[7] P. Bartolomeo, R. Perri and G. Gainotti, The influence of limb crossing on left tactile extinction, *Journal of Neurology, Neurosurgery and Psychiatry* **75** (2004), 49–55.

[8] A. Beaton and M. McCarthy, Auditory neglect after right frontal lobe and right pulvinar thalamic lesions: Comments on Hugdahl, Wester, and Asbjørnsen (1991) and some preliminary findings, *Brain and Language* **44** (1993), 121–126.

[9] A. Beaton and M. McCarthy, On the nature of auditory neglect: A reply to Hugdal and Wester, *Brain and Language* **48** (1995), 351–358.

[10] C. Becchio and C. Bertone, The ontology of neglect, *Consciousness And Cognition* **14** (2005), 483–494.

[11] M. Behrmann, P. Ebert and S.E. Black, Hemispatial neglect and visual search: a large scale analysis, *Cortex* **40** (2004), 247–263.

[12] D.N. Bellas, R.A. Novelly, B. Eskenazi and J. Wasserstein, The nature of unilateral neglect in the olfactory sensory system, *Neuropsychologia* **26** (1988), 45–52.

[13] D.N. Bellas, R.A. Novelly, B. Eskenazi and J. Wasserstein, Unilateral displacement in the olfactory sense: A manifestation of the unilateral neglect syndrome, *Cortex* **24** (1988b), 267–275.

[14] A. Bellmann, R. Meuli and S. Clarke, Two types of auditory neglect, *Brain* **124** (2001), 676–687.

[15] M.B. Bender, Disorders of perception, C.C. Thomas, ed, Springfield, IL, 1952.

[16] M.B. Bender and S.P. Diamond, An analysis of auditory perceptual defects with observations on the localization of the dysfunction, *Brain* **88** (1965), 675–686.

[17] M.B. Bender and D.S. Feldman, Extinction of taste sensation on double simultaneous stimulation, *Neurology* **2** (1952), 195–202.

[18] G. Berlucchi, V. Moro, C. Guerrini and S.M. Aglioti, Dissociation between taste and tactile extinction on the tongue after right brain damage, *Neuropsychologia* **42** (2004), 1007–1016.

[19] A. Berti, A. Allport, J. Driver, Z. Dienes, J. Oxbury and S. Oxbury, Levels of processing for visual stimuli in an extinguished field, *Neuropsychologia* **5** (1992), 403–415.

[20] A. Berti and F. Frassinetti, When far becomes near: remapping of space by tool use, *Journal of Cognitive Neuroscience* **12** (2000), 415–420.

[21] N. Beschin, M. Cazzani, R. Cubelli, S. Della Sala and L. Spinazzola, Ignoring left and far: an investigation of tactile neglect, *Neuropsychologia* **34** (1996), 41–49.

[22] E. Bisiach and C. Luzzatti, Unilateral neglect of representational space, *Cortex* **14** (1978), 129–133.

[23] E. Bisiach, L. Cornacchia, R. Sterzi and G. Vallar, Disorders of perceived auditory lateralization after lesions of the right hemisphere, *Brain* **107** (1984), 37–52.

[24] N. Bolognini, F. Rasi, M. Coccia and E. Ladavas, Visual search improvement in hemianopic patients after audio-visual stimulation, *Brain* **128** (2005), 2830–2842.

[25] G. Bottini, E. Paulesu, M. Gandola, S. Loffredo, P. Scarpa, R. Sterzi, I. Santilli, C.A. Defanti, G. Scialfa, F. Fazio and G. Vallar, Left caloric vestibular stimulation ameliorates right hemianesthesia, *Neurology* **65** (2005), 1278–1283.

[26] D. Bueti, M. Costantini, B. Forster and S.M. Aglioti, Uni- and cross-modal temporal modulation of tactile extinction in right brain damaged patients, *Neuropsychologia* **42** (2004), 1689–1696.

[27] L.J. Buxbaum, M.K. Ferraro, T. Veramonti, A. Farnè, J. Whyte, E. Ladavas, F. Frassinetti and H.B. Coslett, Hemispatial neglect: Subtypes, neuroanatomy, and disability, *Neurology* **62** (2004), 749–756.

[28] G.A. Calvert, M.J. Brammer, E.T. Bullmore, R. Campbell, S.D. Iversen and A.S. David, Response amplification in sensory-specific cortices during crossmodal binding, *Neuroreport* **10** (1999), 2619–2623.

[29] R.P. Carlyon, R. Cusack, J.M. Foxton and I.H. Robertson, Effects of attention and unilateral neglect on auditory stream segregation, *Journal of Experimental Psychology: Human Perception and Performance* **27** (2001), 115–127.

[30] S. Chokron, P. Colliot, P. Bartolomeo, F. Rhein, E. Eusop, P. Vassel and T. Ohlmann, Visual, proprioceptive and tactile performance in left neglect patients, *Neuropsychologia* **40**(12) (2002), 1965–1976.

[31] G. Cocchini, R. Cubelli, S. Della Sala and N. Beschin, Neglect without extinction, *Cortex* **35** (1999), 285–313.

[32] A. Cowey, M. Small and S. Ellis, Left visuospatial neglect can be worse in far than in near space, *Neuropsychologia* **32** (1994), 1059–1066.

[33] R. Cubelli, P. Nichelli, V. Bonito, A. De Tanti and M.G. Inzaghi, Different patterns of dissociation in lateral spatial neglect, *Brain Cognition* **15** (1991), 139–159.

[34] R. Cusack, R.P. Carlyon and I.H. Robertson, Neglect between but not within auditory objects, *Journal of Cognitive Neuroscience* **12** (2000), 1056–1065.

[35] J. Danckert and S. Ferber, Revisiting unilateral neglect, *Neuropsychologia*, in press.

[36] G. Denes, C. Semenza, E. Stoppa and A. Lis, Unilateral spatial neglect and recovery from hemiplegia: a follow-up study, *Brain* **105**(pt 3) (1982), 543–552.

[37] D. Denny-Brown and B.Q. Bamker, Amorphosynthesis from left parietal lesions, *Archives of Neurology and Psychiatry* **71** (1954), 302–313.

[38] D. Denny-Brown, J.S. Meyer and G. Horenstein, The significance of perceptual rivalry resulting from parietal lesion, *Brain* **75** (1952), 433–471.

[39] L.Y. Deouell and N. Soroker, What is extinguished in auditory extinction? *NeuroReport* **11** (2000), 3059–3062.

[40] L.Y. Deouell, S. Bentin and N. Soroker, Electrophysiological evidence for an early (pre-attentive) information processing deficit in patients with right hemisphere damage and unilateral neglect, *Brain* **123** (2000), 353–365.

[41] E. de Renzi, P. Faglioni and G. Scotti, Hemispheric contribution to exploration of space through the visual and tactile modality, *Cortex* **6** (1970), 191–203.

[42] E. de Renzi, M. Gentilini and C. Barcieri, Auditory neglect, *Journal of Neurology, Neurosurgery, and Psychiatry* **52** (1989), 613–617.

[43] E. de Renzi, M. Gentilini and F. Pattacini, Auditory extinction following hemisphere damage, *Neuropsychologia* **22**(6) (1984), 733–744.

[44] M.T. de Schotten, M. Urbanski, H. Duffau, E. Volle, R. Lévy, B. Dubois and P. Bartolomeo, Direct Evidence for a Parietal-Frontal Pathway Subserving Spatial Awareness in Humans, *Science* **309** (2005), 2226–2228.

[45] G. di Pellegrino, G. Basso and F. Frassinetti, Spatial extinction on double asynchronous stimulation, *Neuropsychologia* **35**(9) (1997), 1215–1223.

[46] F. Doricchi and F. Tomaiuolo, The anatomy of neglect without hemianopia: a key role for parietal-frontal disconnection? *Neuroreport* **14**(17) (2003), 2239–2243.

[47] R.L. Doty and J.E. Cometto-Muñiz, Trigeminal chemosensation, in: *Handbook of olfaction and gestation*, R.L. Doty, ed., Marcel Dekker, New York, 2003, pp. 981–999.

[48] J. Driver and P.W. Halligan, Can visual neglect operate in object-centred co-ordinates? An affirmative single-case study, *Cogn Neuropsychol* **8** (1991), 475–496.

[49] J. Driver and J.B. Mattingley, Parietal neglect and visual awareness, *Nature Neuroscience* **1** (1998), 17–22.

[50] J. Driver and P. Vuilleumier, Perceptual awareness and its loss in unilateral neglect and extinction, *Cognition* **79** (2001), 39–88.

[51] J.R. Duhamel, C.L. Colby and M.E. Goldberg, Ventral intraparietal area of the macaque: congruent visual and somatic response properties, *Journal of Neurophysiology* **79** (1998), 126–136.

[52] M. Eimer, A. Maravita, J. Van Velzen, M. Husain and J. Driver, The electrophysiology of tactile extinction: ERP correlates of unconscious somatosensory processing, *Neuropsychologia* **40** (2002), 2438–2447.

[53] A. Farnè and E. Ladavas, Dynamic size-change of hand peripersonal space following tool use, *Neuroreport* **11**(8) (2000), 1645–1649.

[54] A. Farne and E. Ladavas, Auditory peripersonal space in humans, *Journal of Cognitive Neuroscience* **14**(7) (2002), 1030–1043.

[55] A. Farnè, L.J. Buxbaum, M. Ferraro, F. Frassinetti, J. Whyte, T. Veramonti, V. Angeli, H.B. Coslett and E. Ladavas, Patterns of spontaneous recovery of neglect and associated disorders in acute right brain-damaged patients, *Journal of Neurology Neurosurgery And Psychiatry* **75**(10) (2004), 1401–1410.

[56] A. Farnè, M.L. Dematté and E. Ladavas, Neuropsychological evidence of modular organization of the near peripersonal space, *Neurology* **65**(11) (2005), 1754–1758.

[57] S. Ferber and H.O. Karnath, Parietal and occipital lobe contributions to perception of straight ahead orientation, *Journal of Neurology Neurosurgery and Psychiatry* **67** (1999), 572–578.

[58] B. Fierro, F. Brighina, M. Oliveri, A. Piazza, V. La Bua, D. Buffa and E. Bisiach, Contralateral neglect induced by right posterior parietal rTMS in healthy subjects, *Neuroreport* **11** (2000), 1519–1521.

[59] F. Frassinetti, F. Pavani and E. Làdavas, Acoustical vision of neglected stimuli! Interaction among spatially converging audio-visual inputs in neglect patients, *Journal of Cognitive Neuroscience* **14** (2002), 62–69.

[60] F. Frassinetti, M. Rossi and E. Ladavas, Passive limb movements improve visual neglect, *Neuropsychologia* **39**(7) (2001), 725–733.

[61] F. Frassinetti, N. Bolognini, D. Bottari, A. Bonora and E. Ladavas, Audiovisual integration in patients with visual deficit, *Journal of Cognitive Neuroscience* **17**(9) (2005), 1442–1452.

[62] T. Fuji, R. Fukatsu, I. Kimura, S.-I. Saso and K. Kogure, Unilateral spatial neglect in visual and tactile modalitites, *Cortex* **27** (1991), 339–343.

[63] G. Gainotti, C. De Bonis, A. Daniele and C. Caltagirone, Contralateral and ipsilateral tactile extinction in patients with right and left focal brain damage, *International Journal of Neuroscience* **45**(1–2) (1989), 81–89.

[64] S. Geeraerts, K. Michiels, C. Lafosse, E. Vandenbussche and K. Verfaillie, The relationship of visual extinction to luminance-contrast imbalances between left and right hemifield stimuli, *Neuropsychologia* **43**(4) (2005), 542–553.

[65] S. Giaquinto, S. Buzzelli, L. Di Francesco et al., On the prognosis of outcome after stroke, *Acta Neurologica Scandinavica* **100** (1999), 202–208.

[66] M.H. Giard and F. Peronnet, Auditory–visual integration during multimodal object recognition in humans: A behavioral and electrophysiological study, *Journal of Cognitive Neuroscience* **11** (1999), 473–490.

[67] E.E. Gordon, V. Drenth, L. Jarvis et al., Neurophysiologic syndromes in stroke as predictors of outcome, *Archives of Physical Medicine And Rehabilitation* **59** (1978), 399–403.

[68] M.S.A. Graziano and C.G. Gross, The representation of extrapersonal space: a possible role for bimodal visual-tactile neurons, The Cognitive Neurosciences, M.S. Gazzaniga, ed., MIT Press, Cambridge, MA, 1995.

[69] M.S.A. Graziano, L.A.J. Reiss and C.G. Gross, A neuronal representation of the location of nearby sounds, *Nature* **397** (1999), 428–430.

[70] C. Guariglia, A. Padovani, P. Pantano and L. Pizzamiglio, Unilateral neglect restricted to visual imagery, *Nature* **364** (1993), 235–237.

[71] Guide for the Uniform Data Set for Medical Rehabilitation (Including the FIMSM Instrument). Buffalo, NY: State University of New York at Buffalo, 1996.

[72] P.W. Halligan and J.C. Marshall, Left neglect for near but not far space in man, *Nature* **350** (1991), 498–500.

[73] P.W. Halligan and J.C. Marshall, Left visuo-spatial neglect: a meaningless entity? *Cortex* **28** (1992), 525–535.

[74] P.W. Halligan and J.C. Marshall, When two is one: a case study of spatial parsing in visual neglect, *Perception* **22** (1993), 309–312.

[75] P.W. Halligan, G.R. Fink, J.C. Marshall and G. Vallar, Spatial cognition: evidence from visual neglect, *Trends In Cognitive Science* **7** (2003), 125–133.

[76] B. Heldmann, G. Kerkhoff, A. Struppler, P. Havel and T. Jahn, Repetitive peripheral magnetic stimulation alleviates tactile extinction, *Neuroreport* **11** (2000), 3193–3198.

[77] K.M. Heilman, R.T. Watson and E. Valenstein, Neglect I: clinical and anatomic issues, in: *Patient-based approaches to cognitive neuroscience*, M.J. Farah and T.E. Feinberg, eds, MIT Press, Cambridge (MA), 2000.

[78] C.C. Hilgetag, H. Theoret and A. Pascual-Leone, Enhanced visual spatial attention ipsilateral to rTMS-induced 'virtual lesions' of human parietal cortex, *Nature Neuroscience* **4** (2001), 953–957.

[79] H. Hjaltason, G. Caneman and R. Tegner, Visual and tactile rod bisection in unilateral neglect, *Cortex* **29** (1993), 588–593.

[80] H. Hjaltason, R. Tegner, K. Tham, M. Levander and K. Ericson, Sustained attention and awareness of disability in chronic neglect, *Neuropsychologia* **34**(12) (1996), 1229–1233.

[81] K. Hugdahl, K. Wester and A. Asbejornsen, Auditory neglect after right frontal lobe and right pulvinar thalamic lesion, *Brain and Language* **41** (1991), 465–473.

[82] M. Husain and C. Kennard, Distractor-dependent frontal neglect, *Neuropsychologia* **35**(6) (1997), 829–841.

[83] M. Husain and C. Rorden, Non-spatially lateralized mechanisms in hemispatial neglect, *Nature Review of Neuroscience* **4**(1) (2003), 26–36.

[84] A.W. Inhoff, R.D. Rafal and M.J. Posner, Bimodal extinction without cross-modal extinction, *Journal of Neurology Neurosurgery And Psychiatry* **55**(1) (1992), 36–39.

[85] H.O. Karnath, Subjective body orientation in neglect and the interactive contribution of neck muscle proprioception and vestibular stimulation, *Brain* **117** (1994), 1001–1012.

[86] H.O. Karnath, S. Ferber and M. Himmelbach, Spatial awareness is a function of the temporal not the posterior parietal lobe, *Nature* **411** (2001), 950–953.

[87] H.O. Karnath, M. Himmelbach and W. Kuker, The cortical substrate of visual extinction, *Neuroreport* **14**(3) (2003), 437–442.

[88] N. Katz, A. Hartman-Maeir, H. Ring and N. Soroker, Functional disability and rehabilitation outcome in right hemisphere damage patients with and without unilateral spatial neglect, *Archives of Physical Medicine And Rehabilitation* **80** (1999), 379–384.

[89] G. Kerkhoff, Spatial hemineglect in humans, *Progress In Neurobiology* **63** (2001), 1–27.

[90] G. Kerkhoff, F. Aartinger and W. Ziegler, Contrasting spatial hearing deficits in hemianopia and spatial neglect, *NeuroReport* **10** (1999), 3555–3560.

[91] A.J. King and A.R. Palmer, Cells responsive to free-field auditory stimuli in guinea-pig superior colliculus: Distribution and response properties, *Journal of Physiology* **342** (1983), 361–381.

[92] G. Kobal, S. Van Toller and T. Hummel, Is there directional smelling? *Experientia* **45** (1989), 130–132.

[93] E.I. Knudsen, Auditory and visual maps of space in the optic tectum of the owl, *Journal of Neuroscience* **2** (1983), 1177–1194.

[94] E. Ladavas, Functional and dynamic properties of visual peripersonal space in humans, *Trends in Cognitive Science* **6** (2002), 17–22.

[95] E. Ladavas, M. Carletti and G. Gori, Automatic and voluntary orienting of attention in patients with visual neglect: horizontal and vertical dimensions, *Neuropsychologia* **32** (1994), 1195–1208.

[96] E. Ladavas, G. di Pellegrino, A. Farnè and G. Zeloni, Neuropsychological evidence of an integrated visuo-tactile representation of peripersonal space in humans, *Journal of Cognitive Neuroscience* **10** (1998), 581–589.

[97] E. Ladavas, R. Paladini and R. Cubelli, Implicit associative priming in a patient with left visual neglect, *Neuropsychologia* **31** (1993), 1307–1320.

[98] E. Ladavas, F. Pavani and A. Farnè, Auditory peripersonal space in humans: A case of auditory-tactile extinction, *Neurocase* **7** (2001), 97–103.

[99] E. Ladavas, G. Zeloni and A. Farne, Visual peripersonal space centred on the face in humans, *Brain* **121**(Pt 12) (1998), 2317–2326.

[100] S.K. Mannan, D.J. Mort, T.L. Hodgson, J. Driver, C. Kennard and M. Husain, Revisiting previously searched locations in visual neglect: role of right parietal and frontal lesions in misjudging old locations as new, *Journal of Cognitive Neuroscience* **17**(2) (2005), 340–354.

[101] C.A. Marzi, M. Girelli, C. Miniussi, N. Smania and A. Maravita, Electrophysiological correlates of conscious vision: evidence from unilateral extinction, *Journal of Cognitive Neuroscience* **12**(5) (2000), 869–877.

[102] J.B. Mattingley, J.G. Phillips and J.L. Bradshaw, Impairments of movement execution in unilateral neglect: a kinematic analysis of directional bradykinesia, *Neuropsychologia* **32**(9) (1994), 1111–1134.

[103] J.B. Mattingley, Spatial extinction and its relation to mechanism of normal attention, H.O. Karnath, D. Milner and G. Vallar, eds., Oxford University Press, 2002.

[104] R.D. McIntosh, Y. Rossetti and A.D. Milner, Prism adaptation improves chronic visual and haptic neglect: a single case study, *Cortex* **38**(3) (2002), 309–320.

[105] M.A. Mesulam, A cortical network for directed attention and unilateral neglect, *Annals of Neurology* **10** (1981), 309–325.

[106] A.D. Milner, Neglect, extinction, and the cortical streams of visual processing, in: *parietal lobe contributions to orientation in 3D space*, P. Thier and H. O. Karnath, eds, Springer-Verlag, Berlin, 1997.

[107] A.D. Milner and R.D. McIntosh, The neurological basis of visual neglect, *Current Opinion in Neurology* **18**(6) (2005), 748–753.

[108] V. Moro, M. Zampini and S.M. Aglioti, Changes in spatial position of hands modify tactile extinction but not disownership of controlesional hand in two right brain-damaged patients, *Neurocase* **10**(6) (2004), 437–443.

[109] D.J. Mort, P. Malhotra, S.K. Mannan, C. Rorden, A. Pambakian, C. Kennard and M. Husain, The anatomy of visual neglect, *Brain* **126**(Pt 9) (2003), 1986–1997.

[110] M. Moscovitch and M. Behrmann, Coding of spatial information in the somatosensory system: evidence from patients with neglect following parietal lobe damage, *Journal of Cognitive Neuroscience* **6** (1994), 151–155.

[111] M. Oliveri, E. Bisiach, F. Brighina, A. Piazza, V. La Bua, D. Buffa and B. Fierro, rTMS of the unaffected hemisphere transiently reduces contralesional visuospatial hemineglect, *Neurology* **57** (2001), 1338–1340.

[112] M. Oliveri, P.M. Rossini, R. Traversa, P. Cicinelli, M.M. Filippi, P. Pasqualetti, F. Tomaiuolo and C. Caltagirone, Left frontal transcranial magnetic stimulation reduces contralesional extinction in patients with unilateral right brain damage, *Brain* **122** (1999), 1731–1739.

[113] E. Olson, M. Stark and A. Chatterjee, Evidence for a unimodal somatosensory attention system, *Experimental Brain Research* **151**(1) (2003), 15–23.

[114] J.V. Pardo, T.D. Wood, P.A. Costello, P.J. Pardo and J.T. Lee, PET study of the localization and laterality of lingual somatosensory processing in humans, *Neuroscience Letters* **234** (1997), 23–26.

[115] F. Pavani, A. Farnè and E. Làdavas, Poor hand-pointing to sounds in right brain-damaged patients: not just a problem of spatial-hearing, *Brain Cognition* **59** (2005), 215–224.

[116] F. Pavani, E. Ladavas and J. Driver, Selective deficit of auditory localisation in patients with visuospatial neglect, *Neuropsychologia* **40** (2002), 291–301.

[117] F. Pavani, F. Meneghello and E. Làdavas, Deficit of auditory space perception in patients with visuospatial neglect, *Neuropsychologia* **39** (2001), 1401–1409.

[118] F. Pavani, M. Husain, E. Ladavas and J. Driver, Auditory deficits in visuospatial neglect patients, *Cortex* **40** (2004), 347–365.

[119] F. Pavani, E. Ladavas and J. Driver, Gaze direction modulates auditory spatial deficits in stroke patients with neglect, *Cortex* **41** (2005), 181–188.

[120] A. Peru, V. Moro, L. Sattibaldi, J.S. Morgant and M.S. Aglioti, Gravitational influences on reference frames for mapping somatic stimuli in brain-damaged patients, *Experimental Brain Research* **10** (2005).

[121] B. Pinek, J.-R. Duhamel, C. Cavè and M. Brouchon, Audio-spatial deficit in humans: Differential effects associated with left versus right hemisphere parietal damage, *Cortex* **25** (1989), 175–186.

[122] L. Pisella and J.B. Mattingley, The contribution of spatial remapping impairments to unilateral visual neglect, *Neuroscience and Biobehavioral Reviews* **28**(2) (2004), 181–200.

[123] S. Pitzalis, F. Di Russo, F. Figliozzi and D. Spinelli, Underestimation of contralateral space in neglect: a deficit in the "where" task, *Exp Brain Res* **159** (2004), 319–328.

[124] L. Pizzamiglio, G. Vallar and F. Doricchi, Gravitational inputs modulate visuospatial neglect, *Experimental Brain Research* **117** (1997), 341–345.

[125] L. Pizzamiglio, G. Vallar and F. Doricchi, Gravity and hemineglect, *Neuroreport* **7** (1995), 370–371.

[126] J. Porter, T. Anand, B. Johnson, R.M. Khan and N. Sobel, Brain mechanisms for extracting spatial information from smell, *Neuron* **47** (2005), 581–592.

[127] M.I.Posner, J.A. Walker, F.J. Friedrich and R.D. Rafal, Effects of parietal injury on covert orienting of attention, *Journal of Neuroscience* **4**(7) (1984), 1863–1874.

[128] S.Z. Rapcsak, C.R. Cimino and K.M. Heilman, Altitudinal neglect, *Neurology* **38**(2) (1988), 277–281.

[129] P. Remy, M. Zilbovicius, J.D. Degos, A.C. Bachoud-Levy, G. Rancurel, P. Cesaro and Y. Samson, Somatosensory cortical activations are suppressed in patients with tactile extinction: a PET study, *Neurology* **52** (1999), 571–577.

[130] R. Ricci and A. Chatterjee, Sensory and response contributions to visual awareness in extinction, *Experimental Brain Research* **157** (2004), 85–93.

[131] G. Rizzolatti, C. Scandolara, M. Matelli and M. Gentilucci, Afferent properties of periarcuate neurons in macaque monkeys. II Visual responses, *Behavioral Brain Research* **2** (1981), 147–163.

[132] G. Rizzolatti, M. Matelli and G. Pavesi, Deficits in attention and movement following the removal of postarcuate (area 6) and prearcuate (area 8) cortex in macaque monkeys, *Brain* **106**(Pt 3) (1983), 655–673.

[133] G. Rizzolatti, G. Luppino and M. Matelli, The organization of the cortical motor system: new concepts, *Electroencephalography and Clinical Neurophysiology* **106** (1998), 283–296.

[134] T. Ro and A. Farnè, Within-modal anti-extinction in multimodal "neglect", *Cognitive Neuroscience Society Abstracts* **103E** (2001), 139.

[135] I.H. Robertson, T. Manly, N. Beschin, R. Daini, H. Haeske-Dewich, V. Homberg, M. Jehkonen, G. Pizzamiglio, A. Shiel and E. Weber, Auditory sustained attention is a marker of unilateral spatial neglect, *Neuropsychologia* **35** (1997), 1527–1532.

[136] G. Rode, Y. Rossetti and D. Boisson, Prism adaptation improves representational neglect, *Neuropsychologia* **39** (2001), 1250–1254.

[137] C. Rorden, M. Fruhmann Berger and H.O. Karnath, Disturbed line bisection is associated with posterior brain lesions, *Brain Research Cognitive Brain Research* **19** (2005).

[138] R.M. Ruff, N.A. Hersch and K.H. Pribram, Auditory spatial deficit in the personal and extrapersonal frames of reference due to cortical lesions, *Neuropsychologia* **19** (1981), 435–443.

[139] M.L. Rusconi, A. Maravita, G. Bottini and G. Vallar, Is the intact side really intact? Perseverative responses in patients with unilateral neglect: a productive manifestation, *Neuropsychologia* **40**(6) (2002), 594–604.

[140] H. Shikata, D.B. McMahon and P.A. Breslin, Psychophysics of taste lateralization on anterior tongue, *Perception and Psychophysics* **62** (2000), 684–694.

[141] N. Smania and S. Aglioti, Sensory and spatial components of somaesthetic deficits following right brain damage, *Neurology* **45** (1995), 1725–1730.

[142] N. Soroker, N. Calamaro, J. Glicksohn and M.S. Myslobodsky, Auditory inattention in right-hemisphere-damaged patients with and without visual neglect, *Neuropsychologia* **35** (1997), 249–256.

[143] B.E. Stein and M.O. Arigbede, Unimodal and multimodal response properties of neurons in the cat's superior colliculus, *Experimental of Neurology* **36** (1972), 179–196.

[144] B.E. Stein and M.A. Meredith, *The merging of the Senses*, MIT Press, Cambridge, MA, 1993.

[145] S.P. Stone, P. Patel, R.J. Greenwood and P.W. Halligan, Measuring visual neglect in acute stroke and predicting its recovery: the visual neglect recovery index, *Journal of Neurology Neurosurgery and Psychiatry* **55** (1992), 431–436.

[146] H. Tanaka, K. Hachisuka and H. Ogata, Sound lateralisation in patients with left or right cerebral hemispheric lesions: Relation with unilateral visuospatial neglect, *Journal of Neurology, Neurosurgery and Psychiatry* **67** (1999), 481–486.

[147] M. Tinazzi, G. Ferraria, M. Zampini and S.M. Aglioti, Neuropsychological evidence that somatic stimuli are spatially coded according to multiple frames of reference in a stroke patient with tactile extinction, *Neuroscience Letters* (2000), 133–136.

[148] N. Valenza, M.L. Seghier, S. Schwartz, F. Lazeyras and P. Vuilleumier, Tactile awareness and limb position in neglect: Functional magnetic resonance imaging, *Annals of Neurology* **55** (2004), 139–143.

[149] G. Vallar, Spatial hemineglect in humans, Trends In Cognitive, *Science* **2** (1998), 87–97.

[150] G. Vallar and D. Perani, The anatomy of unilateral neglect after right-hemisphere stroke lesions. A clinical/CT-scan correlation study in man, *Neuropsychologia* **24**(5) (1986), 609–622.

[151] G. Vallar, G. Bottini, M.L. Rusconi and R. Sterzi, Exploring somatosensory hemineglect by vestibular stimulation, *Brain* **116**(Pt 1) (1993), 71–86.

[152] G. Vallar, C. Guariglia, D. Nico and E. Bisiach, Spatial hemineglect in back space, *Brain* **118** (1995), 467–471.

[153] G. Vallar, M.L. Rusconi, L. Bignamini, G. Geminiani and D. Perani, Anatomical correlates of visual and tactile extinction in humans: a clinical CT scan study, *Journal of Neurology Neurosurgery and Psychiatry* **57** (1994), 464–470.

[154] C. Villardita, Tactile exploration of space and visual neglect in brain-damaged patients, *Journal of Neurology* **234** (1987), 292–297.

[155] G. von Békésy, Olfactory analogue to directional hearing, *Journal of Applied Physiology* **19** (1964), 369–373.

[156] G. von Békésy, Rhythmical variations accompanying gustatory stimulation observed by means of localization phenomena, *Journal of General Physiology* **47** (1964), 809–825.

[157] P. Vuilleumier, N. Valenza, E. Mayer, A. Reverdin and T. Landis, Near and far visual space in unilateral neglect, *Annals of Neurology* **43**(3) (1998), 406–410.

Stimulus- and goal-driven biases of selective attention following unilateral brain damage: Implications for rehabilitation of spatial neglect and extinction

Jacqueline C. Snow[a,b,*] and Jason B. Mattingley[a]
[a]*Cognitive Neuroscience Laboratory, University of Melbourne, Victoria 3010, Australia*
[b]*School of Psychology, University of Birmingham, Edgbaston, Birmingham B15 2TT, UK*

Received 7 March 2006
Revised 13 May 2006
Accepted 22 June 2006

Abstract. In this review we address the question of whether selective attentional mechanisms within the ipsilesional field are intact in unilateral lesion patients with spatial neglect and extinction. We consider how a lesion-induced bias in the neural representation of salience critically disrupts the integration of goal-driven and stimulus-driven prioritization signals. This has important consequences for selectivity both within the 'impaired' contralesional field within the 'intact' ipsilesional field. Examples are drawn from the neuropsychological literature and recent experiments conducted within our own laboratory. The implications of ipsilesional spatial selection deficits for rehabilitation are discussed.

1. Introduction

Patients suffering unilateral brain damage often display ongoing deficits in spatial cognition and behaviour. In florid cases of neglect and extinction, suprathreshold stimuli arising within the contralesional field fail to be selected for attention and awareness, while attention is biased toward stimuli arising within the ipsilesional field [10,15,41,58]. Even for 'recovered' patients, a sub-clinical spatial bias often persists well beyond the acute phase post-stroke [3,49,78,120,122]. Such lateralized spatial biases invariably lead to difficulties in complex tasks of daily living in which a multitude of stimuli compete for limited capacity attentional resources [82].

In terms of visuospatial function in patients with neglect and extinction, the general picture that has emerged from the neuropsychological literature is a relatively dichotomous one: unilateral brain damage leads to impaired attentional function within the contralesional field and relatively intact functioning within the ipsilesional field [37,42,100,116]. Not surprisingly, the bulk of previous research in this area has focussed on characterising the precise nature of the *contralesional* impairments. The impetus for exploring contralesional deficits has been further strengthened by the intimate relationship between attention and awareness, and our ongoing search for possible 'neural correlates of consciousness' [26,48,59].

In contrast to the contralesional impairments seen in neglect and extinction, the 'intact' ipsilesional field has received less systematic research. Relatively few studies have *specifically* investigated attentional function within the ipsilesional field. In cases where ipsilesional

*Corresponding author: Dr. Jacqueline C. Snow, School of Psychology, University of Birmingham, Edgbaston, Birmingham B15 2TT, UK. Tel.: +44 0121 4147369; E-mail: j.c.snow@bham.ac.uk.

stimulus conditions have been incorporated, they have often served as a convenient within-subject control with which to compare contralesional performance, rather than as an interest in their own right. Nonetheless, current behavioural research and theoretical accounts of neglect and extinction clearly imply that attention is biased toward the ipsilesional field.

2. Selectivity within the ipsilesional field

In patients with unilateral brain damage, the ipsilesional field is predominantly considered to benefit from 'increased attention' [40,43,58,116], or even 'hyperattention' [50,62,108,116]. Similarly, the ipsilesional manifestation of attentional bias has often been viewed as being productive or 'positive' in its effect on perception and action, whereas that of the contralesional side has been characterised as defective, or 'negative' [105, 116]. Accordingly, influential theories of neglect have often regarded the condition as reflecting '*enhanced attention*' toward the ipsilesional field [56–58].

Evidence for attentional enhancement is commonly obtained within the context of formal neuropsychological testing [4,82]. For example, patients perform remarkably well in response to stimuli positioned within the ipsilesional hemispace. Accuracy for detecting ipsilesional targets on cancellation tasks such as Albert's Lines [1], Star cancellation [36,123], and the Balloons Test [29], is typically very high [74]. Further, patients with right hemisphere (RH) damage and left neglect choose to begin cancellation with ipsilesional (right-sided) targets, unlike healthy observers, who typically begin with targets on the left [34,78].

Similarly, in the experimental domain, a number of studies have documented behavioural performance consistent with the notion of enhanced attention toward the ipsilesional field. In visual search, RH-damaged patients show a characteristic early orienting of attention toward the ipsilesional side of the array [34], and an ipsilesional deviation of eye and head movements [9,50]. These patients also demonstrate an increased number of fixations, and show a prolonged inspection time for ipsilesional targets [9]. For example, Karnath and colleagues [50] investigated gaze-, head-, and eye-in-head movements made by four patients with left-neglect while they searched for a target letter within a random array of letters positioned around a small spherical room. Relative to controls, neglect patients showed a strong ipsilesional bias in gaze-, head-, and eye-in-head positions during spontaneous search

of the arrays. The patients were able to orient toward the contralesional side of the array when requested to by the experimenter, suggesting that the ipsilesional attention bias could not merely be attributed to a primary motoric bias [50].

Other experimental support for an ipsilesional attentional enhancement in unilateral brain damaged patients comes from studies using speeded reaction time (RT) tasks. In healthy observers, RTs and accuracy are best when the stimuli appear close to fixation, and gradually decline as targets appear further from the central fixation point. For patients with extinction, however, detection performance is consistently better when target stimuli appear further toward the ipsilesional periphery [23,61,108], suggesting attention is maximal within the ipsilesional field. Further, the RT-advantage for ipsilesional targets is comparatively greater for RH-damaged patients with severe left-neglect, than for those without neglect [64]. Findings such as these have led to speculation that the severity of ipsilesional spatial bias may correspond with stronger lateralised 'attentional enhancements' [5].

3. Mechanisms of prioritisation and selection in the healthy brain

A major problem hindering detailed investigation of attentional function within the ipsilesional hemispace in unilateral brain-damaged patients is that in the neuropsychological domain the term 'attention' is typically used rather loosely to refer to a host of different functions. Perhaps not surprisingly, attentional accounts of neglect span a range of 'levels' along the processing continuum, from stimulus input to response production, and tend to be couched in broad terms [4,6,12,55, 56,58,91,98].

'Attention' is increasingly recognized, however, as an umbrella term that carries little specificity about the large number of neural or cognitive operations it encompasses. For example, in the neuroscience domain, component processes of attention include (a) neural mechanisms of competition between potential sources of information, including both stimulus-driven and goal-driven *prioritization*, (b) mechanisms of *selection* that extract only the most relevant or important information from the environment, and (c) *feedback enhancement* and elaboration processes that operate post-selection [45,46,53,114].

We propose here that an understanding of the neural mechanisms of prioritization and selection is critical for characterising the spatial deficits suffered by patients with extinction and neglect. The following section gives a basic overview of recent knowledge on mechanisms of selection in the healthy brain, before considering how these processes might be impaired in patients with unilateral brain damage, their consequences for behaviour, and decisions regarding rehabilitation strategies.

Because of limits in the amount of information that can be attended at any given moment, stimuli that are *most* relevant to behaviour must be prioritised for attentional selection and awareness, while those of lesser importance must be ignored or suppressed. The healthy brain is able to determine which information is most relevant for selection by integrating and comparing inputs from two different prioritization systems: a 'bottom-up', stimulus-driven system, and a 'top-down', goal-driven system [30,46].

Stimulus-driven prioritization is the result of competitive neural interactions that arise as sensory information is processed across successive stages of the visual processing hierarchy. Stimulus-driven mechanisms bias neural competition in favour of stimuli that have distinguishing physical characteristics within a given context, such as their colour, orientation, brightness, or motion [8,86,125,126]. Once a stimulus begins to dominate neural responses within one visual area, this stimulus benefits from a competitive advantage at progressively higher processing levels, thereby increasing the likelihood that it will be selected [24,25,127]. Conversely, goal-driven signals enable selection to be biased flexibly by our current goals and intentions [30, 31,126]. Goal-driven biasing signals are thought to originate from a distributed network of brain areas, predominantly within the frontal and parietal lobes [21, 83]. At the neural level, these feedback signals bias processing within almost all visual processing areas [25, 53,114,128].

In the healthy brain, stimulus-driven and goal-driven systems interact to determine where, and on what, attention is focused [21,46]. A stimulus representation may therefore gain a competitive advantage either as a result of stimulus-driven contextual distinctiveness, or via modulatory feedback signals (i.e., due to behavioural relevance or salience). Adaptive behaviour requires that selection is able to shift flexibly between internally driven goals, and external stimuli and events [8,46,51,127]. Ideally, selection should favour the *most* relevant information, and be prevented from returning to stimuli that are irrelevant, or that have previously been explored. Information from these different control mechanisms may, in fact, be coded within the same neural populations [75,96,97]. For example, recent evidence suggests that in brain areas such as V4 and MT, stimulus-driven and goal-driven sources of prioritization may ultimately be indistinguishable [75, 113,114].

In the context of unilateral brain damage these two systems have potentially important consequences for understanding the influence of biased feedback signals on selectivity. Current views on the way in which goal-driven and stimulus-driven signals are integrated for the purpose of *selection* are largely based on theoretical or computational models of attention [46,92,112,124]. Several such models propose that incoming stimulus-based and goal-driven signals converge within an integrated 'salience map' [46,47,92,118,124]. A salience map is a theoretical construct intended to provide a possible mechanism for resolving competition between a number of stimulus-driven and goal driven inputs, for the purpose of selection [35,46,47]. Several brain regions have been identified in monkeys that possess neural response properties similar to those of a salience map, including the parietal lobe [14,35,60], frontal eye fields [110,111], pulvinar [52,102], and superior colliculus [32].

The brain regions most commonly affected in neglect and extinction patients are the ventral parietal, superior temporal, and inferior frontal regions within the RH [20,44,85,117]. Some authors within the clinical research domain have followed leads from neuroscience research to propose a neural explanation for neglect and extinction. Based on physiological data from monkeys, and a recent computational model of spatial representation in the parietal cortex, Driver and colleagues [27,92,93] have posited that a loss of neurons in areas such as the parietal lobe produces a spatial imbalance in the representation of salience across the visual field. Specifically, although neurons within each parietal lobe have predominantly contralateral receptive fields, the *number* of neurons that represent progressively more eccentric locations appears to follow a gradient. Increasing numbers of neurons within each parietal lobe represent regions further toward the opposite visual field, with the frequency of representation reaching an 'off-centre-peak' around 10–20° of retinal eccentricity [27,93]. In other words, the spatial location most *strongly* represented by each parietal lobe is not the body midline, but rather, the periphery. Given that the relative spatiotopic activity of parietal neurons corresponds to the location of behavioural selection and enhancement [14], a unilateral lesion-induced imbalance in the number of neurons that code salience should cause selection to be biased in favour of stimuli at ipsilesional locations.

Contrary to previous accounts, therefore, we argue here that RH-damaged patients show a marked lack of selectivity at ipsilesional locations. Specifically, a relative imbalance in the salience afforded to stimuli across the visual field following unilateral damage is likely to have important consequences for the balance between stimulus-driven and goal-driven prioritization signals. As outlined above, information about stimulus-based conspicuity and goal-driven behavioural relevance may be coded within the same neural populations in ventral stream areas, and these areas may be 'blind' to the source of the prioritization signal [75,96,97,113, 114]. If unilateral brain damage causes a lateralized bias in the representation of salience across the visual field [27,92,93], this may disrupt normal mechanisms of prioritization, such that ipsilesional stimuli are selected whether they are behaviourally relevant or not. This (ipsilesional) selection bias is also likely to have flow-on effects post-selection due to neural feedback processes that operate to enhance stimulus representations in early perceptual areas [25,52,87,114]. For patients with RH damage, therefore, brain areas coding salience may receive goal-driven prioritization signals, but these signals are likely to be ineffective in driving selection in an adaptive manner [109].

4. Recent behavioural investigations of selectivity within the ipsilesional field

It is now well established that, in the healthy brain, selection of relevant information and filtering of distractors is controlled by both spatial and 'non-spatial' mechanisms. 'Non-spatial' control mechanisms include: (a) feature-based selectivity, and (b) the constraints imposed by capacity limits on processing in cognitively demanding situations ('load-based' selectivity). We have recently conducted several studies examining these non-spatial aspects of selectivity in patients with unilateral brain damage.

In one such study, we investigated whether RH-damaged patients demonstrate intact goal-driven selectivity for feature-based information. In the healthy brain, goal-driven feedback signals operate not only to selectively prioritise information at relevant *spatial* locations, but also to selectively enhance or suppress certain *feature-based* properties of visual stimuli, depending on their relevance to performance [11,17,18,

76,80,115]. A range of visual stimulus properties can be used to guide feature-based selection, from colour, orientation, and shape, to more complex stimulus properties, such as letter identity or facial identity [25,28, 107].

We examined whether patients with unilateral brain damage resulting in lateralized spatial biases are able to use goal-driven cues to modulate feature-based selectivity, as seen in healthy observers. In the standard flanker paradigm, responses are determined on the basis of featural properties of the target along a single pre-specified featural dimension (e.g., an 'A' or 'B' on the dimension of letter identity). To examine the influence of goal-driven effects on flanker processing, we added a second dimension, so that stimuli were defined by their congruence along two orthogonal dimensions (e.g., the letter 'A' or 'B', presented in red or green) [19,22,77, 84]. Importantly, only one dimension of the target stimulus was relevant to observer's behavioural responses on each trial: the 'task-relevant' dimension. The properties of the target on the other 'task-irrelevant' dimension were to be ignored (see Fig. 1). In our task, on half of the trials participants responded to the identity of the target and ignored its colour. On the remaining trials, participants responded to the target's colour and ignored its identity.

Studies using this paradigm with healthy observers, both from our own laboratory and from others, demonstrate that multidimensional flankers influence RTs to a central target, but only as a function of their congruence with the target on the *task-relevant* dimension (see Fig. 1(c)) [19,77,84]. As illustrated in Fig. 1, task-irrelevant feature-based dimensions of flankers do not affect target RTs. In the healthy brain, therefore, behavioural goals are used to bias selection in favour of task-relevant features by constraining the processing of task-irrelevant, feature-based information at ignored locations.

We then conducted the same multidimensional flanker task in a group of six patients who had suffered a first-episode, unilateral RH stroke, and a group of healthy age- and sex-matched controls. We reasoned that if 'enhanced attention' improves selectivity for ipsilesional events, our patients should show flanker compatibility effects from *only* the task-relevant dimension of flanking distractors on the right side. Conversely, if spatial bias leads to an unselective increase in the salience of ipsilesional stimuli, whether relevant to the current task or not, then all feature-based properties of ignored flanker stimuli on the ipsilesional side should affect performance at the central target location.

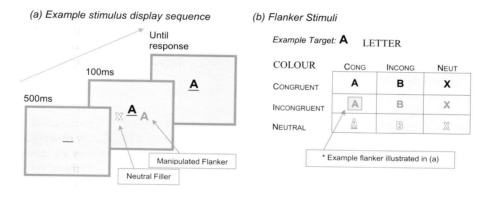

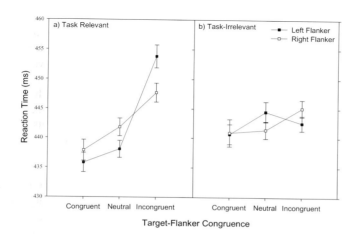

Fig. 1. Example display and target-flanker congruency conditions for the multidimensional flanker task. (a) Each trial began with a central underscore (500 ms) followed by a central target, flanked on either side by a distractor. Distractors disappeared after 100 ms, whereas the central target remained on the screen until response. In the experiment, target and flanker stimuli could be red, green, or yellow in colour; however in (a) and (b) coloured stimuli are illustrated in black, grey, and white, respectively. A single flanker was always neutral (the left one in this example) with respect to the target on both the letter and colour dimensions; this served as a filler to maintain a balanced, competitive display. The opposite 'manipulated flanker' could be congruent, incongruent or neutral with respect to the central target letter on either the letter or colour dimension. (b) Matrix of the 9 different types of flanker stimuli, positioned according to their compatibility with a central target stimulus. If the participant was instructed to report the letter identity of the central target, then the manipulated flanker in this example would be congruent with the target on the task-relevant dimension, but incongruent on the task-irrelevant dimension. (c) Performance of young healthy observers from our own laboratory on the multidimensional flanker task. Only the task-relevant dimension of flankers interferes with RTs to the central target. The task-irrelevant featural dimension does not influence RTs. Flanker effects are equivalent for both left and right-sided flankers. (*Figure adapted with permission from Snow and Mattingley [109]*).

All six patients showed signs of significant rightward attentional bias, and consequent left inattention on standard clinical measures of neglect. Performance of patients and controls in the target response task is displayed in Fig. 2. Both groups showed a similar pattern of performance for the *task-relevant flanker dimension*. Left- and right-sided flankers that were incongruent with the target slowed RTs significantly relative to neutral flankers. For the *task-irrelevant flanker dimension*, the age-matched control group showed an identical pattern of performance to that of young healthy controls (see Fig. 1), in that task-irrelevant features did not facilitate or interfere with response times to the central target. In contrast, RH-damaged patients exhibited significant interference for the task-irrelevant dimension of incongruent right-sided flankers. These results confirm that patients with spatial bias show a striking breakdown in selective processing of visual features in the *ipsilesional* hemifield. Therefore, rather than spatial bias resulting in 'enhanced' attentional function,

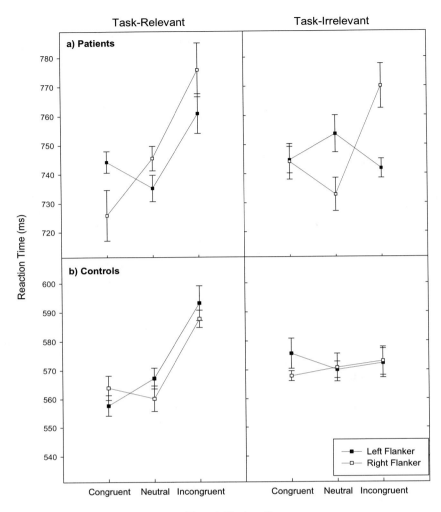

Fig. 2. Mean reaction times (±1 SE) for patients and age-matched controls in the multidimensional flanker task. (a) The upper figures show performance of the patient group, and (b) the lower figures that of the age-matched control group. Left and right panels illustrate the pattern of flanker effects for the Task-Relevant and Task-Irrelevant dimension of flankers, respectively. Data are plotted as a function of congruence, with separate lines for left- and right-sided flankers. Left panels: both patients and controls show significant interference from flanker features that are incongruent with those of the central target on the task-relevant dimension. Right panels: task-irrelevant flanker features had no effect on response times for the control group. Conversely, patients suffer interference from right-sided flanker features, despite being irrelevant to decisions at the target location. (*Figure reproduced, with permission, from Snow and Mattingley [109]*).

RH-damage leads to impairments in selectively inhibiting task-irrelevant information within the ipsilesional field.

In another study, we examined whether ipsilesional distractors are selectively filtered when the task at fixation becomes more difficult. In healthy individuals, filtering of distractors improves when the perceptual difficulty, or 'load', of a central task is increased [39, 65–68,70,94,95,106,129]. If unilateral brain damage causes ipsilesional stimuli to be unselectively prioritised for selection, then distractors arising at this location should be resistant to filtering, despite increased central load.

To investigate this we used a flanker task based on that of Lavie and Robertson [69]. The basic flanker task is illustrated in Fig. 3. Participants were required to indicate whether a central target letter was an 'A' or 'B'. The central target letter was flanked by distractor letters in both the left and right hemifields. The flanker on one side of the target (the manipulated flanker) was congruent, incongruent, or neutral with respect to the target, while the opposite flanker (the filler) was always neutral. The manipulated flanker could appear on either the left or right side of the target. As before, we were interested in the extent to which flanker congruence influenced response times to identify the central target. Critically, we manipulated perceptual load by having observers discriminate the central target from a distractor stimulus: in the low load condition, the distractor was a distinctive "hash mark", while in the high load condition, the distractor was a different but visually similar letter ('R'), chosen to make target detection more difficult. The flankers appeared briefly (100 ms), while the target and central distractor remained on-screen until response.

We tested four patients with unilateral RH lesions who showed rightward spatial attention biases on standard clinical measures of neglect. Representative data from a single parietal patient, S.G., are illustrated in Fig. 4. Reaction times to detect the central target indicated that, as expected, target identification was significantly more difficult in the high- than the low-load condition. Despite this difference in task difficulty between low- and high-load conditions, the interference caused by incongruent ipsilesional flankers was equivalent in both conditions. Ipsilesional distractor processing was therefore unaffected by perceptual load at fixation, suggesting that spatial bias critically affects load-based filtering at the biased location. This result was strikingly similar across all patients tested. For patients with spatial bias, therefore, the normal pattern of selectivity in spatial processing under conditions of increased perceptual load is impaired within the ipsilesional field.

Taken together, our experiments indicate that spatial bias leads to a concomitant reduction in selectivity within the ipsilesional field; this is demonstrated by an inability to flexibly modulate the processing of irrelevant ipsilesional distractors under conditions of increased load in a central task, and a lack of goal-driven selectivity for non-spatial feature-based properties of ipsilesional information. Rather than being 'well-preserved' [37,100,116], therefore, attentional function within the ipsilesional field shows striking signs of impairment. Neglect and extinction may more accurately be conceptualised as a disruption of selectivity affecting selective attention across the *entire* visual field, rather than being a 'unilateral' disruption. It is also worth noting that in the studies outlined above, patients varied in terms of lesion location, and in the extent of their lateralized spatial biases. As a group, the severity of spatial bias generally fell along a continuum; some patients showed mild or fluctuating hemi-inattention and/or extinction, while others showed florid neglect. Further research is required to determine the extent to which the ipsilesional selective deficits following unilateral brain damage are related to the severity of spatial bias, lesion location, and lesion volume.

The notion that selective attention in the ipsilesional hemifield might more accurately be viewed as dysfunctional, rather than intact [40,43,58,105,116], is supported by a number of other commonly observed behavioural patterns in patients with neglect and extinction. For example, many patients show perseverative drawing behaviour and pathological revisiting of ipsilesional targets on cancellation tasks [72,105]. Similarly, neglect patients' line-cancellation performance can be improved if ipsilesional stimuli are erased from the array, rather than merely cancelled [73]. Indeed, in observing that patients with left neglect omit targets in cancellation tasks independently of their position with respect to the midsagittal plane, Marshall and Halligan [74] noted that the deficit suffered by these patients might more aptly be described as 'ipsilateral capture', rather than 'left-neglect'. In addition, the clinical phenomenon of 'allochiria' may reflect dysfunctional selectivity for ipsilesional events; in basic copying tasks details from the contralesional side of a drawing may be faithfully reproduced, but spatially transposed to the ipsilesional side [13,38,71].

Interestingly, patients' RTs to *repeated* peripheral events has often been regarded as reflecting enhanced attention towards the ipsilesional field [6,7,119]. In the healthy brain, attention is prevented from returning to previously explored locations via a mechanism known as 'inhibition of return' (IOR). In experimental tasks, IOR is evidenced by a pattern of prolonged RTs to identify a peripheral target when attention has been drawn to the same location by an irrelevant stimulus (cue) around 800 ms earlier [90]. Vivas, Humphreys and Fuentes [119] used an IOR cueing paradigm with four extinction patients. In contrast to healthy controls, the extinction patients failed to demonstrate the usual pattern of IOR for previously cued targets when these appeared within the ipsilesional field. Rather, patients showed a pattern of facilitated RTs for ipsilesional targets. These results suggest a breakdown in normal mechanisms that operate to disengage or shift attention away from ipsilesional events, and to facilitate exploration of other locations across the visual field.

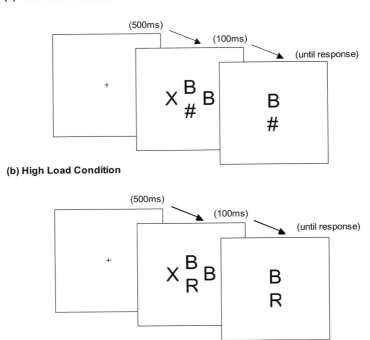

Fig. 3. Example displays for the perceptual load task. Each trial began with a central fixation cross (500 ms), followed by a display consisting of a vertically aligned target/distractor pair, flanked on either side (left and right) by horizontally aligned distractors. The flankers disappeared after 100 ms; the central target/distractor pair remained on-screen until response. On each trial, the central target letter was an "A" or "B", positioned randomly either above or below the fixation point. (a) In the low load condition the central distractor was a hash mark (#). (b) In the high load condition the distractor was an "R". Low- and high-load conditions were blocked throughout the experiment. One flanker (left or right) was always congruent, incongruent, or neutral with respect to the target; the example shown here illustrates a congruent trial in which the target ("B") is flanked to the right by a congruent ("B") distractor. The opposite flanker was always neutral (i.e., an "X"). The neutral flanker again served as a filler to maintain a balanced, competitive display.

5. Implications for rehabilitation of patients with spatial bias

The literature described above, and recent findings from our laboratory, suggest that neglect and extinction should be viewed as disorders in which unilateral brain damage disrupts salience representations, and therefore selection, across the *entire* visual field. The dysfunctional prioritization of ipsilesional events is likely to play a significant causal role in producing and maintaining neglect of contralesional stimuli. This may have consequences not only for our understanding of the nature of the attentional impairments suffered by patients with neglect, but also as a framework for conceptualizing the efficacy of current treatments.

Most treatments for spatial bias can be viewed as falling within one of two categories, based on whether they target stimulus-driven or goal-driven prioritization mechanisms [33,88]. Several treatments appeal to goal-driven mechanisms to ameliorate neglect, by training patients to use cognitive (goal-driven) strategies to overcome their spatial bias. For example, using retraining techniques, patients are encouraged to redirect their gaze, or to direct their attention, toward the contralesional hemifield [99,101]. Although goal-driven treatments can demand long-term training (making them relatively labour-intensive treatment options), lasting improvements have been reported [2,63]. An obvious limitation to goal-driven approaches, however, is that patients must be aware of their lateralized deficits. Indeed, goal-driven strategies may be relatively ineffective in helping patients with severe neglect, or in those who are anosognosic.

Relatively greater success has been achieved using stimulus-driven approaches. In this case, sensory stimulation is used to increase the relative competitive advantage of contralesional events. Examples include vibratory or electric neck muscle stimulation, caloric stimulation of the contralesional ear, contralesional postural rotation of the trunk, optokinetic stimulation,

(a)

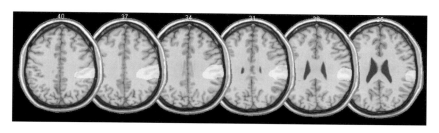

(b)

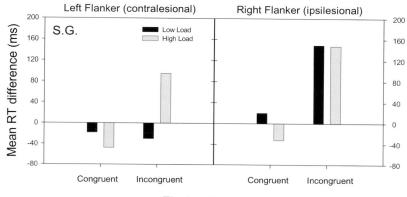

Fig. 4. Brain lesion, and behavioural performance on the load task, for a single representative patient with visual extinction. (a) Lesion maps for patient S.G. plotted onto a normal template brain using MRIcro software [103]. Affected regions (translucent red) are plotted onto axial slices, with numbers above each slice indicating Z-coordinates This patient suffered a right parietal embolic stroke, and showed a strong right-bias and left-neglect on standard clinical cancellation and line-bisection tasks. The data plotted in (b) represent mean (SE) compatibility effects for congruent and incongruent flankers, with reference to the neutral condition, under conditions of low- versus high-perceptual load. The data for contralesional (left) and ipsilesional (right) flanker conditions are plotted separately. The interference from incongruent ipsilesional flankers is not attenuated in the high-load, compared with the low-load condition.

or contralesional limb activation techniques. Although these procedures reportedly induce a bias favouring contralesional selection, the effects tend to be relatively short-lived, and are often confined to the duration of treatment [33,54].

Research from our laboratory suggests that unilateral brain damage results not only in a failure to select contralesional events, but also a high degree of distractibility for information arising within the ipsilesional field. That these patients suffer attentional impairments within *both* visual fields is worth considering in the context of future rehabilitative approaches. In particular, given that the normal integration between stimulus-driven and goal-driven signals may be disrupted, some of the most promising possibilities for rehabilitation may be those that attempt to modulate spatial representations in brain areas involved in *spatial coding* and *selection*, rather than targeting stimulus- or goal-driven prioritization signals that serve as inputs to these areas.

In a recent fMRI study Corbetta and colleagues [20] examined the neural basis of recovery from unilateral neglect. They found that in the acute phase, neglect was not only associated with reduced activity within ipsilesional parietal cortex (a pattern that was mirrored in the visual cortex), but also with abnormally high activation in the contralesional (left) hemisphere. Recovery from neglect was correlated with a reactivation and normalization of activity across these brain areas. Importantly, because unilateral brain damage produced dysfunction in a distributed network of brain areas across both hemispheres [20], treatments for neglect that modulate activity in spatial maps within areas such as the parietal lobe may be expected to have particularly beneficial effects.

One such example is the prismatic adaptation technique, which has been shown to produce ameliorative effects in patients with neglect that last up to 5 weeks, and that generalize across a range of tasks [33,79,81]. Although the effects of prismatic adaptation are likely to be partly stimulus-driven in nature, the misalignment between visual and motor systems is thought to modulate high-level, central, multisensory integration and spatial co-ordinate transformation processes [33,104]. Alternatively, non-invasive neurodisruption techniques such as transcranial magnetic stimulation (TMS) may also be used to modulate activity in brain areas responsible for representing salience and spatial co-ordinate transformations [92,93]. In laboratory animals, neglect has been reversed by producing bilateral lesions in circumscribed regions of the parietal cortex [89]. Similarly, Vuilleumier and colleagues [121] described a patient whose severe left-sided neglect resulting from a unilateral *right*-sided parietal lobe lesion was ameliorated after a subsequent infarct involving the *left* frontal-eye-field. In humans with unilateral brain damage, therefore, repetitive TMS applied to the parietal region of the contralesional (undamaged) hemisphere might be expected to produce similar ameliorative effects (e.g., see [16]).

Knowledge of the neural mechanisms underlying neglect, and how different treatments operate, is critical for determining the best treatment for individual patients. We anticipate that future studies investigating spatial biases in unilateral brain-damaged patients will explore different components of attention in more detail, in both the contralesional and ipsilesional fields. Such developments should serve as a catalyst for developing treatments that produce lasting ameliorative effects.

References

[1] M.L. Albert, A simple test of visual neglect, *Neurology* **23** (1973), 658–664.

[2] G. Antonucci, C. Guariglia, A. Judica, L. Magnotti, S. Paolucci, L. Pizzamiglio and P. Zoccolotti, Effectiveness of neglect rehabilitation in a randomized group study, *Journal of Clinical & Experimental Neuropsychology* **17** (1995), 383–389.

[3] P. Bartolomeo, The novelty effect in recovered hemineglect, *Cortex* **33** (1997), 323–332.

[4] P. Bartolomeo and S. Chokron, *Levels of impairment in unilateral neglect*, Vol. 3, Elsevier Science Publishers, Amsterdam, 2001.

[5] P. Bartolomeo and S. Chokron, Orienting of attention in left unilateral neglect, *Neuroscience & Biobehavioral Reviews* **26** (2002), 217–234.

[6] P. Bartolomeo, S. Chokron and E. Sieroff, Facilitation instead of inhibition for repeated right-sided events in left neglect, *Neuroreport* **10** (1999), 3353–3357.

[7] P. Bartolomeo, E. Sieroff, C. Decaix and S. Chokron, Modulating the attentional bias in unilateral neglect: the effects of the strategic set, *Experimental Brain Research* **137** (2001), 432–444.

[8] D. Beck and S. Kastner, Stimulus context modulates competition in human extrastriate cortex, *Nature Neuroscience* **8** (2005), 1110–1116.

[9] M. Behrmann, S. Watt, S.E. Black and J.J. Barton, Impaired visual search in patients with unilateral neglect: An oculographic analysis, *Neuropsychologia* **35** (1997), 1445–1458.

[10] M.B. Bender and H.L. Teuber, Phenomena of fluctuation, extinction and completion in visual perception, *Archives of Neurology & Psychiatry* **55** (1946), 627–658.

[11] N.P. Bichot, A.F. Rossi and R. Desimone, Parallel and serial neural mechanisms for visual search in macaque area V4, *Science* **308** (2005), 529–534.

[12] E. Bisiach, Mental representation in unilateral neglect and related disorders, *Quarterly Journal of Experimental Psychology A* **46** (1993), 435–461.

[13] E. Bisiach, E. Capitani, C. Luzzatti and D. Perani, Brain and conscious representation of outside reality, *Neuropsychologia* **19** (1981), 543–551.

[14] J.W. Bisley and M.E. Goldberg, Neuronal activity in the lateral intraparietal area and spatial attention, *Science* **299** (2003), 81–86.

[15] W.R. Brain, Visual orientation with special reference to lesions of the right cerebral hemisphere, *Brain* **64** (1941), 244–272.

[16] F. Brighina, E. Bisiach, M. Oliveri, A. Piazza, V. La Bua, O. Daniele and B. Fierro, 1 Hz repetitive transcranial magnetic stimulation of the unaffected hemisphere ameliorates contralesional visuospatial neglect in humans, *Neuroscience Letters* **336** (2003), 131–133.

[17] L. Chelazzi, Neural mechanisms for stimulus selection in cortical areas of the macaque subserving object vision, *Behavioural Brain Research* **71** (1995), 125–134.

[18] L. Chelazzi, E.K. Miller, J. Duncan and R. Desimone, A neural basis for visual search in inferior temporal cortex, *Nature* **363** (1993), 345–347.

[19] A. Cohen and R. Shoup, Perceptual dimensional constraints in response selection processes, *Cognitive Psychology* **32** (1997), 128–181.

[20] M. Corbetta, M.J. Kincade, C. Lewis, A.Z. Snyder and A. Sapir, Neural basis and recovery of spatial attention deficits in spatial neglect, *Nature Neuroscience* **8** (2005), 1603–1610.

[21] M. Corbetta and G.L. Shulman, Control of goal-directed and stimulus-driven attention in the brain, *Nature Reviews Neuroscience* **3** (2002), 201–215.

[22] J. Danckert, P. Maruff, G. Kinsella, S. de Graaff and J. Currie, Attentional modulation of implicit processing of information in spatial neglect, *Neuroreport* **10** (1999), 1077–1083.

[23] E. De Renzi, M. Gentilini, P. Faglioni and C. Barbieri, Attentional shift towards the rightmost stimuli in patients with left visual neglect, *Cortex* **25** (1989), 231–237.

[24] R. Desimone, Visual attention mediated by biased competition in extrastriate visual cortex, in: *Attention, space, and action*, G. Humphreys, J. Duncan and A. Treisman, eds, Vol., Oxford University Press, New York, 1999, pp. 13–30.

[25] R. Desimone and J. Duncan, Neural mechanisms of selective visual attention, *Annual Review of Neuroscience* **18** (1995), 193–222.

[26] J. Driver and J.B. Mattingley, Parietal neglect and visual awareness, *Nature Neuroscience* **1** (1998), 17–22.

[27] J. Driver and P. Vuilleumier, Perceptual awareness and its loss in unilateral neglect and extinction, *Cognition* **79** (2001), 39–88.

[28] J. Duncan, Converging levels of analysis in the cognitive neuroscience of visual attention, *Philosophical Transactions of the Royal Society of London (B): Biological Sciences* **353** (1998), 1307–1317.

[29] J. Edgworth, I.H. Robertson and T. MacMillan, The Balloons Test: A screening test for visual inattention, Thames Valley Test Company, Bury St. Edmunds, United Kingdom, 1998.

[30] H.E. Egeth and S. Yantis, Visual attention: Control, representation, and time course, *Annual Review of Psychology* **48** (1997), 269–297.

[31] C.W. Eriksen and J.E. Hoffman, The extent of processing of noise elements during selective encoding from visual displays, *Perception & Psychophysics* **14** (1973), 155–160.

[32] J.H. Fecteau, A.H. Bell and D.P. Munoz, Neural correlates of the automatic and goal-driven biases in orienting spatial attention, *Journal of Neurophysiology* **92** (2004), 1728–1737.

[33] F. Frassinetti, V. Angeli, F. Meneghello, S. Avanzi and E. Ladavas, Long-lasting amelioration of visuospatial neglect by prism adaptation, *Brain* **125** (2002), 608–623.

[34] G. Gainotti, P. D'Erme and P. Bartolomeo, Early orientation of attention toward the half space ipsilateral to the lesion in patients with unilateral brain damage, *Journal of Neurology, Neurosurgery & Psychiatry* **54** (1991), 1082–1089.

[35] J.P. Gottlieb, M. Kusunoki and M.E. Goldberg, The representation of visual salience in monkey parietal cortex, *Nature* **391** (1998), 481–484.

[36] P. Halligan, B. Wilson and J. Cockburn, A short screening test for visual neglect in stroke patients, *International Disability Studies* **12** (1990), 95–99.

[37] P.W. Halligan, G.R. Fink, J.C. Marshall and G. Vallar, Spatial cognition: Evidence from visual neglect, *Trends in Cognitive Sciences* **7** (2003), 125–133.

[38] P.W. Halligan, J.C. Marshall and D.T. Wade, Left on the right: Allochiria in a case of left visuo-spatial neglect, *Journal of Neurology, Neurosurgery & Psychiatry* **55** (1992), 717–719.

[39] T.C. Handy and G.R. Mangun, Attention and spatial selection: Electrophysiological evidence for modulation by perceptual load, *Perception & Psychophysics* **62** (2000), 175–186.

[40] K.M. Heilman and E. Valenstein, *Clinical neuropsychology*, Oxford University Press, New York, 1993, xix, 726.

[41] K.M. Heilman and E. Valenstein, Mechanisms underlying hemispatial neglect, *Annals of Neurology* **5** (1979), 166–170.

[42] K.M. Heilman, R.T. Watson and E. Valenstein, Neglect and related disorders, in: *Clinical neuropsychology*, K.M. Heilman and E. Valenstein, eds, Vol., Oxford University Press, New York, 1993, pp. 279–336.

[43] K.W. Heilman, E. Valenstein and R.T. Watson, The neglect syndrome, in: *Handbook of clinical neurology*, (Vol. 45), P.J. Vinken, G.W. Bruyn and H.L. Klawans, eds, Elsevier, Amsterdam, 1985, pp. 152–183.

[44] A.E. Hillis, M. Newhart, J. Heidler, P.B. Barker, E.H. Herskovits and M. Degaonkar, Anatomy of spatial attention: Insights from perfusion imaging and hemispatial neglect in acute stroke, *Journal of Neuroscience* **25** (2005), 3161–3167.

[45] J.B. Hopfinger, M.H. Buonocore and G.R. Mangun, The neural mechanisms of top-down attentional control, *Nature Neuroscience* **3** (2000), 284–291.

[46] L. Itti and C. Koch, Computational modelling of visual attention, *Nature Reviews Neuroscience* **2** (2001), 194–203.

[47] L. Itti and C. Koch, A saliency-based search mechanism for overt and covert shifts of visual attention, *Vision Research* **40** (2000), 1489–1506.

[48] N. Kanwisher, Neural events and perceptual awareness, *Cognition* **79** (2001), 89–113.

[49] H.-O. Karnath, Deficits of attention in acute and recovered visual hemi-neglect, *Neuropsychologia* **26** (1988), 27–43.

[50] H.O. Karnath, M. Niemeier and J. Dichgans, Space exploration in neglect, *Brain* **121** (1998), 2357–2367.

[51] S. Kastner, P. De Weerd, R. Desimone and L.G. Ungerleider, Mechanisms of directed attention in the human extrastriate cortex as revealed by functional MRI, *Science* **282** (1998), 108–111.

[52] S. Kastner and M.A. Pinsk, Visual attention as a multilevel selection process, *Cognitive, Affective & Behavioral Neuroscience* **4** (2004), 483–500.

[53] S. Kastner and L.G. Ungerleider, Mechanisms of visual attention in the human cortex, *Annual Review of Neuroscience* **23** (2000), 315–341.

[54] G. Kerkhoff, Modulation and rehabilitation of spatial neglect by sensory stimulation, *Progress in Brain Research* **142** (2003), 257–271.

[55] M. Kinsbourne, Hemi-neglect and hemisphere rivalry, *Advances in Neurology* **18** (1977), 41–49.

[56] M. Kinsbourne, Mechanisms of unilateral neglect, in: *Neurophysiological and neuropsychological aspects of spatial neglect*, M. Jeannerod, ed., Vol., North-Holland, Amsterdam, 1987, pp. 235–258.

[57] M. Kinsbourne, A model for the mechanism of unilateral neglect of space, *Transactions of the American Neurological Association* **95** (1970), 143–146.

[58] M. Kinsbourne, Orientational bias model of unilateral neglect: Evidence from attentional gradients within hemispace, in: *Unilateral neglect: Clinical and experimental studies*, I.H. Robertson and J.C. Marshall, eds, Vol., Lawrence Erlbaum, Hillsdale, NJ, 1993, pp. 63–86.

[59] C. Koch, *The quest for consciousness: A neurobiological approach*, Roberts and Company Publishers, Colorado, 2004.

[60] M. Kusunoki, J. Gottlieb and M.E. Goldberg, The lateral intraparietal area as a salience map: The representation of abrupt onset, stimulus motion, and task relevance, *Vision Research* **40** (2000), 1459–1468.

[61] E. Ladavas, Selective spatial attention in patients with visual extinction, *Brain* **113** (1990), 1527–1538.

[62] E. Ladavas, Spatial dimensions of automatic and voluntary orienting components of attention, in: *Unilateral neglect: Clinical and experimental studies*, I.A. Robertson, J.C. Marshall, C. Code and D. Muller, eds, Vol., Lawrence Erlbaum, Hillsdale, NJ, 1993, pp. 193–210.

[63] E. Ladavas, G. Menghini and C. Umilta, A rehabilitation study of hemispatial neglect, *Cognitive Neuropsychology* **11** (1994), 75–95.

[64] E. Ladavas, A. Petronio and C. Umilta, The deployment of visual attention in the intact field of hemineglect patients, *Cortex* **26** (1990), 307–317.

[65] N. Lavie, Distracted and confused? Selective attention under load, *Trends in Cognitive Sciences* **9** (2005), 75–82.

[66] N. Lavie, Perceptual load as a necessary condition for selective attention, *Journal of Experimental Psychology: Human Perception & Performance* **21** (1995), 451–468.

[67] N. Lavie and S. Cox, On the efficiency of visual selective attention: Efficient visual search leads to inefficient distractor rejection, *Psychological Science* **8** (1997), 395–398.

[68] N. Lavie and E. Fox, The role of perceptual load in negative priming, *Journal of Experimental Psychology: Human Perception and Performance* **26** (2000), 1038–1052.

[69] N. Lavie and I.H. Robertson, The role of perceptual load in neglect: Rejection of ipsilesional distractors is facilitated with higher central load, *Journal of Cognitive Neuroscience* **13** (2001), 867–876.

[70] N. Lavie and Y. Tsal, Perceptual load as a major determinant of the locus of selection in visual attention, *Perception and Psychophysics* **56** (1994), 183–197.

[71] M. Lepore, M. Conson, A. Ferrigno, D. Grossi and L. Trojano, Spatial transpositions across tasks and response modalities: Exploring representational allochiria, *Neurocase* **10** (2004), 386–392.

[72] S.K. Mannan, D.J. Mort, T.L. Hodgson, J. Driver, C. Kennard and M. Husain, Revisiting previously searched locations in visual neglect: Role of right parietal and frontal lesions in misjudging old locations as new, *Journal of Cognitive Neuroscience* **17** (2005), 340–354.

[73] V.W. Mark, C.A. Kooistra and K.M. Heilman, Hemispatial neglect affected by non-neglected stimuli, *Neurology* **38** (1988), 1207–1211.

[74] J.C. Marshall and P.W. Halligan, Does the midsagittal plane play any privileged role in left neglect? *Cognitive Neuropsychology* **6** (1989), 403–422.

[75] J. Martinez-Trujillo and S. Treue, Attentional modulation strength in cortical area MT depends on stimulus contrast, *Neuron* **35** (2002), 365–370.

[76] J. Martinez-Trujillo and S. Treue, Feature-based attention increases the selectivity of population responses in primate visual cortex, *Current Biology* **14** (2004), 744–751.

[77] P. Maruff, J. Danckert, G. Camplin and J. Currie, Behavioral goals constrain the selection of visual information, *Psychological Science* **10** (1999), 522–525.

[78] J. Mattingley, J. Bradshaw, J. Bradshaw and N. Nettleton, Residual rightward attentional bias after apparent recovery from right hemisphere damage: Implications for a multicomponent model of neglect, *Journal of Neurology, Neurosurgery and Psychiatry* **57** (1994), 597–604.

[79] J.B. Mattingley, Visuomotor adaptation to optical prisms: a new cure for spatial neglect? *Cortex* **38** (2002), 277–283.

[80] C.J. McAdams and J.H. Maunsell, Attention to both space and feature modulates neuronal responses in macaque area V4, *Journal of Neurophysiology* **83** (2000), 1751–1755.

[81] R.D. McIntosh, Y. Rossetti and A.D. Milner, Prism adaptation improves chronic visual and haptic neglect: a single case study. see comment, *Cortex* **38** (2002), 309–320.

[82] A. Menon and N. Korner-Bitensky, Evaluating unilateral spatial neglect post stroke: Working your way through the maze of assessment choices, *Topics in Stroke Rehabilitation* **11** (2004), 41–66.

[83] E.K. Miller, The prefrontal cortex and cognitive control, *Nature Reviews Neuroscience* **1** (2000), 59–65.

[84] J.T. Mordkoff, Between-dimension flanker effects: A clarification with encouraging implications, *Psychonomic Bulletin & Review* **5** (1998), 670–675.

[85] D.J. Mort, P. Malhotra, S.K. Mannan, C. Rorden, A. Pambakian, C. Kennard and M. Husain, The anatomy of visual neglect, *Brain* **126** (2003), 1986–1997.

[86] H.-C. Nothdurft, Salience from feature contrast: Additivity across dimensions, *Vision Research* **40** (2000), 1183–1201.

[87] D.H. O'Connor, M.M. Fukui, M.A. Pinsk and S. Kastner, Attention modulates responses in the human lateral geniculate nucleus, *Nature Neuroscience* **5** (2002), 1203–1209.

[88] A. Parton, P. Malhotra and M. Husain, Hemispatial neglect, *Journal of Neurology, Neurosurgery & Psychiatry* **75** (2004), 13–21.

[89] B.R. Payne and R.J. Rushmore, Animal models of cerebral neglect and its cancellation, *Neuroscientist* **9** (2003), 446–454.

[90] M.I. Posner and Y.A. Cohen, Components of visual orienting, in: *Attention and performance X*, H. Bouma and D.G. Bouwhuis, eds, Vol., Erlbaum, Hillsdale, NJ, 1984, pp. 513–556.

[91] M.I. Posner, J.A. Walker, F.J. Friedrich and R.D. Rafal, Effects of parietal injury on covert orienting of attention, *Journal of Neuroscience* **4** (1984), 1863–1874.

[92] A. Pouget, S. Deneve and T.J. Sejnowski, Frames of reference in hemineglect: A computational approach, *Progress in Brain Research* **121** (1999), 81–97.

[93] A. Pouget and J. Driver, Relating unilateral neglect to the neural coding of space, *Current Opinion in Neurobiology* **10** (2000), 242–249.

[94] G. Rees, C. Frith and N. Lavie, Modulating irrelevant motion perception by varying attentional load in an unrelated task, *Science* **278** (1997), 1616–1619.

[95] G. Rees, C. Frith and N. Lavie, Processing of irrelevant visual motion during performance of an auditory attention task, *Neuropsychologia* **39** (2001), 937–949.

[96] J.H. Reynolds and R. Desimone, Interacting roles of attention and visual salience in V4, *Neuron* **37** (2003), 853–863.

[97] J.H. Reynolds, T. Pasternak and R. Desimone, Attention increases sensitivity of V4 neurons, *Neuron* **26** (2000), 703–714.

[98] G. Rizzolatti and A. Berti, Neural mechanisms of spatial neglect, in: *Unilateral neglect: Clinical and experimental studies*, I.A. Robertson and J.C. Marshall, eds, Vol., Erlbaum, Hillsdale, NJ, 1993, pp. 87–105.

[99] I.H. Robertson, Do we need the lateral in unilateral neglect? Spatially nonselective attention deficits in unilateral neglect and their implications for rehabilitation, *Neuroimage* **14** (2001), S85–90.

[100] I.H. Robertson and P.W. Halligan, *Spatial neglect: A clinical handbook for diagnosis and treatment*, Erlbaum, Hove, East Sussex, 1999.

[101] I.H. Robertson, R. Tegner, K. Tham, A. Lo et al., Sustained attention training for unilateral neglect: Theoretical and rehabilitation implications, *Journal of Clinical & Experimental Neuropsychology* **17** (1995), 416–430.

[102] D.L. Robinson and S.E. Petersen, The pulvinar and visual salience, *Trends in Neurosciences* **15** (1992), 127–132.

[103] C. Rorden and M. Brett, Stereotaxic display of brain lesions, *Behavioral Neurology* **12** (2000), 191–200.

[104] Y. Rossetti, G. Rode, L. Pisella, A. Farne, L. Li, D. Boisson and M.T. Perenin, Prism adaptation to a rightward optical deviation rehabilitates left hemispatial neglect, *Nature* **395** (1998), 166–169.

[105] M.L. Rusconi, A. Maravita, G. Bottini and G. Vallar, Is the intact side really intact? Perseverative responses in patients with unilateral neglect: A productive manifestation, *Neuropsychologia* **40** (2002), 594–604.

[106] S. Schwartz, P. Vuilleumier, C. Hutton, A. Maravita, R.J. Dolan and J. Driver, Attentional load and sensory competition in human vision: Modulation of fMRI responses by load at

[107] J.T. Serences, J. Schwarzbach, S.M. Courtney, X. Golay and S. Yantis, Control of object-based attention in human cortex, *Cerebral Cortex* **14** (2004), 1346–1357.

[108] N. Smania, M.C. Martini, G. Gambina, G. Tomelleri, A. Palamara, E. Natale and C.A. Marzi, The spatial distribution of visual attention in hemineglect and extinction patients, *Brain* **121** (1998), 1759–1770.

[109] J.C. Snow and J.B. Mattingley, Goal-driven selective attention in patients with right hemisphere lesions: how intact is the ipsilesional field? *Brain* **129** (2006), 168–181.

[110] K.G. Thompson and N.P. Bichot, A visual salience map in the primate frontal eye field, *Progress in Brain Research* **147** (2005), 251–262.

[111] K.G. Thompson, N.P. Bichot and T.R. Sato, Frontal eye field activity before visual search errors reveals the integration of bottom-up and top-down salience, *Journal of Neurophysiology* **93** (2005), 337–351.

[112] A.M. Treisman and G. Gelade, A feature-integration theory of attention, *Cognitive Psychology* **12** (1980), 97–136.

[113] S. Treue, Neural correlates of attention in primate visual cortex, *Trends in Neurosciences* **24** (2001), 295–300.

[114] S. Treue, Visual attention: The where, what, how and why of saliency, *Current Opinion in Neurobiology* **13** (2003), 428–432.

[115] S. Treue and J.C. Martinez Trujillo, Feature-based attention influences motion processing gain in macaque visual cortex, *Nature* **399** (1999), 575–579.

[116] G. Vallar, Spatial hemineglect in humans, *Trends in Cognitive Sciences* **2** (1998), 87–97.

[117] G. Vallar, M.L. Rusconi, L. Bignamini, G. Geminiani and D. Perani, Anatomical correlates of visual and tactile extinction in humans: A clinical CT scan study, *Journal of Neurology, Neurosurgery & Psychiatry* **57** (1994), 464–470.

[118] R. VanRullen, Visual saliency and spike timing in the ventral visual pathway, *Journal of Physiology* **97** (2003), 365–377.

[119] A.B. Vivas, G.W. Humphreys and L.J. Fuentes, Inhibitory processing following damage to the parietal lobe, *Neuropsychologia* **41** (2003), 1531–1540.

[120] B.T. Volpe, J.E. Ledoux and M.S. Gazzaniga, Information processing in an extinguished visual field, *Nature* **282** (1979), 722–724.

[121] P. Vuilleumier, D. Hester, G. Assal and F. Regli, Unilateral spatial neglect recovery after sequential strokes, *Neurology* **46** (1996), 184–189.

[122] R. Ward, S. Goodrich and J. Driver, Grouping reduces visual extinction: Neuropsychological evidence for weight-linkage in visual selection, *Visual Cognition* **1** (1994), 101–129.

[123] B. Wilson, J. Cockburn and P.W. Halligan, *Behavioural Inattention Test*, Thames Valley Test Company, Bury St. Edmunds, 1987.

[124] J.M. Wolfe, Guided search 2.0: A revised model of visual search, *Psychonomic Bulletin & Review* **1** (1994), 202–238.

[125] J.M. Wolfe and T.S. Horowitz, What attributes guide the deployment of visual attention and how do they do it? *Nature Reviews Neuroscience* **5** (2004), 495–501.

[126] S. Yantis, Control of visual attention, in: *Psychology Press*, H. Attention, Pashler, ed., Vol., London, 1998, pp. 223–256.

[127] S. Yantis, How visual salience wins the battle for awareness, *Nature Neuroscience* **8** (2005), 975–977.

[128] S. Yantis and J.T. Serences, Cortical mechanisms of space-based and object-based attentional control, *Current Opinion in Neurobiology* **13** (2003), 187–193.

[129] D.J. Yi, G.F. Woodman, D. Widders, R. Marois and M.M. Chun, Neural fate of ignored stimuli: Dissociable effects of perceptual and working memory load, *Nature Neuroscience* **7** (2004), 992–996.

Anosognosia for motor and sensory deficits after unilateral brain damage: A review

Giuseppe Vallar[a,b,*] and Roberta Ronchi[c]
[a]*Department of Psychology, University of Milano-Bicocca, Milano, Italy*
[b]*IRCCS Istituto Auxologico Italiano, Milano, Italy*
[c]*Faculty of Psychology, University of Milano-Bicocca, Milano, Italy*

Received 28 December 2005
Revised 15 February 2006
Accepted 22 June 2006

Abstract. *Purpose:* The syndrome of unawareness (anosognosia) for sensory and motor neurological deficits (hemiplegia, hemianaesthesia, and hemianopia), contralateral to the side of a hemispheric lesion, is reviewed.
Content: Main topics include: basic historical facts; the types of patient's interview and specific questions used to reveal the deficits; the clinical patterns of presentation; the associations and dissociations of the different anosognosic manifestations, and their relationships with associated disorders of sensory, memory, and executive-intellectual functions; the hemispheric asymmetry of anosognosia, that, as the syndrome of unilateral spatial neglect, is more frequent and severe after damage to the right cerebral hemisphere; the relationships between spatial neglect and the anosognosias, and their neural correlates; the effects of lateralized sensory stimulations on defective awareness of neurological impairments.
Conclusions: The argument is made that anosognosia for sensory and motor neurological deficits should be considered as a multi-component syndrome, including a number of specific disorders that are due to the impairment of discrete monitoring systems, specific for the different supervised functions. The putative causal role of associated deficits of other parts of the sensory-motor or cognitive (e.g., memory, general intelligence) system is critically discussed. These specific control processes may be physically implemented in brain areas anatomically (and functionally) close to those subserving the monitored function.

1. Introduction

The notion that patients with damage to the cerebral hemispheres may be unaware of their neurological impairments may be traced back to observations made in the second half of the XIX century, although a non-scientific cursory mention of unawareness of disease may be found as early as in the I century by Seneca [1, 2]. Disorders of awareness of neurological disorders reported in the 1880–1900 period comprise cortical blindness, word deafness [3–5], and left hemiplegia [6–8]. Unawareness of disease was definitely included under the rubric of specific neurological disorders, that could not be interpreted in terms of more general intellectual impairments, with the 1914–1918 reports by Josef François Babinski [9–12], who also proposed the term *anosognosia*. The following excerpts from original early reports illustrate the phenomena of anosognosia.

Anosognosia for cortical blindness
"... Since the last accident the patient was not aware of his amaurosis. At the beginning he thought he was in a dark humid hole or cellar and strongly screamed for light and fire... When he was quiet, he said from time to time that he was old, stupid and weak; never he declared to be blind..."
"... but the patient showed generally a sufficient organisation of his thinking, he was also able to express himself correctly and what he said was absolutely not always absurd or stupid. He also had as-

---

*Corresponding author: Giuseppe Vallar, MD, Università degli studi di Milano-Bicocca, Dipartimento di Psicologia, Edificio U6, Piazza dell'Ateneo Nuovo 1 20126-Milano, Italia. E-mail: giuseppe.vallar@unimib.it.

0922-6028/06/$17.00 © 2006 – IOS Press and the authors. All rights reserved

pirations and desires, which were not basically different from those of an old but intellectually unimpaired man" [3].

"... It was now extremely astonishing, that the patient did not notice her massive and later complete loss of her ability to see.... When she was asked directly about her ability to see, she answered in a vague, general way, that it is always so, that one sees better in the youth. She assured in a calm and trustful way that she saw the objects that were shown to her, while the everyday examination proved the opposite.... The patient was not even aware that there was a reason to be worried or sad about this defect...." [4].

Anosognosia for hemiplegia

"... The patient is mildly confused, *he is not aware of his paralysis* (Anton's italics), he thinks to have performed movements with the left arm" [6].

"... about three weeks later, it was followed by a left hemiplegia... left hemianopia, the cutaneous sensation was not impaired... He was completely disoriented in time and place..."

"... that he had no comprehension of his paralysis, he wondered about the fact that he had been dismissed from the army, and he wanted to show how straight he could walk, a sign which persisted from that moment..."

"... It is worthwhile also to mention that our patient had lost all comprehension, even the awareness of his paralysis; this is even more surprising, as the paralysed limbs did not show any sensory impairment..." [8].

"... the patient was lucid and oriented, had no impairment of language, recognized his environment and the physician, used the right hand skilfully and properly, remembered the spatial arrangement of his and of the other rooms, and also knew himself to be ill. During the night, he easily lost orientation, and repeatedly appeared confused. His mood was often irritable, impatient, but generally cheerful, and joking. This was consistent with the peculiar fact that *he never mentioned his palsy*, never drew his attention to it, and did not express embarrassment regarding his handicap. He never attended to his left body half, apparently never missed it, and seemed to have completely forgotten about it..." [13,14].

"... One such patient... hit by left hemiplegia has largely maintained her intellectual and affective faculties, for many months. She remembered well past events, was willing to talk, expressed herself correctly, her ideas were sensible; she was interested in persons known to her and asked about new people; ... No hallucinations, delirium, confusional state, confabulation. What did contrast with the apparent preservation of intelligence of this patient was that she seemed to ignore the existence of a nearly complete hemiplegia, she had been afraid of for many years. Never did she complain about it; never did she even alluded to it. If she was asked to move her right arm, she immediately executed the command. If she was asked to move the left one, she stayed still, silent, and behaved as if the question had been put to somebody else.

I should remark that sensation in the paralysed limbs was defective but not abolished; the patient perceived a little passive displacements, and sometimes complained about pain in the left shoulder. ..." [9].

In his seminal 1942 paper on the body schema and its disorders Gertsmann [15] mentioned three varieties of anosognosia: (i) anosognosia (i.e., the lack of knowledge, complete or incomplete, of hemiplegia, most frequently left-sided); (ii) anosognosia with amnesia for (autosomatamnesia) or imperception of (autosomatagnosia) the affected limbs or side of the body; (iii) anosognosia with, in addition to the experience of absence, associated illusions or distortions concerning the perception of, and confabulations or delusions referring to the affected limbs or side of the body (somatoparaphrenia). Gerstmann [15] also wrote (pp. 899–900): "Indeed, the patients are not as a rule demented; their sensorium, orientation, memory, attention and judgment are good except for the amnestic-agnostic disturbance in the sphere of body awareness and recognition; in other words, the activity of the mind as a whole is uninterrupted. Thus, the *local cerebral lesion* involving a *specific physiological mechanism* causes a certain group of experiences in the field of body consciousness..." [authors' italics].

In sum, the classical reports illustrate a main distinguishing feature of this disorder of monitoring of function, namely its *selectivity, and specificity*. A general mental deterioration was not a main distinctive feature of the behaviour of these patients, and could not, therefore, constitute the main deficit underlying non-awareness. A somatosensory impairment was not necessarily associated with non-awareness of motor deficits, and, as mental deterioration, could not entirely account for the disorder. Finally unawareness of the motor deficit concerned the *left side* of the body. The classical cases suggest the existence of discrete neuropsychological deficits of function monitoring, that can not be readily explained in terms of other associated impairments of related, more or less specific (e.g., somatosensory deficits vs. dementia), functions. Subsequent research has largely confirmed these early observations. This review shall consider unawareness of sensory and motor deficits, brought about by unilateral hemispheric lesions, in both their functional features and their neural correlates.

2. The specificity of anosognosia

2.1. The behavioural assessment

Starting from the early standardized assessments [16–18], anosognosia is investigated by a short interview to the patient [19–25]. The interaction with the patients typically starts with a general question by the examiner about their complaints and deficits, continues with more specific questions concerning the strength of the limbs, tactile sensation or vision, and may conclude with a demonstration of the deficits through routine techniques of neurological examination. These interviews directly assess 1st person knowledge of the deficit. A recent study [26] has contrasted 1st (i.e., how could patients perform various tasks) vs. 3rd person (i.e., how could the examiners perform these tasks, had they been in the patients' present state) awareness of hemiplegia. Up to 50% of right-brain-damaged patients showed an overestimation in the 1st person vs. the 3rd person condition, with no patient exhibiting the opposite (3rd vs. 1st person overestimation). This difference suggests that patients may have some covert or implicit knowledge of their impairment that comes to the fore when awareness of hemiplegia is not assessed with reference to the patients' abilities, but, less directly, with reference to the abilities of someone else. The explicit vs. implicit dissociation is a main general feature of the neglect syndrome, with patients showing evidence of preserved processing of stimuli presented in the neglected side, provided no overt report of them is required [27]. In the case of anosognosia for hemiplegia, some implicit knowledge of the deficit is suggested by the clinical observation that in the wards severely anosognosic patients often do not attempt at raising from bed.

More specifically, a 1st vs. 3rd person difference had been a clinical observation by M.W. Van Hof (see Ref. [28]), followed by an experimental result in a right-brain-damaged patient, FB [28], who showed a productive delusion concerning the left limbs (somatoparaphrenia: the patient claimed that her left hand was her niece's hand) [15], and left hemianaesthesia. FB's left somatosensory deficit recovered when the examiner warned the patient that she was delivering touches to "her niece's hand", namely: FB's ability to perceive tactile stimuli was spared, provided that these were referred to someone else's body, in a 3rd person condition. The conclusion that patients such as FB make use, when aware of left-sided somatosensory deficits, of the preserved (delusional) representation of a body part of another person, rather than of the impaired representation of their own body part, may be extended to the 3rd vs. 1st person modulation of anosognosia, conveyed by the examiner's questions [26].

2.2. Associations and dissociations

Anosognosia for contralesional motor and sensory deficits is frequently associated with right brain damage and is considered a component deficit of the syndrome of unilateral spatial neglect [29]. In studies of series of patients with unilateral brain lesions a significant association between damage to the right hemisphere and anosognosia for left hemiplegia has been found, with some left brain-damaged patients showing anosognosia for right hemiplegia [30]. Similarly, most reported patients with anosognosia for hemianopia have right-sided damage and a left-sided visual deficit, but left-brain-damaged patients with unawareness of right hemianopia are on record [17,31].

Anosognosia, similar to the case of extra-personal neglect, may however occur with no associated sensorimotor deficits, in addition to the specific impairment of which patients are unaware (e.g., hemiplegia for anosognosia for motor deficits), and no general cognitive impairment. Somatosensory deficits (cutaneous sensation and position sense) and anosognosia are frequently associated [16,18,32], but anosognosia for left hemiplegia may occur with no associated deficits in sensation for both touch [17,33], and position sense [33, 34]. Conversely, patients with left-sided defects for touch and position sense may acknowledge the motor disorder. Anosognosia for hemiplegia may also occur independent of both extra-personal visuo-spatial unilateral neglect [17,35,36], and personal neglect or hemiasomatognosia [17,37–39]. Furthermore, double dissociations have been reported for awareness of extra-personal spatial neglect and anosognosia for motor deficits [19]. Finally, also the early clinical observations in individual patients that anosognosia for left hemiplegia may occur in the absence of general intellectual impairment or confusion [40] have been confirmed in series of right brain-damaged patients investigated through psychometric batteries [34,37,41], and in individual case studies [42]. Similarly, anosognosia for a visual loss in the contralateral homonymous half field (or half quadrant) may occur without concomitant anosognosia for hemiplegia or spatial unilateral neglect, and without motor, or somatosensory deficits [17, 31], and a general cognitive impairment [31].

These dissociations constrain the range of interpretations of unawareness of neurological disorders. Since anosognosia of neurological deficits may occur in the absence of associated sensory impairments, and sensory impairments are not systematically associated with unawareness [17,31,36], a general reduction of sensory inputs cannot account for the disorder. Furthermore, it is a clinical fact that patients with severe anosognosia for left hemiplegia deny the impairment also when the arm is brought into the non-neglected right side of vision, and the patient is explicitly required to monitor the arm's function [17,43,44]. A similar argument applies to the role of general cognitive impairment. Accordingly, interpretations in terms of effects of sensory deficits and associated general cognitive impairments [41,45] do not provide an adequate interpretation of the disorder. Anosognosia for hemiplegia and hemianaesthesia can not, therefore, be traced back to the co-occurrence of some other deficits (sensory, or general cognitive, or their association), that prevent the "discovery" of the neurological impairment [41,45].

In the light of all these dissociations, the argument may be put forward that, in different patients, the combination of different impairments (e.g., touch or proprioceptive sensory deficits; higher level cognitive disorders, such as confusion, reduced general intelligence, or defective short-term, working, or episodic long-term memory), may bring about unawareness of disease. According to such a view the deficit is not one of specific function monitoring, but a more generic disorder, whereby single or multiple impairments of other lower (sensory) or higher level (orientation, intelligence, memory) systems may bring about unawareness, with a variety of possible pathological mechanisms. One such view is a generic two-factor theory about the aetiology of monothematic delusions [46], where the first factor is a neuropsychological anomaly that impairs the patient's awareness. This, in the case of hemiplegia, may be somatosensory loss, unilateral neglect, defective intention to move [43], or a specific memory deficit [47]. As for the second factor, memory impairments (amnesia) are suggested as a possible candidate deficit. Such a generic and multi-factor account is not easy to falsify, however, and this may be regarded, by itself, as a weakness of the hypothesis [48].

More specifically, the dissociation between personal neglect and anosognosia rules out interpretations of anosognosia for hemiplegia in terms of a manifestation of a more general disorder of the internal representation (image or schema) of the body [1,15,49–52], since personal neglect is characterized by defective of awareness of the contralesional side of the body [13, 14], that is assessed by requiring patients to reach their contralesional hand [53], or to explore the body [54].

Finally, there are dissociations also within unawareness of neurological deficits. Patients may recognise that they are paralysed in the left upper limb, but deny paralysis of the lower limb [32,37]. One classical patient, Ursula Mercz, denied blindness, but was aware of her mild dysphasia [4]. Another patient was acutely aware of the right hemiplegia, but not of right homonymous hemianopia [55]. These findings suggest that the system that monitors the operation of sensory and motor functions should not be conceived as unitary and monolithic, comprising instead a number of discrete components, that can be selectively disrupted by brain damage. Finally, elaborate positive delusions concerning the contralesional limbs are frequently associated with anosognosia for hemiplegia, as originally suggested [15], but there are reports of somatoparaphrenia without anosognosia for neurological deficits [56,57].

In sum, the hemispheric asymmetry of anosognosia, the dissociations from other components of the neglect syndrome (visuo-spatial extra-personal neglect, personal neglect), from associated sensory deficits, and from general cognitive impairment concur to suggest that the discrete manifestations of unawareness of neurological deficits are due to the impairment of monitoring systems, specific for different functions: Namely, defective awareness of sensory and motor deficits can not be readily explained in terms of the impairment of some other, more or less closely related, function. This conclusion is, by and large, in line with current views concerning the multi-componential neural and functional architecture of systems supporting spatial cognition [29,58].

The existence of some relationship between anosognosia and other components of the neglect syndrome is however suggested not only by the same hemispheric asymmetry of these disorders, and their frequent association, but also by the finding that vestibular stimulation, a manoeuvre which may temporarily improve a number of manifestations of the syndrome of spatial unilateral neglect [59–61], – including left-sided somatosensory [62–65], and motor [66–68] deficits – ameliorates also anosognosia for left hemiplegia [63, 66,69,70]. These observations indicate that the neural processes defective in anosognosia for left motor weakness, and in other aspects of the syndrome of spatial unilateral neglect, are modulated in a similar fashion by specific sensory inputs [59], suggesting a spatial component in the mechanisms underlying anosognosia for contralesional neurological disorders. This may be conceived in terms of a representation of the working *space* of sensorimotor systems, that allows function monitoring and detection of abnormal operation.

The empirical data reviewed earlier indicate that associated sensory or cognitive deficits may not account by themselves for the occurrence of defective awareness of sensory and motor impairments, unless one takes a generic and multi-factorial view [46], where, in different patients, different underlying pathological mechanisms are involved (see other multi-faceted accounts in Refs. [26,71]). Alternatively, defective awareness for sensory and motor disorders may be conceived in terms of monitoring impairments specific for a particular function. The precise pathological mechanisms are not definite, however. One suggestion [Heilman's "feed forward" or "intentional" theory of anosognosia for hemiplegia, see Refs. [43,72]) traces back unawareness of disease to the defective intention to plan and implement movements of the contralesional side of the body at the level of the upper motor neuron. This defective intention leads to the lack of expectations of movement by a "monitor" or "comparator", which, therefore, fails to detect the pathological absence of movement, due to hemiplegia (see also Ref. [73], for an early forward model of movement monitoring). Support for this view comes from a study where one patient with persistent anosognosia failed to contract not only the contralesional, but also the ipsilesional pectoralis muscle when asked to squeeze a dynamometer with his contralesional, paretic hand; by contrast he contracted both muscles when using the ipsilesional hand. Neurologically unimpaired subjects, patients with hemiparesis, a patient with neglect, and a patient with resolved anosognosia for hemiplegia contracted both pectorales when asked to squeeze with each hand [74].

The evidence that vestibular [66–68] and optokinetic [75] stimulations substantially improve both left-sided motor deficits and anosognosia for hemiplegia [63,66,69,70] suggest that, at least in some patients, hemiplegia may be conceived as a higher level deficit of action planning of the contralesional limbs, rather than as a primary motor disorder. In line with this view, left hemiplegia after right brain damage is more frequent than right hemiplegia after left brain damage, and this hemispheric difference extends to visual and somatosensory deficits [76]. These findings suggest that patients with anosognosia for hemiplegia may be not aware of their defective ability to plan and implement movements using the contralesional limbs, rather than of hemiplegia *per se*. Hemiplegia itself would be, at least in part, a higher level impairment of movement planning of the contralesional limbs, which, as spatial neglect itself, is intrinsically characterized by defective awareness [68]. This account is compatible with the "feed forward" or "intentional" theory of anosognosia for hemiplegia [43], that distinguishes between an "intention-motor activation system" and a "monitor or comparator". When the patients, after caloric vestibular stimulation, recover, at least partially, their ability to move their contralesional limbs, and actually execute movements, then the unimpaired monitoring system detects the deficit. A similar account can be in principle applied to anosognosia for somatosensory deficits, since also these disorders have an higher level component, that is temporarily ameliorated by vestibular and other sensory lateralized stimulations [59,65,77]. Figure 1 shows a diagram model, based on Heilman's [43] comparator system, where the functional locus of the component defective in anosognosia for hemiplegia is located close to the monitored motor system. This account may be readily extended to anosognosia for contralesional sensory deficits, with the functional locus of impairment involving perceptual attentional and representational systems. Patient who are not attending the contralesional side would be unable to monitor and detect their inability to report contralesional sensory events (in the visual modality: hemianopia; in the somatosensory modality: hemianaesthesia). In line with this view, similar to the case of hemiplegia, both left hemianopia [78,79], and left hemianaesthesia [63,64, 79,80] may have a higher level component related to neglect, of which they may be a manifestation ("Hemispatial visual inattention masquerading as hemianopia", as in Ref. [78]), rather than be only a primary sensory disorder.

This view of unawareness of sensory and motor deficits contralateral to a hemispheric lesion in terms of the impairment of specific systems, operating in spatial reference frames, concerned with the planning of action and with the perceptual awareness of sensory events in the contralateral side of space, readily accounts for all

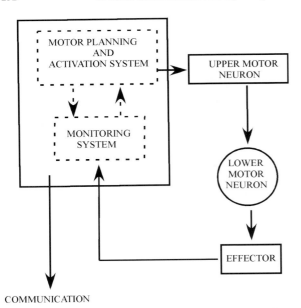

Fig. 1. A possible mechanism for anosognosia for contralesional hemiplegia. A defective activation of the motor system, due to damage to the premotor planning system, leads to lack of feedback concerning the actual execution of the intended action, since such action is not planned at the premotor level of representation (motor neglect). As a consequence, the presence of a motor deficit is not detected [43,72]. Since patients fail to activate the motor system (upper motor neuron) the motor deficit itself may be a higher level impairment, of which patients are unaware as they are unaware of all other manifestations of the neglect syndrome [68]. According to this view, there may be no distinction between the motor programming and the monitoring system, as indicated by the dashed boxes. Finally the system operates in a spatial medium, where actions take place. The hemispheric asymmetry that characterizes anosognosia for hemiplegia may be spatial in nature, similar to that of other manifestations of the neglect syndrome [82].

the dissociations of anosognosia from other possibly co-occurring sensory and cognitive deficits, as well as from other manifestations of the neglect syndrome [29]. Finally, the spatial nature of the monitoring system, based on the fact that actions and events occur in space, may explain the beneficial effects of caloric vestibular stimulation both on anosognosia for left hemiplegia, and on other manifestations of the syndrome of left unilateral spatial neglect [59].

3. The neuroanatomy of anosognosia

Anosognosia for contralesional sensory and motor deficits has long been considered a component part of the neglect syndrome, with right posterior parietal damage being maintained as the canonical lesion site [1,15,81]. More recently, anosognosia, as unilateral spatial neglect, has been associated with a variety of lesions sites, including the frontal and temporal cortices, and subcortical structures, such as the thalamus, the basal ganglia, and the white matter (see Ref. [82], for review). A recent meta-analysis of 85 cases published between 1938 and 2001 [30] confirms that a variety of cortical and subcortical lesions may be associated with anosognosia for hemiplegia, with a fronto-parietal damage being the more frequent combination. In the case of purely subcortical lesions, damage to the basal ganglia and the thalamus is the more frequent lesion site.

Two recent studies further elucidate the anatomical correlates of anosognosia for hemiplegia. In a series of 30 right-brain-damaged patients ($n = 17$ with anosognosia and neglect; $n = 12$ with neglect without anosognosia, one with anosognosia without neglect), Berti et al. [36] found that anosognosia for left hemiplegia was associated with lesions in areas related to the programming of motor acts, particularly Brodmann's premotor areas 6 and 44, motor area 4, and the somatosensory cortex; the dorsolateral premotor cortex and the insula were less frequently damaged. By contrast, in patients with hemiplegia without anosognosia the white matter of the deep centrum semiovale was more frequently involved. One patient, who showed anosognosia without spatial neglect, had a lesion involving the pre-motor cortex. These results provide anatomical support for the view that anosognosia for left hemiplegia is due to the deficit of a specific monitoring component, close to the monitored motor system, both functionally, and anatomically. The system may operate in a spatial medium. The anatomical data of Berti et al. [36] are compatible with this view, since damage to the premotor cortex (BAs 6 and 44) is associated also with unilateral spatial neglect, although less frequently than posterior parietal damage [83,84]. Figure 2 shows the anatomical correlates of anosognosia for left hemiplegia as found in this study [36].

Another study in 27 right-brain-damaged patients with ($n = 14$) and without ($n = 13$) anosognosia for left hemiplegia [85] has suggested the right posterior insula as a critical locus of damage in patients with anosognosia for left motor deficits. There is, however, a relevant methodological difference with the study by Berti et al. [36], that too suggested some role for the insular region. Only patients with a complete left hemiplegia entered this study [36], so that denial concerned a deficit that was likely to be detected by the patient, unless a definite and severe monitoring impairment was present. Karnath et al.'s [85] series com-

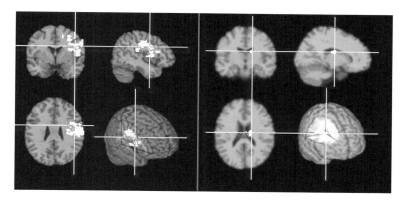

Fig. 2. Anatomical comparison between anosognosic and non-anosognosic right-brain-damaged patients. Left hand-side: The brain areas more frequently damaged in patients with neglect, left hemiplegia, and anosognosia include the premotor cortex (BAs 6, and 44), the motor cortex (BA 4), the post-central gyrus (BAs 1, 2, and 3), and, although less frequently, the dorsolateral prefrontal cortex (BA 46), and the insula. Right hand-side: The brain areas more frequently damaged in patients with neglect, left hemiplegia, and without anosognosia include the white matter of the deep centrum semiovale (reprinted with permission from Ref. [36], Fig. 2, modified).

prised instead patients who had a median score for contralesional paresis of "0" (where "0" stands for complete hemiplegia and "5" for preserved movement), but with a 0–4 range, indicating that also patients with a very mild motor deficit were included. Unfortunately, information concerning the mean severity of the motor weakness was not provided. This study [85], therefore, may have included patients where the diagnosis of anosognosia may be questioned, since the deficit was very mild. Furthermore, as to the suggested role of the posterior insular region, it should be noted that a recent meta-analysis [30], while showing that the insula may be damaged in patients with anosognosia for hemiplegia, does not reveal a special role for this lesion site. Out of 85 patients, 19 had damage involving the insula; by contrast the frontal lobe was damaged in 46 patients, the parietal lobe in 45, the temporal lobe in 32, and the basal ganglia in 22. To summarize, the present available evidence suggests that, while a wide set of cortical and subcortical regions may contribute to the monitoring of motor function, damage to the fronto-parietal cortex seems to be particularly relevant [30], with the recent suggestion of a specific role of lesions to the premotor cortex [36].

Much less data are available concerning anosognosia for somatosensory and visual half-field deficits. In patients with anosognosia for hemianopia the deficit may be produced by lesions involving the visual cortices, the parietal and frontal lobes, the subcortical white matter and subcortical grey nuclei, such as the thalamus [17,64]. In a number of patients the primary sensory visual cortex was largely spared, with lesions clustering more anteriorly, in the posterior parietal region [79,86]. In one study [31], performed in 32 brain-damaged patients, anosognosia for contralesional hemianopia occurred predominantly, but not exclusively, after right-sided lesions, and was not necessarily associated with other anosognosic deficits or spatial neglect. Lesions included multiple visual cortices, the parietal and frontal lobes, the pulvinar, and the lateral geniculate bodies.

4. Concluding remarks

The behavioural dissociations between anosognosia for somatosensory and motor deficits and co-occurring disorders, as well as the selectivity of these impairments of awareness of function, make unlikely interpretations in terms of other pathological, more or less specific, factors. It remains possible, however, that associated sensory impairments, and deficits of memory, executive and cognitive functions may shape anosognosic disorders.

Anatomical and physiological data constrain the behavioural evidence, providing some clues for more specific interpretations. The hemispheric asymmetry of anosognosia for contralesional sensory and motor deficits, with damage to the right cerebral hemisphere playing a major role (see Ref. [30], for anosognosia for hemiplegia, see Ref. [87], for a clinical general review) has long been taken as evidence for some commonality of the pathological underpinnings of unilateral spatial neglect and unawareness of contralesional sensory and motor disorders [82,88]. More specifically, the suggestion has been repeatedly made that anosognosia for hemiplegia may reflect a disordered representation of the body [49,51], underlying motor and sensory neglect, anosognosia and asomatognosia [1]. This time-honoured account has been definitely supported by the finding that the physiological manoeuvre of caloric vestibular stimulation improves on the one hand extra-personal neglect, personal neglect, somatosensory and motor contralesional deficits, and on the other hand anosognosia for hemiplegia [59,65], suggesting that these disorders share some neurofunctional component, modulated by vestibular input.

One recent study investigating the neurological correlates of anosognosia for motor deficits points to the right posterior insular cortex [85]. The role of damage to the insula [85] as a correlate of anosognosia for hemiplegia is in line with the evidence that caloric vestibular stimulation, which temporarily improves anosognosia for hemiplegia [59], activates the insula in humans [89–91], see Ref. [92] for galvanic vestibular stimulation, see also Ref. [93], for related evidence from electrical stimulation in patient with partial epilepsy]. Secondly, activation studies in humans have suggested a role of the anterior insular region and the inferior parietal cortex in monitoring motor actions, the relevant variable being whether or not the subject was performing the action [94]. Activation in the right posterior insula and the right inferior posterior parietal lobe is modulated by the degree of discrepancy between the movement executed by the subject, and the movement seen on the screen [95]. These activation studies, in general, relate the role of the insular region, and of the inferior posterior parietal cortex, to a representation of the body, a body schema [96–98], including the monitoring of the function of body parts. Anatomo-clinical correlation studies show that damage confined to the right posterior insular cortex [99], patient #4], or including the right insula [28], may bring about a disorder of body representation such as somatoparaphrenia, characterized by pathological beliefs concerning the ownership of contralesional body parts. However, interpretations of anosognosia for motor deficits in terms of defective representation of the body should consider that unawareness of hemiplegia may occur independent of not only extra-personal, but also of personal neglect, namely neglect for the contralesional side of the body, whose motor function is not properly monitored [17, 36,53,100].

These instances of double dissociation between anosognosia for hemiplegia and neglect for the contralesional side of the body, as well as for extra-personal space, may be accounted for by fractionating [101] the internal representation of the body, to include specific and discrete components concerned with motor, and somatosensory, function monitoring. The recent anatomo-clinical correlation data by Berti et al. [36] provide a possible neural basis for one specific pathological mechanism. Their finding of an association between damage to the premotor cortex and anosognosia for hemiplegia suggests a view of monitoring systems in terms of multiple components, functionally and anatomically close to the to-be-monitored function. The precise mechanisms whereby such a control takes place remains to be defined. One suggestion is that, although damage to premotor areas impairs the process of motor monitoring, it is still possible, because of some spared premotor activity, to generate a distorted representation of the intended motor act, which is responsible for the false belief of being able to move [36]. Another possibility is that the premotor damage impairs the patients' ability to program and set up plans for motor action by the contralesional limbs. This may be conceived as a deficit of motor intention [43,74], that prevents the organization of movements by the contralesional limbs. According to this view, the motor deficit of patients with anosognosia for hemiplegia is, at least in part, a higher level disorder of motor planning, of which they are not aware [68]. Patients, rather that being unaware of a primary motor deficit, as traditionally maintained (see Ref. [88], for review), are unaware of their inability to set up motor programs by the contralesional limbs, which results in a motor deficit that has a higher level component [76]. The relationship with spatial representations, the right hemisphere, and the syndrome of unilateral spatial neglect [29], may reside in the fact that even simple movements occur in space.

To conclude, the available behavioural and anatomo-clinical evidence suggest that anosognosia for contralesional sensory and motor deficits should be conceived in terms of specific impairments of function monitoring that takes place in a spatial medium. The specific mechanisms of such control processes, and their impairments produced by brain damage, remain to be further explored and elucidated.

Acknowledgements

This study was supported in part by a PRIN 2005 Grant to G.V. We are grateful to Tony Marcel for a helpful and stimulating discussion about 1st vs. 3rd person interviews in anosognosia.

References

[1] M. Critchley, *The parietal lobes*, New York: Hafner, 1953.

[2] C. Papagno and G. Vallar, Anosognosia for left hemiplegia: Babinski's (1914) cases, in: *Classic Cases in Neuropsychology*, (Vol. 2), C. Code, C.-W. Wallesch, Y. Joanette and A.R. Lecours, eds, Hove, East Sussex: Psychology Press, 2003, pp. 171–189.

[3] C. Von Monakow, Experimentelle und pathologisch-anatomische Untersuchungen über die Beziehungen der sogenannten Sehsphäre zu den infracorticalen Opticuscentren und zum N. opticus, *Archiv für Psychiatrie und Nervenkrankheiten* **16** (1885), 151–199.

[4] G. Anton, Über die Selbstwahrnehmung der Herderkrankungen des Gehirns durch den Kranken bei Rindenblindheit und Rindentaubheit, *Archiv für Psychiatrie und Nervenkrankheiten* **32** (1899), 86–127.

[5] G. Anton, Über Herderkrankungen des Gehirnes, welche vom Patienten selbst nicht wahrgenommen werden, *Wiener klinische Wochenschrift* **11** (1898), 227–229.

[6] G. Anton, Beiträge zur klinischen Beurtheilung und zur Localisation der Muskelsinnstörungen im Grosshirne, *Zeitschrift für Heilkunde* **14** (1893), 313–348.

[7] E. Kumbier, H. Haack and S. Herpertz, Überlegungen zum Wirken des Neuropsychiaters Gabriel Anton (1858–1933) [Considerations on the work of the neuropsychiatrist Gabriel Anton (1858–1933)], *Nervenarzt* **76** (2005), 1132–1136, 1138–1140.

[8] A. Pick, Über allgemeine Gedächtnisschwäche als unmittelbare Folge cerebraler Herderkrankung. Beiträge zur Pathologie und pathologischen Anatomie des Centralnervensystems mit Bemerkungen zur normalen Anatomie desselben. Berlin: Karger, 1898.

[9] J. Babinski, Contribution à l'étude des troubles mentaux dans l'hémiplégie organique cérébrale, *Revue Neurologique (Paris)* **27** (1914), 845–848.

[10] J. Babinski, Anosognosie, *Revue Neurologique (Paris)* **31** (1918), 365–367.

[11] J. Babinski, Sur l'anosognosie, *Revue Neurologique (Paris)* **39** (1923), 731–732.

[12] M. Critchley, *The citadel of the senses and other essays*, New York: Raven Press, 1986.

[13] H. Zingerle, Über Störungen der Wahrnehmung des eigenen Körpers bei organischen Gehirnerkrankungen, *Monatsschrift für Psychiatrie und Neurologie* **34** (1913), 13–36.

[14] T. Benke, C. Luzzatti and G. Vallar, Hermann Zingerle's Impaired perception of the own body due to organic brain disorders, An introductory comment, and an abridged translation, *Cortex* **40** (2004), 265–274.

[15] J. Gerstmann, Problem of imperception of disease and of impaired body territories with organic lesions, *Archives of Neurology and Psychiatry* **48** (1942), 890–913.

[16] M. Nathanson, P.S. Bergman and G.G. Gordon, Denial of illness, *Archives of Neurology and Psychiatry* **68** (1952), 380–387.

[17] E. Bisiach, G. Vallar, D. Perani, C. Papagno and A. Berti, Unawareness of disease following lesions of the right hemisphere: anosognosia for hemiplegia and anosognosia for hemianopia, *Neuropsychologia* **24** (1986), 471–482.

[18] J. Cutting, Study of anosognosia, *Journal of Neurology, Neurosurgery, and Psychiatry* **41** (1978), 548–555.

[19] M. Jehkonen, J.P. Ahonen, P. Dastidar, P. Laippala and J. Vilkki, Unawareness of deficits after right hemisphere stroke: double-dissociations of anosognosias, *Acta Neurologica Scandinavica* **102** (2000), 378–384.

[20] S. Maeshima, N. Dohi, K. Funahashi, K. Nakai, T. Itakura and N. Komai, Rehabilitation of patients with anosognosia for hemiplegia due to intracerebral haemorrhage, *Brain Injury* **11** (1997), 691–697.

[21] P. Appelros, G.M. Karlsson, A. Seiger and I. Nydevik, Neglect and anosognosia after first-ever stroke: incidence and relationship to disability, *Journal of Rehabilitation Medicine* **34** (2002), 215–220.

[22] S.E. Starkstein, J.P. Fedoroff, T.R. Price, R. Leiguarda and R.G. Robinson, Anosognosia in patients with cerebrovascular lesions, A study of causative factors, *Stroke* **23** (1992), 1446–1453.

[23] T.E. Feinberg, D.M. Roane, P.C. Kwan, R.J. Schindler and L.D. Haber, Anosognosia and visuoverbal confabulation, *Archives of Neurology* **51** (1994), 468–473.

[24] B. Baier and H.-O. Karnath, Incidence and diagnosis of anosognosia for hemiparesis revisited, *Journal of Neurology Neurosurgery and Psychiatry* **76** (2005), 358–361.

[25] I. Nimmo-Smith, A.J. Marcel and R. Tegnér, A diagnostic test of unawareness of bilateral motor task abilities in anosognosia for hemiplegia, *Journal of Neurology Neurosurgery and Psychiatry* **76** (2005), 1167–1169.

[26] A.J. Marcel, R. Tegner and I. Nimmo-Smith, Anosognosia for plegia: specificity, extension, partiality and disunity of bodily unawareness, *Cortex* **40** (2004), 19–40.

[27] A. Berti, Unconscious processing in neglect, in: *The cognitive and neural bases of spatial neglect*, H.-O. Karnath, A.D. Milner and G. Vallar, eds, Oxford: Oxford University Press, 2002, pp. 313–326.

[28] G. Bottini, E. Bisiach, R. Sterzi and G. Vallar, Feeling touches in someone else's hand, *NeuroReport* **13** (2002), 249–252.

[29] G. Vallar, Spatial hemineglect in humans, *Trends in Cognitive Sciences* **2** (1998), 87–97.

[30] L. Pia, M. Neppi-Modona, R. Ricci and A. Berti, The anatomy of anosognosia for hemiplegia: a meta-analysis, *Cortex* **40** (2004), 367–377.

[31] G.G. Celesia, M.G. Brigell and M.S. Vaphiades, Hemianopic anosognosia, *Neurology* **49** (1997), 88–97.

[32] K.O. Von Hagen and E.R. Ives, Anosognosia (Babinski), imperception of hemiplegia, *Bulletin of the Los Angeles Neurological Society* **2** (1937), 95–103.

[33] R. Willanger, U.T. Danielsen and J. Ankerhus, Denial and neglect of hemiparesis in right-sided apoplectic lesions, *Acta Neurologica Scandinavica* **64** (1981), 310–326.

[34] M. Small and S. Ellis, Denial of hemiplegia: an investigation into the theories of causation, *European Neurology* **36** (1996), 353–363.

[35] R. Willanger, U.T. Danielsen and J. Ankerhus, Visual neglect in right-sided apoplectic lesions, *Acta Neurologica Scandinavica* **64** (1981), 327–336.

[36] A. Berti, G. Bottini, M. Gandola, L. Pia, N. Smania, A. Stracciari, I. Castiglioni, G. Vallar and E. Paulesu, Shared cortical anatomy for motor awareness and motor control, *Science* **309** (2005), 488–491.

[37] A. Berti, E. Ladavas and M. Della Corte, Anosognosia for hemiplegia, neglect dyslexia and drawing neglect: Clinical findings and theoretical considerations, *Journal of the International Neuropsychological Society* **2** (1996), 426–440.

[38] A. Berti, E. Làdavas, A. Stracciari, C. Giannarelli and A. Ossola, Anosognosia for motor impairment and dissociations with patients' evaluation of the disorder: theoretical considerations, *Cognitive Neuropsychiatry* **3** (1998), 21–44.

[39] K.J. Meador, D.W. Loring, T.E. Feinberg, G.P. Lee and M.E. Nichols, Anosognosia and asomatognosia during intracarotid amobarbital inactivation, *Neurology* **55** (2000), 816–820.

[40] R.W. Gilliatt and R.T.C. Pratt, Disorders of perception and performance in a case of right-sided cerebral thrombosis, *Journal of Neurology, Neurosurgery, and Psychiatry* **15** (1952), 264–271.

[41] D.N. Levine, R. Calvanio and W.E. Rinn, The pathogenesis of anosognosia for hemiplegia, *Neurology* **41** (1991), 1770–1781.

[42] A. Venneri and M.F. Shanks, Belief and awareness: reflections on a case of persistent anosognosia, *Neuropsychologia* **42** (2004), 230–238.

[43] K.M. Heilman, Anosognosia: Possible neuropsychological mechanisms, in: *Awareness of deficit after brain injury*, G.P. Prigatano and D.L. Schacter, eds, New York: Oxford University Press, 1991, pp. 53–62.

[44] J.C. Adair, R.L. Schwartz, D.L. Na, E. Fennell, R.L. Gilmore and K.M. Heilman, Anosognosia: examining the disconnection hypothesis, *Journal of Neurology, Neurosurgery, and Psychiatry* **63** (1997), 798–800.

[45] D.N. Levine, Unawareness of visual and sensorimotor defects: a hypothesis, *Brain and Cognition* **13** (1990), 233–281.

[46] M. Davies, A. Aimola Davies and M. Coltheart, Anosognosia and the two-factor theory of delusions, *Mind & Language* **20** (2005), 209–236.

[47] K. Carpenter, A. Berti, S. Oxbury, A.J. Molyneux, E. Bisiach and J.M. Oxbury, Awareness of and memory for arm weakness during intracarotid sodium amytal testing, *Brain* **118** (1995), 243–251.

[48] K.R. Popper, *The logic of scientific discovery*, London: Hutchinson, 1959.

[49] H. Hécaen and M.L. Albert, *Human neuropsychology*, New York: John Wiley, 1978.

[50] J.M. Nielsen, *Agnosia, apraxia, and their value in cerebral localization*, 2 ed. New York: Hafner, 1946.

[51] M. Roth, Disorders of the body image caused by lesions of the right parietal lobe, *Brain* **72** (1949), 89–111.

[52] P.H. Sandifer, Anosognosia and disorders of body scheme, *Brain* **69** (1946), 122–137.

[53] E. Bisiach, D. Perani, G. Vallar and A. Berti, Unilateral neglect: personal and extrapersonal, *Neuropsychologia* **24** (1986), 759–767.

[54] G. Cocchini, N. Beschin and M. Jehkonen, The Fluff Test: A simple task to assess body representation neglect, *Neuropsychological Rehabilitation* **11** (2001), 17–31.

[55] M. M. Gassel and D. Williams, Visual function in patients with homonymous hemianopia. Part II. Oculomotor mechanisms, *Brain* **86** (1963), 1–36.

[56] P.W. Halligan, J.C. Marshall and D.T. Wade, Three arms: a case study of supernumerary phantom limb after right hemisphere stroke, *Journal of Neurology, Neurosurgery, and Psychiatry* **56** (1993), 159–166.

[57] P.W. Halligan, J.C. Marshall and D.T. Wade, Unilateral somatoparaphrenia after right hemisphere stroke: a case description, *Cortex* **31** (1995), 173–182.

[58] P.W. Halligan, G.R. Fink, J.C. Marshall and G. Vallar, Spatial cognition: evidence from visual neglect, *Trends in Cognitive Sciences* **7** (2003), 125–133.

[59] G. Vallar, C. Guariglia and M.L. Rusconi, Modulation of the neglect syndrome by sensory stimulation, in: *Parietal lobe contributions to orientation in 3D space*, P. Thier and H.-O. Karnath, eds, Heidelberg: Springer-Verlag, 1997, pp. 555–578.

[60] G. Kerkhoff, Modulation and rehabilitation of spatial neglect by sensory stimulation, *Progress in Brain Research* **142** (2003), 257–271.

[61] Y. Rossetti and G. Rode, Reducing spatial neglect by visual and other sensory manipulations: non-cognitive (physiological) routes to the rehabilitation of a cognitive disorder, in: *The cognitive and neural bases of spatial neglect*, H.-O. Karnath, A.D. Milner and G. Vallar, eds, Oxford: Oxford University Press, 2002, pp. 375–396.

[62] G. Vallar, G. Bottini, M.L. Rusconi and R. Sterzi, Exploring somatosensory hemineglect by vestibular stimulation, *Brain* **116** (1993), 71–86.

[63] G. Vallar, R. Sterzi, G. Bottini, S. Cappa and M.L. Rusconi, Temporary remission of left hemianaesthesia after vestibular stimulation, *Cortex* **26** (1990), 123–131.

[64] G. Vallar, G. Bottini, R. Sterzi, D. Passerini and M.L. Rusconi, Hemianesthesia, sensory neglect and defective access to conscious experience, *Neurology* **41** (1991), 650–652.

[65] G. Bottini, E. Paulesu, M. Gandola, S. Loffredo, P. Scarpa, R. Sterzi, I. Santilli, C.A. Defanti, G. Scialfa, F. Fazio and G. Vallar, Left caloric vestibular stimulation ameliorates right hemianesthesia, *Neurology* **65** (2005), 1278–1283.

[66] G. Rode, N. Charles, M.T. Perenin, A. Vighetto, M. Trillet and G. Aimard, Partial remission of hemiplegia and somatoparaphrenia through vestibular stimulation in a case of unilateral neglect, *Cortex* **28** (1992), 203–208.

[67] G. Rode, M.T. Perenin, J. Honoré and D. Boisson, Improvement of the motor deficit of neglect patients through vestibular stimulation: evidence for a motor neglect component, *Cortex* **34** (1998), 253–261.

[68] G. Vallar, G. Bottini and R. Sterzi, Anosognosia for left-sided motor and sensory deficits, motor neglect, and sensory hemiinattention: is there a relationship? *Progress in Brain Research* **142** (2003), 289–301.

[69] S.F. Cappa, R. Sterzi, G. Vallar and E. Bisiach, Remission of hemineglect and anosognosia during vestibular stimulation, *Neuropsychologia* **25** (1987), 775–782.

[70] V.S. Ramachandran, Anosognosia in parietal lobe syndrome, *Consciousness and Cognition* **4** (1995), 22–51.

[71] P. Vuilleumier, Anosognosia: the neurology of beliefs and uncertainties, *Cortex* **40** (2004), 9–17.

[72] K.M. Heilman, A.M. Barrett and J.C. Adair, Possible mechanisms of anosognosia: a defect in self-awareness, *Philosophical Transactions of the Royal Society of London* **B353** (1998), 1903–1909.

[73] A.G. Greenwald, Sensory feedback mechanisms in performance control: with special reference to the ideo-motor mechanism, *Psychological Review* **77** (1970), 73–99.

[74] M. Gold, J.C. Adair, D.H. Jacobs and K.M. Heilman, Anosognosia for hemiplegia: an electrophysiologic investigation of the feed-forward hypothesis, *Neurology* **44** (1994), 1804–1808.

[75] G. Vallar, C. Guariglia, D. Nico and L. Pizzamiglio, Motor deficits and optokinetic stimulation in patients with left hemineglect, *Neurology* **49** (1997), 1364–1370.

[76] R. Sterzi, G. Bottini, M.G. Celani, E. Righetti, M. Lamassa, S. Ricci and G. Vallar, Hemianopia, hemianaesthesia, and hemiplegia after left and right hemisphere damage: a hemispheric difference, *Journal of Neurology, Neurosurgery, and Psychiatry* **56** (1993), 308–310.

[77] A. Maravita, J. McNeil, P. Malhotra, R. Greenwood, M. Husain and J. Driver, Prism adaptation can improve contrale-

[78] C.A. Kooistra and K.M. Heilman, Hemispatial visual inattention masquerading as hemianopia, *Neurology* **39** (1989), 1125–1127.

[79] G. Vallar, P. Sandroni, M.L. Rusconi and S. Barbieri, Hemianopia, hemianesthesia and spatial neglect. A study with evoked potentials, *Neurology* **41** (1991), 1918–1922.

[80] G. Vallar, M.L. Rusconi and C. Guariglia, Nonsensory components of somatosensory deficits contralateral to hemispheric lesions in humans, in: *Touch, temperature, and pain in health and disease: mechanisms and assessments*, J. Boivie, P. Hansson and U. Lindblom, eds, Seattle, WA: IASP Press, 1994, pp. 85–95.

[81] S.M. McGlynn and D.L. Schacter, Unawareness of deficits in neuropsychological syndromes, *Journal of Clinical and Experimental Neuropsychology* **11** (1989), 143–205.

[82] E. Bisiach and G. Vallar, Unilateral neglect in humans. in: *Handbook of neuropsychology*, F. Boller, J. Grafman and G. Rizzolatti, eds, 2 ed, Amsterdam: Elsevier Science, B.V., 2000, pp. 459–502.

[83] G. Vallar, Extrapersonal visual unilateral spatial neglect and its neuroanatomy, *Neuroimage* **14** (2001), S52–S58.

[84] G. Vallar, The anatomical basis of spatial hemineglect in humans, in: *Unilateral neglect: clinical and experimental studies*, I.H. Robertson and J.C. Marshall, eds, Hove: Lawrence Erlbaum, 1993, pp. 27–59.

[85] H.-O. Karnath, B. Baier and T. Nagele, Awareness of the functioning of one's own limbs mediated by the insular cortex? *Journal of Neuroscience* **25** (2005), 7134–7138.

[86] P.J. Koehler, L.J. Endtz, J.T. Velde and R.E.M. Hekster, Aware or non-aware. On the significance of awareness for localization of the lesion responsible for homonymous hemianopia, *Journal of the Neurological Sciences* **75** (1986), 255–262.

[87] A. Carota, F. Staub and J. Bogousslavsky, Emotions, behaviours and mood changes in stroke, *Current Opinion in Neurology* **15** (2002), 57–69.

[88] E. Bisiach and G. Geminiani, Anosognosia related to hemiplegia and hemianopia, in: *Awareness of deficit after brain injury*, G.P. Prigatano and D.L. Schacter, eds, New York: Oxford University Press, 1991, pp. 17–39.

[89] G. Bottini, R. Sterzi, E. Paulesu, G. Vallar, S.F. Cappa, F. Erminio, R.E. Passingham, C.D. Frith and R.S.J. Frackowiak, Identification of the central vestibular projections in man: a positron emission tomography activation study, *Experimental Brain Research* **99** (1994), 164–169.

[90] G. Bottini, H.-O. Karnath, G. Vallar, R. Sterzi, C.D. Frith, R.S. Frackowiak and E. Paulesu, Cerebral representations for egocentric space: Functional-anatomical evidence from caloric vestibular stimulation and neck vibration, *Brain* **124** (2001), 1182–1196.

[91] M. Dieterich, S. Bense, S. Lutz, A. Drzezga, T. Stephan, P. Bartenstein and T. Brandt, Dominance for vestibular cortical function in the non-dominant hemisphere, *Cerebral Cortex* **13** (2003), 994–1007.

[92] S.B. Eickhoff, P.H. Weiss, K. Amunts, G.R. Fink and K. Zilles, Identifying human parieto-insular vestibular cortex using fMRI and cytoarchitectonic mapping, *Human Brain Mapping* **27** (2005), 611–621.

[93] P. Kahane, D. Hoffmann, L. Minotti and A. Berthoz, Reappraisal of the human vestibular cortex by cortical electrical stimulation study, *Annals of Neurology* **54** (2003), 615–624.

[94] C. Farrer and C.D. Frith, Experiencing oneself vs another person as being the cause of an action: the neural correlates of the experience of agency, *Neuroimage* **15** (2002), 596–603.

[95] C. Farrer, N. Franck, N. Georgieff, C.D. Frith, J. Decety and M. Jeannerod, Modulating the experience of agency: a positron emission tomography study, *Neuroimage* **18** (2003), 324–333.

[96] G. Vallar and C. Papagno, Pierre Bonnier's (1905) cases of bodily aschématie, in: *Classic cases in neuropsychology*, (Vol. 2), C. Code, C.-W. Wallesch, Y. Joanette and A.R. Lecours, eds, Hove, East Sussex: Psychology Press, 2003, pp. 147–170.

[97] A. Benton and A.B. Sivan, Disturbances of the body schema, in: *Clinical neuropsychology*, K.M. Heilman and E. Valenstein, eds, 3 ed., New York: Oxford University Press, 1993, pp. 123–136.

[98] T. Chaminade, A.N. Meltzoffa and J. Decety, An fMRI study of imitation: action representation and body schema, *Neuropsychologia* **43** (2005), 115–127.

[99] C. Cereda, J. Ghika, P. Maeder and J. Bogousslavsky, Strokes restricted to the insular cortex, *Neurology* **59** (2002), 1950–1955.

[100] J.C. Adair, D.L. Na, R.L. Schwartz, E.M. Fennell, R.L. Gilmore and K.M. Heilman, Anosognosia for hemiplegia: test of the personal neglect hypothesis, *Neurology* **45** (1995), 2195–2199.

[101] G. Vallar, Left spatial hemineglect: An unmanageable explosion of dissociations? No. *Neuropsychological Rehabilitation* **4** (1994), 209–212.

Diagnostic issues

What do eye-fixation patterns tell us about unilateral spatial neglect?

Sumio Ishiai*
Department of Rehabilitation, Sapporo Medical University, School of Medicine, Sapporo, Japan

Received 1 September 2005
Revised 13 February 2006
Accepted 22 June 2006

Abstract. *Purpose:* Eye-fixation patterns, which include ocular searching and fixation, may change with tasks, stimuli, and instructions. This article reviews our studies over 18 years on eye-fixation patterns of neglect patients and aims to elucidate the visuospatial processing of unilateral spatial neglect.
Methods: We recorded eye-fixation patterns when patients with neglect bisected a line in various conditions.
Results: Patients with neglect rarely searched to the left side when bisecting a line of the ordinary length (e.g., 200 mm). They persisted in fixating a right-side point, at which they later marked the subjective midpoint. They made no effective comparison between the leftward and rightward extents not only for a whole line but also for its explored right segment. Where they 'favored' to fixate as the subjective midpoint depended strongly upon the location of the right endpoint in space. Their representational image of a line was also estimated with modified line bisection tasks performed on a touch-panel display.
Conclusions: For patients with neglect, the representational image of a line may be formed on the basis of the attended segment between the right endpoint and the favored point of fixation. The line bisection task, if combined with recording of eye-fixation, would further contribute to elucidation of the mechanisms underlying neglect.

1. Introduction

Patients with left unilateral spatial neglect orient the eyes and the head toward the right side in the acute stage of illness [9,10]. They may regain the spontaneous posture to look straight ahead in their course, while the gaze is often magnetized to right-side stimuli and ocular exploration tends to be restricted to right space [15]. However, forced orientation of the gaze to the left side hardly eliminates neglect. Patients with neglect bisect a horizontal line placing the mark to the right of the objective center. Such rightward errors cannot be corrected into the normal range even after they have been cued to the left endpoint to see the whole extent of the line [27,43]. Also, patients with neglect may fail to complete the left side of each object when copying a complex scene [36,45]. In this case, they omit the left parts of the right-side objects even though their gaze travels over the unfinished spaces to find the left-side objects [12].

In the cancellation tasks, patients with neglect omit targets on the left side exploring less into left space. For example, they cross out right-side lines and omit left-side lines on the sheet of the line cancellation test [1]. It is unlikely that they fail to cross out a line they find and fixate. Occasional omissions on the right side [44,48] suggest that targets in the searched area may be omitted if they are not fixated. In the cancellation tasks, which involve 'many' targets, fewer fixations on the left side may be directly linked to less cancellation of the left-side targets. In the exploration task to find a single target, the duration of ocular searching was reported to be shorter on the left side than on the right side, which was related to neglect severity [8]. Also, in the search for the non-existing target in the random array of letters,

---

*Address for correspondence: Sumio Ishiai, MD, Department of Rehabilitation, Sapporo Medical University School of Medicine, S1W16, Chuo-ku, Sapporo, 060-8543, Japan. Tel.: +81 11 611 2111; Fax: +81 11 618 5220; E-mail: ishiai@sapmed.ac.jp.

the distribution of exploration time was deviated to the right side in the body-centered space [32].

Patients with neglect usually identify a single object as 'what' it is. They correctly name a figure of a complete daisy, never stating that it is a right-half daisy [28]. They believe that their own copy lacking the left-side petals is a complete daisy. By contrast, we found that when shown a right-half flower prepared by the examiner, most of the patients with neglect were able to discriminate between the left-lacking flowers and the complete flowers [28]. When copying a complete flower, however, they typically omitted the left-side petals and never noticed the left-side incompleteness. The strong engagement of attention to the right side while copying may result in the lack of leftward shift of gaze or attention in such a small area (about six degrees of visual angle).

We expected that eye-fixation patterns, which includes ocular searching and fixation, would change depending upon whether the visual stimulus is a single object or contains multiple elements and whether the task requires simple observation of the stimulus or exploration of targets or visuospatial processing with manual responses. Studies on eye-fixation patterns would contribute to elucidating where patients with neglect look at in the visual scene, which part(s) they utilize for visuospatial processing, and how their representational image is formed in the brain.

A 'line' is defined by two endpoints and has no other conspicuous point between them [34,37]. A line is an object without specific meaning, and its length, location, and direction can be changed freely in space. Wherever we fixate on a line except the two endpoints, the line extends to either side along its direction. If the line is not so long, healthy subjects are able to detect both endpoints easily. However, this simple perception seems difficult for patients with neglect when they are presented with a horizontal line. They usually bisect a line of the ordinary length (e.g., 200 mm) to the right of the objective midpoint [13,15,35]. It is more difficult for them to find the left endpoint than to find the right endpoint. However, they, as healthy subjects, may see a line extending to either side when fixating a point on the line. In the line bisection task, we are able to estimate the point where patients with neglect fixate on the line only when they are marking the subjective midpoint. Recording of eye-fixation pattern with a device such as an eye camera is necessary to elucidate how they explore a line and where they fixate on it [20]. This article reviews our studies over 18 years on eye-fixation patterns of neglect patients and tries to elucidate the visuospatial processing of unilateral spatial neglect.

2. Simple observation vs. exploration

Except in the early stage of illness, patients with left neglect may direct their gaze or face forwardly when they have nothing to do. Rightward tendency of gaze becomes obvious when they search objects, find novel stimuli, or perform spatial tasks [9,15]. Firstly, we analyzed the distribution of fixation duration when hemianopic patients with chronic neglect and those without neglect were asked to look at a horizontal line or a rectangle freely but carefully [18]. The left hemianopic patients without neglect moved the eyes leftward and saw the whole figure in the right intact visual field. The distribution of fixation duration had a peak near the left extreme of the figure. By contrast, the patients with left hemianopia and neglect did not show such a leftward tendency of fixation. Their fixation fell on either side of the figures, and the percentage fixation duration on the left half of the figures was not significantly different between the patients with neglect and the healthy control subjects. In other words, the patients with neglect did not show rightward deviation of fixation when observing a horizontal line or a rectangle with no spatial task to perform.

We recorded the eye-fixation pattern when patients with left hemianopia and neglect observed two old Japanese 'Ukiyoe' pictures that depicted persons going over the bridge in the rain and a boat on the river [19]. One of the pictures had the original right-left orientation, and the other was the one reversed horizontally (Fig. 1). Except for a mild case, the patients with neglect fixated and commented on the right-side elements only. None of them noticed that the two pictures were the horizontally reversed ones. Also in the condition of picture observation, we asked the patients to look at the picture freely but carefully. Rightward tendency of fixation may have become apparent as the figures of persons on the right side attracted attention of the patients. However, patients with neglect may explore into left space, if a picture has no feature on the right side [47] or a multi-object figure contains a meaningful relationship between the right and left elements [33]. Although eye-fixation patterns of patients with neglect may change with figure contents, they probably report little about the elements they fail to fixate.

3. Eye-fixation in line bisection

A line extends to either side along its direction wherever we fixate a point on the line except the two end-

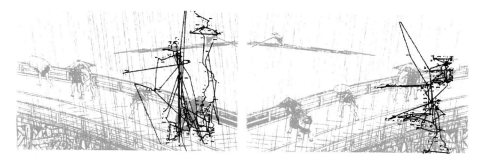

Fig. 1. Eye-fixation patterns when a patient with neglect observed old Japanese 'Ukiyoe' pictures.

points. When simply observing a horizontal line, some patients with neglect may not choose a rightward point to fixate on it as reported in the above study [18]. When patients with typical neglect are asked to bisect a line (e.g., about 200 mm in length), however, they place the subjective midpoint to the right of the objective center [13,15,35]. The simplest explanation of rightward bisection is that patients with neglect ignore the left extent and bisect the attended right extent. Until up to our eye-fixation study [20], nothing was known about how they explore a horizontal line and where they place the subjective midpoint on the line segment perceived in the attentive right visual field.

We investigated the relationship between the subjective midpoint and the attended extent, observing eye-fixation patterns and marking process [20]. Control patients who had left hemianopia but not neglect saw the whole line, searching to the left endpoint, and bisected it correctly or slightly to the hemianopic left side. By contrast, patients with neglect never searched to the left side. Once they fixated a certain point on the right part of the line, they persisted with this point and marked the subjective midpoint there (Fig. 2). Accordingly, the subjective midpoint was marked, not at the center of the line segment perceived in the attentive right visual field, but at the left extreme point of it. However, the patients with neglect were proved to understand the meaning of line bisection, as they were able to appreciate the deviation of the subjective midpoint in the right visual field when forced to fixate the left endpoint of the line after bisection. The results were interpreted to mean that patients with neglect may see a representational image of a line extending equally to either side of the point of the persistent fixation, where they later place the subjective midpoint.

We consider that absence of leftward searching is characteristic of patients with typical neglect when they are asked to 'bisect a line'. However, changes of instruction may affect their searching behavior. Barton

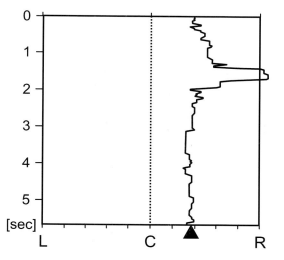

Fig. 2. Eye-fixation pattern when a patient with neglect bisected a 200-mm line. The horizontal axis corresponds to the line extent: R, C, and L indicate the right endpoint, the center or the objective midpoint, and the left endpoint of the line respectively. The arrowhead indicates the location of the subjective midpoint. The vertical axis indicates the time from the presentation of the line to the placement of the subjective midpoint.

et al. [2] investigated ocular searching during line bisection when they asked the subjects to 'examine the entire line and then to touch the midpoint'. In their patients with neglect, the authors found more heterogeneous patterns of ocular searching compared with our study [20]. It was not uncommon that the patients searched leftward beyond the point where the subjective midpoint was later placed, which may have reflected the instruction for the patients to examine the entire line. Also with the ordinary instruction to bisect a line, it is possible that patients with chronic neglect, who have received rehabilitation for neglect, may search toward the left endpoint before marking the subjective midpoint. We recorded eye-fixation patterns of such a patient who searched leftward in some bisections [26]. In the remaining trials, however, he showed the charac-

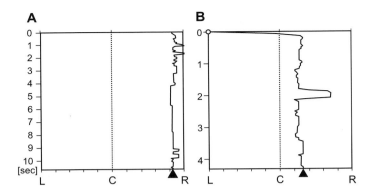

Fig. 3. Eye-fixation patterns of a patient with neglect in the ordinary line bisection test (A) and the line bisection test with cueing (B, the cued fixation on the left endpoint is circled).

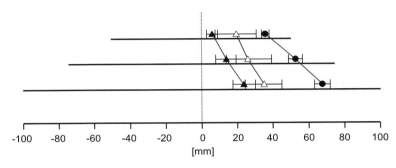

Fig. 4. Bisection errors for a patient with left unilateral spatial neglect (Case 3 from Ishiai et al. [24]). The mean locations of the subjective midpoint with standard deviations are shown separately for the 100-, 150-, and 200-mm lines. The horizontal axis indicates rightward deviations from the true center. Closed circles = line bisection without cueing, black triangles = line bisection with cueing, white triangles = representational bisection.

teristic pattern of eye-fixation without leftward searching.

4. Line bisection and cueing

Absence of leftward searching prevents patients with neglect from forming an appropriate representational image for the left extent of a line, especially when they have left visual field defect. A strategy to ensure their seeing the whole line in the attentive right visual field is cueing to the left endpoint. Patients with neglect often show a decrease of rightward errors of bisection after they identified a letter at the left endpoint [41,43]. However, the technique of cueing cannot eliminate neglect. We recorded eye-fixation patterns when patients with neglect were forced to fixate the left endpoint of a line and then placed the subjective midpoint [27].

To avoid possible interference of the presence of a letter [41], a line with no additional stimuli was used, and fixation at the left endpoint was monitored with the eye camera. After cueing to the left endpoint, patients with neglect swiftly moved the eyes to the right and fixated a point on the right part of the line, where they later placed the subjective midpoint (Fig. 3). The information about the left part perceived at the time of cueing may have been utilized insufficiently for the estimation of the subjective midpoint. We considered that rightward bias of attention may predominate to determine the point of fixation on the line after cueing. If patients with neglect see the representational line image that extended equally to either side of the persistent fixation, they would feel no need to search again to the left endpoint after cueing.

Recently, we reconsidered the visuospatial process of line bisection after cueing [24]. Although the left

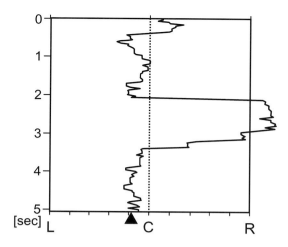

Fig. 5. Eye-fixation pattern when a patient with neglect bisected a 150-mm line presented in the right hemispace.

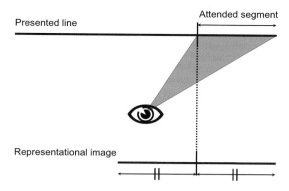

Fig. 6. Representational image when patients with neglect bisect a line. They rarely search leftward and persist with a rightward point on the line, where they later place the subjective midpoint. Accordingly, they attened mostly to the right segment between the subjective midpoint and the right endpoint. Our interpretation of the results is that patients with neglect see a representational image that extends equally toward either side of the subjective midpoint. This image may be formed on the basis of the information about the attended right segment.

part of a line falls in the inattentive or defective field of vision after cueing, its mental representation may be at least partially stored. By contrast, the right part continues to be perceived in the attentive right visual field. When bisecting a line after cueing, patients with neglect seem to bisect the extent that consists of the mental representation on the left side and the real line segment on the right side. In a new representational line bisection task, patients with neglect were presented a line on a touch panel display, until they touched the left endpoint. A blank display followed, and they pointed to the subjective midpoint. The rightward errors in the representational bisection were greater than or equivalent to those in the ordinary line bisection with cueing (Fig. 4). The effect of line length in which the errors became greater for the longer lines was equally found in the line bisection with cueing and the representational bisection. It is therefore unlikely that after cueing to the left endpoint, rightward bisection errors of patients with neglect are caused by simple over-attention to the right segment of the physical line. Left neglect may occur for the mental representation formed at the time of cueing or seeing the whole extent.

In our first eye-fixation study in line bisection [20], we found that some patients showed small leftward errors for the 150-mm lines in the midline or the right hemispace presentation. Also in these trials, the pattern of eye-fixation was the same as in the typical trials with rightward bisection errors (Fig. 5). Some patients may show leftward errors in the line bisection test, while they neglect the left side in the other tests [44]. We reported a right-hemisphere damaged patient who constantly erred leftward when bisecting the lines of the ordinary length (e.g., 200 mm) [22]. This patient showed small but constant leftward deviations when bisecting 100-, 150-, and 200-mm lines without cueing. The direction of bisection errors changed toward the right side, when he bisected the lines after pointing to the left endpoint. In other words, leftward cueing increased 'rightward' errors of bisection. The rightward errors in the left-cue condition were greater for the longer lines, although the leftward errors in the no cue condition were nearly the same for the three lengths. Accordingly, cueing to the left endpoint was effective in that it improved the patient's leftward representation of the lines and induced neglect errors according to the lengths. In the no cue condition, the paradoxical leftward errors may have occurred as the patient neglected the shortness of the leftward extent.

We recorded the eye-fixation patterns when this patient bisected lines in the same conditions a week after the above study. He continued to bisect the lines with small leftward errors. In the no cue condition, his initial fixation fell on the slightly leftward point on the line, and no leftward search occurred. The patient thereby bisected the lines with small leftward errors. In the left-cue condition, the fixation moved from the left endpoint to the right of the objective center, and thereafter no leftward search occurred. These eye-fixation data also indicated that the patient's leftward error of bisection was an expression of 'left' but not right neglect.

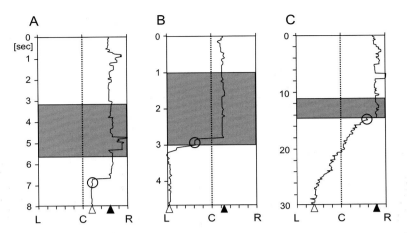

Fig. 7. Eye-fixation patterns when patients with neglect bisected a 200-mm line and then searched for the left endpoint. The initial fixation in search for the left endpoint is circled. R, C, and L indicate the right endpoint, the center, and the subjective midpoint of the line. The black arrowhead indicates the location of the subjective midpoint, and the white arrowhead indicates the location of the subjective left endpoint. The grey areas show the period of drawing the mark of the subjective midpoint.

5. Representational image when patients with neglect bisect a line

In the eye-fixation study in line bisection [20], our interpretation of the results was that patients with neglect see the representational image that extends equally toward either side of the subjective midpoint (Fig. 6). This representational image is the one they see at the time when they place the subjective midpoint. We expected that this image may affect leftward searches for the left endpoint after line bisection. Nine patients were asked to mark the center of a line and then to search for and mark the point that they believed to be the left endpoint of the line [29]. Until up to the placement of the subjective midpoint, the eye-fixation pattern was the same as we found in the first study [20]. They persisted in fixating a point on the right part of the line and placed the mark without searching leftward. They then searched leftward beyond the subjective midpoint. The initial fixation after a leftward saccade always fell near the point located to the left of the subjective midpoint by the distance between the subjective midpoint and the right endpoint of the line (Fig. 7). The search further to the left of this point was laborious and frequently fell short of the true left endpoint. We considered that they initially shifted fixation to the left endpoint of the hypothesized line representation, which may have been determined mainly by the location of the fixation when they marked the subjective midpoint.

In the visual scene where the subjective midpoint or the printed center is present, patients with neglect may compare the left and right extents from the reference

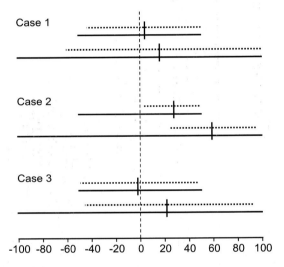

Fig. 8. Estimation of the representational image by asking patients with neglect to point to the left or right endpoint on the blank display after bisection of lines. Vertical bars indicate the mean location of the subjective midpoint, and the representational images are drawn as dotted lines between the mean locations of the reproduced right and left endpoints.

point [17,30,31,46]. Recently, we asked patients with neglect to point to the left or right endpoint on the blank display after bisection of a line, and tried to estimate their representational image. They were presented a line on a touch panel display. The moment they touched the subjective midpoint without cueing, the line disappeared. After a delay of two seconds, during which the examiner specified the side, they pointed to the right or left endpoint on the blank display according to their representational image. We expected that as in the first eye movement study in line bisection, they would see a representational line image, which extends equally to either side of the subjective midpoint (Fig. 6), and point to the right or left endpoint according this image. Patients with neglect placed the right endpoint almost correctly. The patients with neglect following the temporo-parietal lesions placed the left endpoint near the left extreme of the expected representational line image (Fig. 8).

Bisiach et al. [4,5] reported a neglect disorder implying a horizontal anisometry of spatial representation. The patients with neglect bisected an actual line and a virtual line between the two points, and then they set the endpoints of the imaginary line on the basis of its printed center. The left endpoint was placed farther from the printed center than the right endpoint. Ishiai [17] recorded the eye-fixation pattern when two patients with neglect performed a symmetric positioning task similar to the task of Bisiach et al. On the test sheet, the central mark and the right point were printed. The patients were asked to place the left point so that the left and right points should be equally distant from the central mark. In this task, the patients shifted the fixation leftward to the location where they later placed the subjective left point. When leftward overextension occurred as reported earlier, the gaze and the hand moved together further to the left side of the ideal left point. In this stage, no rightward search occurred. An exaggerated "perceptual-motor interaction" in neglect was considered to misdirect responses toward the neglected side when the task elicited a leftward orientation. Overextension of the left distance may result partly from overrepresentation on the left side of the map [4,5]. Less use of the information about the perceived right point may result from impairments in spatial remapping [42] or spatial working memory [16] after saccades. The visuospatial processing for the line extension or the symmetric positioning task is extremely different from that for the line bisection task. The recording of the eye-fixation pattern clearly demonstrated such difference. We therefore consider that at least elimination of the reference point showing the midpoint is necessary to estimate the representational image when patients with neglect bisect a line. Again, spatial representation of a line may vary with seemingly small modification of tasks [17].

6. Favoring the location of the subjective midpoint not comparing the rightward and leftward extents

In the eye-movement studies, we have repeatedly maintained that patients with neglect make no or little use of the information about the left extent when bisecting a line without cueing [17,20,29]. However, most current explanations for line bisection error presuppose that the task examines the ability of neglect patients to compare the right and left extents of a line [38]. The concept of perceptual distortion explains that the leftward portion of a line is 'perceived' as laterally compressed relative to the rightward extent [3,14,39,40]. The psychophysical approach tried to estimate the subjective length when patients with neglect bisect lines of various lengths with corresponding error sizes [6,7]. The power function used in these estimations adopted the objective length of lines as independent variable. Marshall and Halligan [35] hypothesized that for a line of the ordinary length (e.g., 200 mm) patients with neglect might approach the subjective midpoint from the right side because of an initial rightward shift of attention [11] at the moment of line presentation. Rightward bisection error would follow such an approach from the right side to the pathologically expanded 'indifference zone', in which neglect patients judge the leftward and rightward lengths to be equal. Our eye-fixation studies, as stated above, revealed that at least leftward searches rarely occur to permit such comparison between the leftward and rightward extents. However, the possibility has not been ruled out that patients with neglect approach the subjective midpoint after early rightward orientation of attention. When a line printed on a sheet of paper is presented manually, they may trace the line toward the point from which analysis of eye movements will be started.

To eliminate any potential interference from manual presentation, we adopted a liquid crystal display (LCD) monitor with a cordless tablet for the line bisection test [23]. Four patients with neglect bisected 200-, 100-, and 25-mm lines that appeared across the center of the LCD monitor. The fixation immediately before line presentation was located on average near the center of the lines. Three of the patients approached the subjective midpoint directly from the left side in more than 70% of the 200- and 100-mm trials. The subjective midpoint frequently deviated leftward on the 'attended' segment between the leftmost point of fixation and the right endpoint, while it was displaced rightward on the total extent (Fig. 9). The remaining patient searched

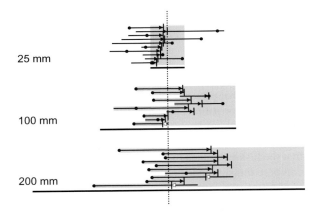

Fig. 9. Location of the fixation before line presentation (black dots), the searched extent between the leftmost and rightmost points of fixation (narrow lines), and the subjective midpoint (vertical bars) for all trials. The line extent perceived in the right attentive field of vision is indicated as grey areas. The arrowheads show the direction of final approach to the subjective midpoint. The vertical grey dotted line indicates the center of the monitor or the objective midpoint of the stimulus lines.

beyond the right endpoint and in turn approached the subjective midpoint from the right side in about half of the trials. In the 200- and 100-mm trials, the subjective midpoint divided the attended right segment nearer to the right endpoint.

On the attended right extent of a line, patients with neglect may place the subjective midpoint toward the side from which they approached that point. However, contrary to the hypothesis by Marshall and Halligan [35], the approach from the right endpoint was observed infrequently. Also, the length of the attended right segment and the deviation of the subjective midpoint on it varied widely. The results indicate that patients with neglect may make no effective comparison between the leftward and rightward extents not only for a whole line but also for its attended right segment. The fixation immediately before line presentation, which often corresponded to the left extreme point of fixation on the line, may hardly affect selection of the location to place the subjective midpoint.

Patients with neglect may bisect lines with leftward errors in some particular conditions. Most frequently, they bisect very short lines (e.g., 25 mm) to the left of the objective center. Marshall and Halligan [35] reported 'cross-over' of the direction of line bisection errors at short length. They supposed that patients with neglect might perceive the whole extent in one fixation and approach the midpoint from the left side. Our study [23] for the first time included 25-mm lines in the recording of eye fixation, when four patients with neglect bisected lines. Three of them, who showed typical leftward errors in the bisection of the 25-mm lines, initially searched leftward beyond the left endpoint. They then approached the subjective midpoint from the left side (Fig. 9). These results supported Marshall and Halligan's hypothesis for the very short lines [35]. As the whole extent of the lines fell in the right attentive visual field, the proportion between the rightward and leftward extents was rather consistent compared with those found for the longer lines. However, such bisection of the 25-mm lines also may not result from the active comparison of the rightward and leftward extents.

Leftward bisection errors appear to represent 'right' neglect for the extent of very short 25-mm lines. Neglect may be hypothesized to occur in representational process of a line or estimation of the midpoint on the formed image, or both. We devised a line image task using a computer display with a touch panel and approached the representational image of a line to be bisected [21]. Three patients with typical left neglect were presented with a line and forced to see its whole extent with cueing to the left endpoint. After disappearance of the line, they pointed to the right endpoint, the left endpoint, or the subjective midpoint according to their representational image. The line image between the reproduced right and left endpoints was appropriately formed for the 200-mm lines. However, the images for the shorter 25- and 100-mm lines were longer than the physical lengths with overextension to the left side (Fig. 10). The image for a fully perceived line may be represented far enough into left space even when left neglect occurs after a lesion that involves the right parietal lobe. The patients with neglect placed the subjective midpoint rightward from the center of the stimulus line for the 100- and 200-mm lines and leftward for the 25-mm lines. This crossover of bisection errors disappeared when the displacement of the subjective midpoint was measured from the center of the representational line image. Left neglect may occur consistently in estimation of the subjective midpoint on the representational image, which may be explained by a simple rightward bias of attentional distribution.

This explanation may be applicable to the bisection of 25-mm lines without cueing, as we found that patients with neglect usually searched beyond the left endpoint for such lines [23]. It is possible that patients with neglect might perceive the leftward extent of the very short lines when they searched to find the left endpoint. At the moment of placing the mark, however, patients with neglect may see the representational image that

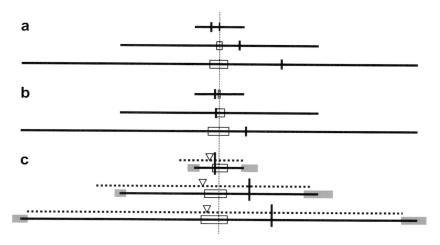

Fig. 10. (a) Ordinary line bisection task, (b) line bisection task with cueing, and (c) line image task after cueing. Vertical bars indicate the subjective midpoint, and the vertical dotted line show the center of the lines. Boxes around the center of the lines represent the normal ranges (mean ± two standard deviations) of the subjective midpoint, which were obtained from the individual means of 10 healthy control subjects. In the line image task (c), the normal ranges for the reproduced right and left endpoints are also depicted as grey areas. The representational images are drawn as horizontal dotted lines between the mean locations of the reproduced right and left endpoints. Downward triangles show the center of the representational images. The subjective midpoint (vertical bars) was always placed to the right of the representational center (Downward triangles), while it was shifted to the left of the objective center (vertical dotted line) for the 25-mm lines.

extend to the actual right endpoint but farther beyond the left endpoint. Also for very short lines, it is unlikely that patients with neglect may compare the left and right extents to determine the subjective midpoint.

Patients with neglect appear to be quite satisfied with their response, when asked if their mark is placed at the center of the line [46]. Even when they were able to respond correctly in the task to point to the longer side of the bisected line, their bisection performance did not improve in the following trials. Also, we examined three patients with neglect in the perceptual judgment task where they were asked to point to the longer right or left segment of the pretransected 200-mm lines [25]. They were able to detect the deviation of the transections that were placed 10 mm or more to the right or left of the true center. The same patients erred more than 30 mm when bisecting 200-mm lines. In a new line bisection task by fixation, the patients were presented a line and asked to fixate its center. The subjective midpoint was determined by asking if the point briefly indicated by the examiner correspond to their estimation of the center. Their bisection by fixation was also deviated 30 mm or more to the right of the true center. These findings also suggest that where to bisect may be related not to active comparison between the leftward and rightward extents but to rather consistent fixation at a favorable rightward point.

7. Favoring a rightward point with major reference to the right endpoint

Swift rightward shift of gaze from the initial fixation, and less contribution of the perceived leftward extent to formation of the representational image and placement of the subjective midpoint itself [23] suggest that the location of the right endpoint may be a major determinant factor of line bisection for patients with neglect. Koyama et al. [34] investigated the line bisection performance when patients with neglect bisected lines of two lengths (100- and 200-mm) in three positions relative to the body midline. In patients with severe neglect, length had little effect on the placement of the subjective midpoint, while location of the right endpoint in the egocentric space mainly determined the subjective midpoint. Ishiai et al. [24] examined patients with neglect in the condition where the right endpoint was placed at a fixed point and the line length was varied. When asked to bisect lines without cueing, they placed the subjective midpoint nearly the same distance to the left of the right endpoint irrespective of line length (Fig. 11). The length effect appeared when they bisected lines presented in the same condition after cueing to the left endpoint. McIntosh et al. [38] also manipulated the right and left endpoints to quantify the influence of each endpoint on determination of the subjective midpoint. They provided a representative data of patients with severe neglect in which the

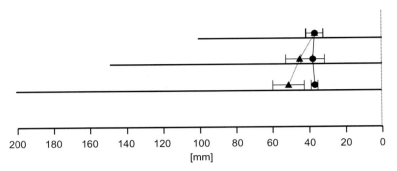

Fig. 11. Bisection errors in the right condition for a patient with neglect (Case 3 from Ishiai et al. [24]). The mean locations of the subjective midpoint with standard deviations are shown separately for the 100-, 150-, and 200-mm lines. The horizontal axis indicates the distance from the right endpoint to the subjective midpoint. Closed circles = line bisection without cueing, black triangles = line bisection with cueing.

left endpoint had no influence upon the location of the subjective midpoint.

8. Conclusion

Eye-fixation patterns of patients with unilateral spatial neglect may vary widely with tasks, stimuli, and instructions. Accordingly, we should approach the mechanisms of left neglect in line bisection by analyzing the visuospatial processing when patients with neglect bisect a line. When bisecting a line without cueing, they rarely search leftward and make no effective comparison between the leftward and rightward extents not only for the whole line but also for its explored right segment. They may see the line as extending equally to either side of their subjective midpoint. Any point on the line except the two endpoints could be selected or favored as the subjective midpoint. For patients with neglect, the right endpoint and the favored point of fixation on the line may contribute to formation of its representational image. Unlike healthy subjects, the left endpoint appears to have little determinant value. Moreover, where patients with neglect 'favor' to fixate as the subjective midpoint seems to depend strongly upon the location of the right endpoint in space. The favorite point or the subjective midpoint varies widely with patients and spatial attributes of a line. Analysis of bisection errors gives us only a small amount of information about visuospatial processing of neglect patients. However, the line bisection task, if combined with recording of eye-fixation, would further contribute to elucidation of the mechanisms underlying neglect.

Acknowledgements

This work was supported by a Grant in Aid for Scientific Research (C) to Sumio Ishiai from the Ministry of Education, Science, Sports, and Culture, Japan.

References

[1] M.L. Albert, A simple test of visual neglect, *Neurology* **23** (1973), 658–664.
[2] J.J.S. Barton, M. Behrmann and S. Black, Ocular search during line bisection. The effects of hemi-neglect and hemianopia, *Brain* **121** (1998), 1117–1131.
[3] E. Bisiach, L. Pizzamiglio, D. Nico and G. Antonucci, Beyond unilateral neglect, *Brain* **119** (1996), 851–857.
[4] E. Bisiach, R. Ricci and M.N. Mòdona, Visual Awareness and anisometry of spatial representation in unilateral neglect: a panoramic investigation by means of a line extension task, *Consciousness and Cognition* **7** (1998), 327–355.
[5] E. Bisiach, M.L. Rusconi, V.A. Peretti and G. Vallar, Challenging current accounts of unilateral neglect, *Neuropsychologia* **32** (1994), 1431–1434.
[6] A. Chatterjee, Cross-over, completion and confabulation in unilateral spatial neglect, *Brain* **118** (1995), 455–465.
[7] A. Chatterjee, M. Mennemeier and K.M. Heilman, The psychophysical power law and unilateral spatial neglect, *Brain Cogn* **25** (1994), 92–107.
[8] F. Chédru, M. Leblanc and F. Lhermitte, Visual searching in normal and brain-damaged subjects (contribution to the study of unilateral inattention), *Cortex* **9** (1973), 94–110.
[9] R.P. Friedland and E.A. Weinstein, Hemi-inattention and hemisphere specialization: introduction and historical review. in: *Advances in Neurology, Vol. 18, Hemi-inattention and hemisphere specialization*, E.A. Weinstein and R.P. Friedland, eds, Raven Press, New York, 1977, pp. 1–31.
[10] M. Fruhmann-Berger and H.-O. Karnath, Spontaneous eye and head position in patients with spatial neglect, *J Neurol* **252** (2005), 1194–1200.
[11] G. Gainotti, P. D'Erme and P. Bartolomeo, Early orientation of attention toward the half space ipsilateral to the lesion in

patients with unilateral brain damage, *J Neurol Neurosurg Psychiatry* **54** (1991), 1082–1089.
[12] G. Gainotti, P. D'Erme, D. Monteleone and M.C. Silveri, Mechanisms of unilateral spatial neglect in relation to laterality of cerebral lesions, *Brain* **109** (1986), 599–612.
[13] P.W. Halligan and J.C. Marshall, How long is a piece of string? A study of line bisection in a case of visual neglect, *Cortex* **24** (1988), 321–328.
[14] P.W. Halligan and J.C. Marshall, Spatial compression in visual neglect: a case study, *Cortex* **27** (1991), 623–629.
[15] K.M. Heilman, R.T. Watson and Valenstein E, Neglect and related disorders, in: *Clinical neuropsychology*, 3rd ed, K.M. Heilman and E. Valenstein, eds, Oxford University Press, New York, 1993, pp. 279–336.
[16] M. Husain, S. Mannan, T. Hodgson, E. Wojciulik, J. Driver and C. Kennard, Impaired spatial working memory across saccades contributes to abnormal search in parietal neglect, *Brain* **124** (2001, 941–952.
[17] S. Ishiai, Perceptual and motor interaction in unilateral spatial neglect, in: *The cognitive and neural bases of spatial neglect*, H.-O. Karnath, D. Milner and G. Vallar, eds, Oxford University Press, Oxford, 2002, pp. 181–193.
[18] S. Ishiai, T. Furukawa and H. Tsukagoshi, Eye-fixation patterns in homonymous hemianopia and unilateral spatial neglect, *Neuropsychologia* **25** (1987), 675–679.
[19] S. Ishiai, T. Furukawa and H. Tsukagoshi, Eye-fixation patterns in homonymous hemianopia and unilateral spatial neglect: a study with eye camera, (in Japanese), *Clinical Neurology* **27** (1987), 643–641.
[20] S. Ishiai, T, Furukawa and H. Tsukagoshi, Visuospatial processes of line bisection and the mechanisms underlying unilateral spatial neglect, *Brain* **112** (1989), 1485–1502.
[21] S. Ishiai, Y. Koyama, N. Nakano, K. Seki, K. Nishida and K. Hayashi, Image of a line is not shrunk but neglected. Absence of crossover in unilateral spatial neglect, *Neuropsychologia* **42** (2004), 251–256.
[22] S. Ishiai, Y. Koyama and K. Seki, Significance of paradoxical leftward error of line bisection in left unilateral spatial neglect, *Brain Cogn* **45** (2001), 238–248.
[23] S. Ishiai, Y. Koyama, K. Seki, K. Hayashi and Y. Izumi, Approaches to subjective midpoint of horizontal lines in unilateral spatial neglect, *Cortex* (2006), 685–691.
[24] S. Ishiai, Y. Koyama, K. Seki and M, Izawa, Line versus representational bisections in unilateral spatial neglect, *J Neurol Neurosurg Psychiatry* **69** (2000), 745–750.
[25] S. Ishiai, Y. Koyama, K. Seki and T. Nakayama, What is line bisection in unilateral spatial neglect? Analysis of perceptual and motor aspects in line bisection tasks, *Brain Cogn* **36** (1998), 239–252.
[26] S. Ishiai, K. Seki, Y. Koyama and S. Gono, Ineffective leftward search in line bisection and mechanisms of left unilateral spatial neglect, *J Neurol* **243** (1996), 381–387.
[27] S. Ishiai, K. Seki, Y. Koyama and R. Okiyama, Effects of cueing on visuospatial processing in unilateral spatial neglect, *J Neurol* **242** (1995), 367–373.
[28] S. Ishiai, K. Seki, Y. Koyama and T. Yokota, Mechanisms of unilateral spatial neglect in copying a single object, *Neuropsychologia* **34** (1996), 965–971.
[29] S. Ishiai, M. Sugishita, K. Mitani and M, Ishizawa, Leftward search in left unilateral spatial neglect, *J Neurol Neurosurg Psychiatry* **55** (1992), 40–44.
[30] S. Ishiai, M. Sugishita, S. Watabiki, T. Nakayama, M. Kotera and S. Gono, Improvement of left unilateral spatial neglect in a line extension task, *Neurology* **44** (1994), 294–298.
[31] S. Ishiai, S. Watabiki, E. Lee, T. Kanouchi and N. Odajima, Preserved leftward movement in left unilateral spatial neglect due to frontal lesions, *J Neurol Neurosurg Psychiatry* **57** (1994), 1085–1090.
[32] H.-O. Karnath, M. Niemeier and J. Dichgans, Space exploration in neglect, *Brain* **121** (1998), 2357–2367.
[33] L.D. Kartsounis and E.K. Warrington, Unilateral visual neglect overcome by cues implicit in stimulus arrays, *J Neurol Neurosurg Psychiatry* **52** (1989),1253–1259.
[34] Y. Koyama, S. Ishiai, K. Seki and T. Nakayama, Distinct processes in line bisection according to severity of left unilateral spatial neglect, *Brain Cogn* **35** (1997), 271–281.
[35] J.C. Marshall and P.W. Halligan, When right goes left: an investigation of line bisection in a case of visual neglect, *Cortex* **25** (1989), 503–515.
[36] J.C. Marshall and P.W. Halligan, Visuo-spatial neglect: a new copying test to assess perceptual parsing, *J Neurol* **240** (1993), 37–40.
[37] J.C. Marshall and P.W. Halligan, Within- and between-task dissociations in visuo-spatial neglect: a case study, *Cortex* **31** (1995), 367–376.
[38] R.D. McIntosh, The eyes have it: ocular exporation and line bisection in neglect, *Cortex* (2006), 692–698.
[39] A.D. Milner and M. Harvey, Distortion of size perception in visuospatial neglect, *Current Biology* **5** (1995), 85–89.
[40] A.D. Milner, M. Harvey, R.C. Roberts and S.V. Foster, Line bisection errors in visual neglect: misguided action or size distortion? *Neuropsychologia* **31** (1993), 39–49.
[41] P. Nichelli, M. Rinaldi and R. Cubelli, Selective spatial attention and length representation in normal subjects and in patients with unilateral spatial neglect, *Brain Cogn* **9** (1989), 57–70.
[42] L. Pisella and J.B. Mattingley, The contribution of spatial remapping impairments to unilateral visual neglect. *Neuroscience and Biobehavioral Reviews* **28** (2004), 181–200.
[43] M.J. Riddoch and G.W. Humphreys, The effect of cueing on unilateral neglect, *Neuropsychologia* **21** (1983), 589–599.
[44] I.H. Robertson, P.W. Halligan, C. Bergego, V. Homberg, L. Pizzamiglio, E. Weber and B.A. Wilson, Right neglect following right hemisphere damage? *Cortex* **30** (1994), 199–213.
[45] K. Seki and S. Ishiai, Diverse patterns of performance in copying and severity of unilateral spatial neglect, *J Neurol* **243** (1996), 1–8.
[46] K. Seki, S. Ishiai, Y. Koyama and S. Sato, Unassociated responses to two related task demands: a negative factor for improvement of unilateral spatial neglect, *Neuropsychologia* **37** (1999), 75–82.
[47] X. Seron, F. Coyette and R. Bruyer, Ipsilateral influence on contralateral processing in neglect patients, *Cogn Neuropsychol* **6** (1989), 475–498.
[48] S. Weintraub and M.-M. Mesulam, Right cerebral dominance in spatial attention: further evidence based on ipsilateral neglect, *Arch Neurol* **44** (1987), 621–625.

A battery of tests for the quantitative assessment of unilateral neglect[1]

Philippe Azouvi[a,*], Paolo Bartolomeo[b], Jean-Marie Beis[c], Dominic Perennou[d], Pascale Pradat-Diehl[e] and Marc Rousseaux[f]

[a]*Service de Médecine Physique et de Réadaptation, Université de Versailles-Saint-Quentin, et INSERM UPMC 731, AP-HP, Hôpital Raymond Poincaré, Garches, France*
[b]*INSERM U 610, Hôpital de la Salpétrière, Paris, France*
[c]*Institut Régional de Réadaptation, Nancy, France*
[d]*Service de Rééducation Neurologique, CHU and INSERM ERM 207, Dijon, France*
[e]*Service de Médecine Physique et de Réadaptation, INSERM UPMC 731, AP-HP Hôpital de la Salpétrière, Paris, France*
[f]*Service de Rééducation Neurologique, CHRU, Lille, France*

Received 8 March 2006
Revised 13 June 2006
Accepted 22 June 2006

Abstract. *Purpose*: The lack of agreement regarding assessment methods is responsible for the variability in the reported rate of occurrence of unilateral neglect (UN) after stroke. In addition, dissociations have been reported between performance on traditional paper-and-pencil tests and UN in everyday life situations.
Methods: In this paper, we present the validation studies of a quantitative test battery for UN, including paper-and-pencil tests, an assessment of personal neglect, extinction, and anosognosia, and a behavioural assessment, the Catherine Bergego Scale (CBS). The battery was given to healthy subjects ($n = 456 - 476$) and to patients with subacute stroke, either of the right or the left hemisphere.
Results: In healthy subjects, a significant effect of age, education duration and acting hand was found in several tasks. In patients with right hemisphere stroke, the most sensitive paper and pencil measure was the starting point in the cancellation task. The whole battery was more sensitive than any single test alone. An important finding was that behavioural assessment was more sensitive than any other single test. Neglect was two to four times less frequent, but also less severe and less consistent after left hemisphere stroke.
Conclusion: Assessment of UN should rely on a battery of quantitative and standardised tests. Some patients may show clinically significant UN in everyday life while obtaining a normal performance on paper-and-pencil measures. This underlines the necessity to use a behavioural assessment of UN.

Keywords: Unilateral neglect, assessment, stroke

*Corresponding author: Prof. Philippe Azouvi, MD, PhD, Department of Physical Medicine and Rehabilitation, Raymond Poincare Hospital, 92380 Garches, France. Tel.: +33 14 710 70 74; Fax: +33 1 47 10 77 25; E-mail: philippe.azouvi@rpc.aphp.fr.
[1]For the French collaborative study group on assessment of unilateral neglect (GEREN/GRECO).

1. Introduction: why a quantitative test battery for unilateral neglect?

Unilateral neglect (UN) is a failure to attend to the contralesional side of space. It is a puzzling disorder commonly encountered after stroke, particularly of the right hemisphere. The study of UN is of considerable interest for neuroscientists interested in spatial cognition or attention [38]. However, UN also has major practical significance for clinicians and rehabilitation professionals dealing with stroke patients. Indeed, UN may affect many daily living skills and has been found associated with poor functional recovery from stroke. Denes et al. [30] found that neglect was the worst prognostic factor for functional recovery in hemiplegia, when compared to other cognitive disorders, such as aphasia, intellectual deterioration, or disturbed emotional reactions. These findings have been subsequently largely reproduced by other authors, who showed that neglect had an adverse influence upon functional outcome, improvement on rehabilitation, length of hospital stay and discharge to home [2, 3,25,45,53], although contradictory results have been reported [35,54].

In most severe cases, after a large right hemisphere stroke, UN is obvious and can be detected by simple observation of the patient in his bed. However, in most patients, UN is not clinically apparent and specific testing is needed to reveal the disorder. Specific testing is also necessary to give objective measures of the severity of neglect and to monitor recovery during rehabilitation. However, objective assessment of neglect is not easy, for at least two reasons. Firstly, it is now widely accepted that UN is not, at least from a clinical point of view, a unitary disorder [14]. Clinical manifestations of UN may vary from one patient to the other, and in a given patient, according to time and nature of assessment. The different clinical manifestations of UN, that can dissociate one from each other, include viewer- or object-centred neglect, neglect for near or far extrapersonal space, personal neglect, representational neglect, motor neglect, directional hypokinesia [43]. However, most commonly used tests only take into account visual or visuo-motor aspects of UN in the near peripersonal space [42]. Secondly, UN is not an all-or-nothing phenomenon. Neglect can vary in a given patient according to the test used, its nature, its complexity, but also according to extraneous factors, such as fatigue, motivation, or mood status.

Assessment of UN. A great number of clinical tests of UN have been reported in the literature. However, despite a large amount of research, there is still no consensus among clinicians regarding the methods of identifying neglect and monitoring changes after treatment [22,59]. A recent review [51] identified 62 assessment tools for UN. Only 28 of them were standardised, thus allowing objective quantified measurement of the disorder. In a recent systematic review of published reports, Bowen et al. [22] found that the frequency of occurrence of neglect in patients with right brain damage ranged from 13% to 82%. The assessment method used was one of the main factors explaining the discrepancies between the different studies. Thirty studies were included in this latter review, most of them using a battery of paper-and-pencil tests. Only one study [46] did not specify how UN was assessed. Nineteen studies used a battery of up to 7 different tests. The most frequently used single task was a cancellation task. Figure copying was also commonly used. Only occasionally did the assessment of UN involve an ecological assessment of neglect in everyday life.

Many clinicians are familiar with several simple bedside screening tests, such as object copying [33,52], or drawing. However, such tests are not very sensitive and are difficult to score in a quantitative way. Cancellation tasks are more sensitive and may give quantitative scores. There are several versions, but all of them require the patient to find and cancel target items displayed on an A4 paper sheet. In the classical line cancellation task [1], there are no distractor, only lines to cancel. In most other tests, such as the bells test [34], or the star cancellation test [71], distractors are mixed with targets in a pseudo-random fashion, thus improving the sensitivity of the task. Line bisection is another widely used test. Patients with UN tend to show a rightward deviation of the subjective midpoint [64]. The sensitivity of line bisection depends on the length of the line to bisect, longer lines being more sensitive [16]. With short lines, neglect patients show a paradoxical leftward deviation ("crossover effect") [39]. Other clinical tests have been proposed, such as the overlapping figures test [32], in which patients are asked to name four overlapping figures, two on the right and two on the left of a fifth centrally located figure, and reading and writing tasks. These different tests assess visual or visuo-motor aspects of UN in the close peripersonal space. Personal neglect can be assessed by asking the patient to comb his hair, shave or put on make-up [15, 50,73], or to reach his left arm with his right hand [18]. The Fluff test has been recently proposed as a simple test for studying personal neglect [27]. This latter test requires patients to remove, with one's eyes closed, 24 2-cm diameter circles attached with velcro to the front of their clothes. Neglect in the far extrapersonal space can be assessed by requiring a patient to describe objects in the room around him, or to bisect lines or cancel items located outside hand reach, for example with a laser pointer [40]. However, these tests cannot easily be replicated across different settings. Representational neglect is addressed by asking the patient to describe from memory a familiar place [17], although such a procedure cannot be scored quantitatively. Rode and Perenin [61] devised a simple test that permits to obtain a quantitative score of representational neglect for French patients. Patients have to generate a mental image of the map of France and to cite as many cities they can mentally visualize on the right and the left of an imaginal line. Motor neglect is usually observed by therapists who remark the lack of spontaneous use of the contralesional limb. However, there is no simple way to quantitatively score motor neglect or directional hypokinesia in a routine clinical setting. A few standardised assessment batteries including various clinical tests have been published. The Behavioural Inattention Test (BIT) [37,71] is a comprehensive and well validated one, including both paper and pencil and behavioural tests.

Ecological assessment of UN. Although paper-and-pencil tests are useful for rapid clinical screening, they fail to consider the patient's actual performance in his everyday life. Some patients obtain a normal performance on conventional tests, while showing a directional bias in daily life skills. Such dissociations have been attributed to the relative sparing of voluntary orientation of attention (involved in conventional tests) contrasting with an impairment of automatic orienting which allows attention to be automatically captured by relevant stimuli in everyday life [10,65]. There is a need for standardised ecological measures of neglect to quantify the extent of neglect in everyday life, to adapt rehabilitation to the individual patient's limitations, to monitor changes and to assess the effectiveness of rehabilitation. This last point is of great importance for rehabilitation studies, which are often limited by the lack of evidence of any therapeutic effect on everyday life skills [20,21,58]. The need for controlled rehabilitation studies including a meaningful activity level measures has been emphasised in a recent meta-analysis [20].

Several ecological assessment measures have been proposed in the literature, either based on the simulation of realistic conditions, or on a questionnaire attempting to measure patients' subjective account of everyday difficulties [69,71,73]. Towle and Lincoln [69] proposed a questionnaire on neglect in everyday life, including 19 questions each with a dichotomous score. The questionnaire is filled out by the patient or a relative. The Behavioural Inattention Test includes nine behavioural subtests, based on the simulation of realistic conditions, such as reading a menu, a newspaper article, a road map, sorting coins, setting or reading the time [71].

Performance on these subtests has been found significantly correlated with a checklist score completed by an occupational therapist. This battery demonstrated good inter-rater and test-retest reliability. However, it did not seem to be more sensitive than paper-and-pencil tests. An Italian team has devised a semi-structured scale of both personal and extrapersonal neglect [56, 72,73]. Extrapersonal neglect is assessed by asking the patients to serve tea or to distribute cards to four persons around a square table, to describe complex figures and objects in a room. Personal neglect is assessed by requiring to use common objects (razor or powder, comb, glasses). Inter-rater reliability is good [72]. Only extrapersonal subtests were significantly correlated with paper-and-pencil tests. A modified version of the personal subscale has been proposed, the comb and razor test, with a more precise quantitative scoring system [15,50]. The Baking Tray Task consists of 16 wooden cubes, that the patient is required to place as evenly as possible over a 75×100 cm board, "as if they were buns on a baking tray" [68]. Patients with UN tend to place the cubes preferentially on the right part of the board.

Although these different tasks are all simulations of real-life situations, they do not provide any objective information on the patient's behaviour in his actual everyday environment. Most of these ecological tests still represent quite artificial situations which may rely more on voluntary rather than automatic orienting of attention. Moreover, they do not take into account anosognosia. Considering the above mentioned limitations and difficulty of assessment of UN, a collaborative study was decided in the French-speaking community, with the objective to design and validate a test battery of UN, that could be both psychometrically sound and easy to complete within a rehabilitation setting. This battery ("Batterie d'évaluation de la négligence spatiale", BEN) comprises two different parts. The first one includes traditional clinical and "paper and pencil" tests of neglect and related disorders, the second one is a standardised observational scale, aimed at providing an ecological assessment of neglect in the patient's everyday life.

2. Paper-and pencil tests of the French test battery for UN ("Batterie d'évaluation de la négligence spatiale", BEN)

2.1. Materials and methods

2.1.1. Subjects

As a first step, normative data were collected in a group of healthy individuals ($n = 456$ to 576 depending on the task) [62]. The objective was to determine norms and a pathological threshold for each task, and to assess the effect on performance of five factors: gender; age (four age groups: 20–34; 35–49; 50–64; 65–80); education duration ($\leqslant$8 years; 9–12 years; $\geqslant$13 years); handedness; and acting hand (half of the subjects performed the task with their preferred hand, half of them with their non-dominant hand).

Two groups of patients were included, at the subacute stage after a stroke either in the right ($n = 206$) [6] or the left ($n = 89$) [11] hemisphere. For patients with left hemisphere stroke, only non-verbal subtests were given, to control for any confounding effect of associated language impairments. Nevertheless, 11 patients with left hemisphere stroke were excluded from the study due to severe aphasia with major comprehension deficits. The main characteristics of the two groups are displayed on Table 1. It appeared that, as compared to the general stroke population, these patients were relatively younger, probably due to a selection bias related to the fact that most of them were recruited through specialised stroke rehabilitation units, and not from geriatric wards. These patients should be regarded as representative of stroke patients referred to a rehabilitation facility. Not surprisingly, the majority of patients also had motor deficits (hemiparesis or hemiplegia). Severity of motor impairments (which reflects overall stroke severity) was assessed with a four-level scale, ranging from 0 (no motor deficit) to 3 (severe hemiplegia). The amount of patients with severe hemiplegia was quite similar in both groups (see Table 1). In addition, patients were classified in four groups according to stroke localisation (anterior; posterior; anteroposterior; subcortical) as assessed with CT and/or MRI scans by examiners blind to neuropsychological assessment. Anatomic data were not available for 49 patients in the right hemisphere group and for seven patients in the left hemisphere group.

2.1.2. Methods: Paper-and pencil tests of the BEN

Most of paper-and-pencil tests included in the battery were adapted from the existing literature, with their authors' permission. In addition to these traditional tests, personal UN and related disorders, such as anosognosia and extinction were also addressed.

2.1.2.1. Paper-and-pencil tests of extrapersonal neglect

The bells test [34]. Subjects were asked to circle 35 targets (black-ink drawings of bells), presented on a horizontal A4 paper sheet, along with 280 distractors in

Table 1
Characteristics of patients included in the validation studies of paper-and-pencil tests of the BEN (Azouvi et al., 2002; Beis et al., 2004); RH = right hemisphere; LH = left hemisphere

	RH stroke	LH stroke
Number of patients	206	78
Gender (% male)	60.7%	58.9%
Age	55.9 (15.3)	54.6 (15.7)
% right handers	87.8%	83.2%
Time since onset (weeks)	11.1 (13.8)	10.8 (12.4)
% ischaemic stroke	65.5%	69.3%
% severe hemiplegia	21.4%	24.3%
Stroke localisation		
Anterior	7 (4.4%)	7 (9.8%)
Posterior	29 (18.5%)	9 (12.6%)
Antero-posterior	92 (58.6%)	35 (49.3%)
Subcortical	29 (18.5%)	20 (28.2%)

a pseudo-random array. The total number of omissions and the difference between left- and right-sided omissions were recorded. In addition, a special care was given to identifying the subject's starting point. Targets were equally distributed in seven columns (three left, three right, and one central) numbered from 1 to 7 starting from the left. The starting point was operationally defined as the number (1–7) of the column including the first circled bell.

Figure copying [33,52]. Subjects were asked to copy on a horizontal A4 sheet a drawing including (from the left to the right) a tree, a fence, a house with a left-sided chimney, and a second tree. Following Ogden [52], a five-level scale was used, ranging from 0 (no omission) to 4 (omission of the left tree and of at least the left part of another item).

Clock drawing. Patients were required to place the 12 hours in a circle drawn by the examiner. A three-level scale was used, with a score of 0 in case of a normal symmetrical performance, of 1 in case of omissions of a part of left-sided hours and of 2 in case of omission or rightward displacement of all left-sided hours.

Line bisection. Patients were asked to mark the middle of four lines of two different lengths (5-cm and 20-cm), presented separately centred on an A4 horizontal sheet. Deviation from the true middle was measured in mm, positively for rightward deviation, negatively for leftward deviation.

Overlapping Figures Test [32]. Test stimuli consisted of two figures overlapping on the right and two on the left side of a card, all of them overlapping a fifth centrally located figure. Patients were asked to name all the figures they could detect. The total number of omitted figures, and the difference between left- and right-sided omissions across five trials were recorded.

Reading [70]. Patients were asked to read a short 12-line text, horizontally printed on an A4 sheet. The total

Table 2
Performance of healthy controls on the BEN (adapted from Rousseaux et al., 2001)

Test variables	Maximal possible score	Mean (SD)	Range	Percentile 5/95
Bells test ($n = 576$)				
Omissions (total number)	35	2.06 (1.49)	0 / 10	0 / 6
Omissions (left minus right)	15	−0.05 (1.39)	−6 / 5	−2 / 2
Starting point	7	1.88 (1.49)	1 / 7	1 / 5
Figure copying ($n = 487$)	4	0.04 (0.21)	0 / 2	0 / 0
Clock drawing ($n = 457$)	2	0.01 (0.09)	0 / 1	0 / 0
Bisection (mm) ($n = 457$)				
20-cm lines	100	−0.95 (4.15)	−16 / 15	−7.2 / 6.5
5-cm lines	25	−0.17 (1.45)	−7 / 5	−2.5 / 2
Text reading ($n = 457$)				
Omissions (total number)		0.04 (0.26)	0 / 3	0 / 0
Omissions (left minus right)		0.02 (0.26)	−1 / 3	0 / 0
Writing (left margin, cm) ($n = 456$)		3.0 (2.54)	0 / 25	0.79 / 7.72

number of words omitted, and the difference between left- and right-sided omissions within the first five lines were recorded.

Writing. Patients were asked to write, on three separate lines, their first and last names, address, and profession (or the current date if they had no profession). The score was the maximal left margin width (in cm).

2.1.2.2. Assessment of gaze orientation and personal neglect

Spontaneous gaze and head orientation was assessed with a four-level scale [60] ranging from 0: no deviation, to 3: permanent rightward deviation of gaze and head.

Personal neglect was assessed following Bisiach et al. [18] methodology. Patients were asked to reach their left hand with the right hand, first with eyes open, then with eyes closed. A four-level scale was used, ranging from 0: normal performance, to 3: no attempt to reach the target.

2.1.2.3. Assessment of related disorders

Awareness of motor and visual deficits was assessed following Bisiach et al. methodology [19], using a four-level scale, both for motor and visual impairments (range: 0 = perfect awareness to 3 = the patient never admitted having some impairment, despite its demonstration by the examiner).

Visual extinction and hemianopia were tested clinically by wiggling fingers for two seconds in one or both visual fields (six trials). Extinction was considered as present when a patient failed at least once to report a contralesional stimulus during bilateral simultaneous presentation, while accurately detecting unilateral stimuli.

2.2. Results

2.2.1. Performance of healthy controls

Some tasks showed a ceiling effect due to a nearly perfect performance: clock drawing, overlapping figures, reading, head and gaze deviation, personal neglect, and visual extinction. For these tasks, any deviation from optimal performance should be considered as abnormal. The other tasks showed a more variable pattern of performance, allowing the determination of a pathological threshold that was arbitrary set below the fifth percentile of the control group. The main results of the performance of the control group are displayed in Table 2.

There was no significant effect of gender, for any task. However, performance in several tasks appeared to be significantly affected by age, education, and by the acting hand [62]. In the bells test, the total number of omissions was significantly higher in older or less educated people. The difference between left and right omissions was also significantly associated with education (more left-sided omissions for lower education levels and more right-sided omissions for higher education duration). Although only a minority of subjects showed one omission in the Figure copying test, the effect of education was significant, due to less omissions in the highest education group. There was a mild, but significant, leftward deviation in line bisection. This deviation was significantly influenced by the acting hand (larger leftward deviation with the left hand), but only for short lines (5-cm). Other factors, including age, gender or handedness, had no significant influence on performance in line bisection. Finally, the left margin in the writing test was significantly larger in older persons, when using the left hand or in left-handers.

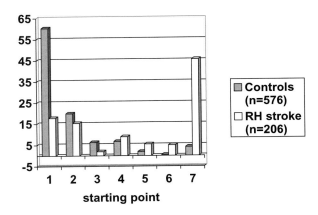

Fig. 1. Starting point in the bells test for controls and patients with right hemisphere (RH) stroke. The bells are equally pseudo-randomly distributed across seven virtual columns. The X-axis shows the number of the columns from left (1) to right (7), and the Y-axis shows the amount (%) of subjects who began the task by circling a bell in each of the corresponding column.

2.2.2. Patients with right hemisphere stroke

The main result was that test sensitivity greatly varied from one test to another (Table 3) [6]. The amount of patients with neglect on each individual subtest ranged from 19.0% to 50.5%. However, more than 85% of patients showed UN on at least one test. The two most sensitive tests were the bells test and the reading test. In the bells test, the most sensitive measure was not the number of omissions, but rather the spatial location of the starting point spontaneously used by the patient. While 80% of controls used a left to right scanning strategy, a majority of patients used a reverse pattern, starting with a right-sided target (Fig. 1).

In the line bisection test, a length effect was found. Indeed, longer lines (20-cm) were nearly twice as sensitive than shorter (5-cm) ones. Bisection of short lines was the less sensitive test in the battery. A paradoxical leftward deviation (cross-over effect) was found in some patients, more frequently with short lines.

To assess the relationships between the different tests, a correlation matrix was calculated for paper-and-pencil measures. The great majority of correlation coefficients was positive and significant ($p < 0.0001$), and about one third of these coefficients had a value of 0.50 or more.

2.2.3. Patients with left hemisphere stroke

Neglect was clearly less frequent and less severe in the left hemisphere group [11]. As indicated in Table 3, paper-and-pencil tests revealed right neglect in 3.8% to 13.2% of patients, depending on the task. However, as far as 43.5% of patients demonstrated some degree of UN on at least one task. Personal neglect was just as frequent as extrapersonal neglect (9 and 13% with eyes open and eyes closed respectively), and was nearly as frequent as after right hemisphere stroke (16% and 13%). Anosognosia for motor and visual deficits was much less frequent than after right hemisphere stroke. Inter-tests correlations were low (<0.50).

2.3. Discussion

In healthy controls, there was a significant effect of age and/or education for the bells test, figure copying and writing, suggesting that these factors should be taken into account in the assessment of a patient suspect of UN. A significant effect of the acting hand was found only in line bisection. In this latter test, controls showed a mild but significant leftward deviation, a phenomenon known as "pseudo-neglect" [23,24,44]. This effect was larger with the left hand and with short lines, a result in accordance with a meta-analysis [44]. The effect of handedness is debated in the literature, and the lack of effect found in the present study should be taken with caution, due to the relatively low number of left-handed individuals ($n = 49$).

The battery was found sensitive to detect UN in patients with right hemisphere stroke. Indeed, more than 85% of patients showed UN on at least one test. An important finding was that an assessment across several different tests was more sensitive than any single test alone. This finding, in accordance with previous reports [41,52], suggests that a normal performance on one test alone is not sufficient to rule out the presence of UN. The two most sensitive tests were the bells test and the reading test, both including a strong visual component that has been suggested to exacerbate UN [9]. However, it should be emphasised that the number of left-sided omissions should not be considered as the sole marker of UN. The pattern of visual scanning used by the patient should be taken into consideration. Indeed, in the bells test, the most sensitive measure was the spatial location of the first circled bell. Contrary to controls, who used preferentially a left to right scanning strategy, a majority of patients started with a right-sided target. This supports the assumption that an early automatic orientation of attention toward the ipsilesional half of space is a major component of unilateral neglect [29,32,49]. Previous studies found that a rightward orientation bias was the only detectable residual impairment in patients who had apparently recovered from neglect [26,49]. In the line bisection tests, a length effect was found, in accordance with previous studies

Table 3
Performance of patients (adapted from Azouvi et al., 2002 and Beis et al., 2004). LH = left hemisphere; RH = right hemisphere

Test variables	Cut-off	LH stroke		RH stroke	
		Mean (SD)	% pathologic	Mean (SD)	% pathologic
Bells test					
Omissions (total number)	> 6	3.7 (2.5)	12.8	8.4 (9.4)	41.3
Omissions (left minus right)	> 2	0.5 (2.1)	11.7	3.1 (4.4)	44.9
Starting point	> 5			4.6 (2.4)	
Figure copying	> 0	0.4 (1.2)	10.4	1.2 (1.6)	42.7
Clock drawing	> 0	0.2 (0.6)	13.2	0.4 (0.6)	27.8
Bisection (mm)					
20-cm lines	> 6.5	0.4 (19.7)	6.4	10.1 (19.4)	37.7
5-cm lines	> 2.0	0.2 (2.9)	3.8	0.6 (3.7)	19.0
Text reading					
Omissions (total number)	> 0			11.9 (25.3)	46.8
Omissions (left minus right)	> 0			5.6 (11.4)	41.2
Writing (left margin, cm)	> 7.7			6.8 (5.0)	34.3
Gaze and eye deviation			12		32
Personal neglect					
Eyes open			9		16
Eyes closed			13		13
Anosognosia					
For hemiplegia			6		17
For hemianopia			10		46

showing a linear increase in rightward displacement as a function of line length in most neglect patients [16, 39]. The cross-over effect for short lines has been reported in previous studies [39,48], although its mechanism remains a matter of debate. Nevertheless, these results suggest that bisection of short lines should not be recommended as a screening test for neglect.

Neglect was clearly less frequent and less severe in the left hemisphere group, in accordance with a large amount of previous studies, although this has been a matter of debate [1,7,22,31,41,52,54,66]. The present data showed that, depending on the criteria used, right UN was two to four times less frequent than left UN. Neglect was not only less frequent, it was only much less severe in the left hemisphere group as compared to patients suffering from a right hemisphere stroke. An other difference between right and left UN was that paper-and-pencil tests were significantly correlated one with each other in the right hemisphere group, while there were only poor inter-tests correlations in the left hemisphere group. This finding suggests that right neglect is a somewhat elusive phenomenon, with less clinical consistency than left UN. In opposition with the findings obtained with paper-and-pencil tests, there was no such asymmetry with personal neglect that was not significantly more frequent after right hemisphere stroke. It should be acknowledged that the two groups were not systematically matched in terms of stroke size and severity, and that a few patients ($n = 11$), presumably with the most severe strokes, had to be excluded from the left hemisphere group due to comprehension deficits. Moreover, data on stroke localisation showed that the right hemisphere group tended to present more frequent antero-posterior and posterior strokes. Nevertheless, the two groups appeared to be quite similar in terms of associated motor impairments, suggesting that differences in stroke severity could not readily account for the dramatic differences in the frequency and severity of UN.

3. Behavioural assessment of UN: the Catherine Bergego Scale (CBS)

3.1. Materials and methods

3.1.1. Subjects

Several studies have been conducted successively with the CBS. Most of them were conducted in patients with subacute right hemisphere stroke in a rehabilitation setting. The first, preliminary study, included 18 patients, with the objective to assess inter-rater reliability. Further studies on psychometric properties of the scale have been conducted on two successive groups of patients with subacute-chronic right hemisphere stroke ($n = 50$ and $n = 83$ respectively) [4,5]. The CBS was also used in a subgroup of 69 patients in two participating centres of the previously mentioned validation study of the BEN [6].

Two of us (DP, PA) have more recently investigated behavioural aspects of right neglect in patients suffering from a left hemisphere stroke (unpublished data). Fifty-four patients suffering from a first-ever left hemisphere stroke were included. They were all right-handed. Time since stroke onset was 65.9 days ($SD = 40.5$). Stroke was ischaemic in 71.7% of cases.

3.1.2. Methods

The Catherine Bergego Scale (CBS) is based on a direct observation of the patient's functioning in ten real-life situations, such as grooming, dressing, or wheelchair driving [4,5,13]. For each item, a four-point scale is used, ranging from 0 (no neglect) to 3 (severe neglect). A total score is then calculated (range: 0–30). Arbitrary cut-off points were drawn in the CBS, to distinguish different levels of impairment. Patients with a total score of 0 were considered as having no UN, a score ranging from 1 to 10 was considered as mild behavioural UN, a score 11–20 as a moderate UN and a score 21–30 as a severe UN. To assess patients' awareness of neglect-related everyday difficulties, a parallel form of the CBS has been designed as a questionnaire, with the same ten items previously described. An anosognosia score can be computed by recording the difference between the observer's and the patient's scores.

3.1.3. Statistical analyses

Reliability was assessed by computing Cohen's kappa coefficients on each of the ten items of the scale, and the correlation coefficient between the total scores given by two independent examiners [13]. Concurrent validity was assessed by comparison of behavioural assessment with the CBS to the results of conventional paper-and-pencil tests. Correlation coefficients between the CBS total score and conventional measures were computed. To further address the relationships between conventional and behavioural assessment, a stepwise multiple regression analysis was performed in the 69 patients from the validation study of the BEN. The total score on the CBS was used as dependent variable, and paper and pencil measures as explicative variables.

Internal consistency of the scale was established by measuring Spearman rank correlation between the scores on each individual question and the total score. The internal structure of the scale was assessed by two different methods on the data from 83 right hemisphere stroke patients from our department [5]. Firstly, a principal component analysis with varimax rotation was computed. In a second step, a Rasch analysis was computed (Bigsteps software) [47]. Rasch analysis is a method specifically designed for evaluating characteristics of rating scales with the expectation of unidimensionality [57,67]. Briefly, the Rasch model has been designed to assess the validity of ordinal scales and to permit the transformation of raw discontinuous scores into an equal interval measure.

3.2. Results

Inter-rater reliability was found satisfactory in the first group of patients ($n = 18$) who were scored simultaneously by two independent raters [13]. The kappa coefficients for the ten items of the scale ranged from 0.59 to 0.99, demonstrating a fair to high inter-rater reliability [13]. In addition, the total scores of the two examiners were strongly correlated one with each other (Spearman rank order correlation coefficient = 0.96, $p < 0.0001$) [13].

Spearman's correlation coefficients between the scores on each individual question and the CBS total score were all significant, ranging between 0.58 to 0.88 [4]. A principal component analysis with varimax rotation ($n = 83$) extracted only one factor with an eigenvalue higher than 1, explaining 65.8% of total variance. All items of the CBS obtained a high loading on this factor (range: 0.77–0.84). Rasch analysis revealed that the ten items defined a common, single ability continuum with widespread measurement range and quite regular item distribution, and showed a satisfactory reliability [5].

In our three different studies [5,6,13], the three following items were found to be the most sensitive of the scale: neglect of left limbs, collisions while moving, and neglect in dressing. Behavioural assessment with the CBS was compared to the results of conventional paper-and-pencil tests. In our different studies previously mentioned, the total CBS score correlated significantly and relatively strongly with most paper-and-pencil tests. Bisection of short lines was the only test that did not correlate with behavioural neglect. The strongest correlations were obtained with the bells test with correlation coefficients always above 0.7 [4,5]. However, an important finding was that the CBS was constantly found to be more sensitive than conventional tests [4–6]. This point was addressed in the previously mentioned validation study of the BEN [6]. In this latter study, the highest incidence of UN found with any individual paper-and-pencil test was 50%, while 76% of patients demonstrated neglect on at least one item of the CBS. Six patients performed within the normal range on the bells test and nevertheless showed a moderate to severe behavioural neglect on the CBS [6]. A stepwise multiple regression analysis found that four variables, from three paper-and-pencil tasks, significantly predicted the total CBS score (R square = 0.79, $F(4,57) = 54.2$, $p < 0.00001$): the total number of omissions and the starting point in the bells test, figure copying and clock drawing. These three tasks in combination revealed neglect in 148 patients (71.84%), and missed only 29 neglect patients (16.38%), most of whom had a mild neglect [6].

Patient's self-assessment with the CBS was significantly lower than the examiner's score ($t(66) = -4.4$, $p < 0.0001$), indicating some form of anosognosia of neglect-related difficulties in everydaylife [6]. The difference was of 5 or more in 25 patients (37.3%). Anosognosia for behavioural neglect correlated significantly, although moderately, with anosognosia for motor and visual impairment ($r = 0.29$ and 0.37 respectively, $p < 0.05$). The anosognosia score correlated strongly with neglect severity, as assessed with the CBS ($r = 0.82$, $p < 0.0001$), or with paper and pencil tests (r ranging from 0.47 to 0.70, $p < 0.0001$), except for short-line bisection [6]. However, individual analysis revealed dissociations between anosognosia and neglect, some patients with moderately severe neglect obtaining anosognosia scores close to 0.

The study with the CBS in patients with left hemisphere stroke (unpublished data) revealed that 41 (77.3%) patients showed at least some neglect on one item of the scale (i.e. had a CBS score of 1 or more). However, only three (5.4%) had a CBS score higher than 10, corresponding to a clinically significant behavioural UN. This should be compared to the much higher rate of clinically significant neglect in patients with right hemisphere stroke (36%) [6]. The items from the CBS that obtained the highest scores (more severe neglect) were neglect of right limbs, neglect in dressing and mouth cleaning after eating, all corresponding to personal neglect. In opposition, items related to extrapersonal neglect, such as collisions while walking or wheelchair driving, obtained lower scores (Fig. 2). The CBS score was significantly correlated with the bells test ($r = 0.41$ with total omissions and 0.34 with right minus left omissions, both ps < 0.01), although the correlation coefficients were of lower magnitude than those observed in studies with right brain damaged patients (above 0.7). The CBS did not significantly correlate with line bisection. There were also significant correlations with functional disability, particularly with independence in basic activities of daily living (the Functional Independence Measure (FIM) [36] ($r = -0.48$, $p < 0.01$) and with posture and balance (Postural Assessment for Stroke Scale, PASS) [12] ($r = -0.55$, $p < 0.001$). Similarly to the findings obtained after right hemisphere stroke, the CBS score was significantly correlated with the presence of lesions in the left parietal cortex.

3.3. Discussion

These results suggest that the CBS is reliable and valid, and that the ten items define a homogeneous construct. The discrepancies between paper-and-pencil and behavioural assessments are very important to consider. We have repeatedly found that behavioural assessment was more sensitive to the presence of UN than any single paper-and-pencil test. This suggests that the diagnosis of UN should not be ruled out based on the performance on paper-and-pencil tests alone, without a careful examination of how the patient behaves in his real environment. In addition, it should also be mentioned that the CBS has been used in a rehabilitation trial in severe neglect patients, and was found sensitive to change, and useful to monitor patients' improvement after rehabilitation [63].

The CBS is also useful to assess anosognosia of neglect in everyday life. Although anosognosia significantly correlated with UN, double dissociations were found between both disorders, in accordance with previous studies [19,28] Moreover, the data presented here suggest that anosognosia is not a unitary phenomenon [55] and that anosognosia for motor, visual or cognitive deficits can be dissociated from each other.

Findings from the study with left hemisphere stroke patients again suggested that right UN is much less severe than left UN. Clinically significant behavioural neglect (about 5% of patients) is much less frequent than after right hemisphere stroke. It seems that right UN is, like left UN, significantly associated with functional and balance impairments. These results may also raise the intriguing possibility of a qualitative difference between right and left neglect, with right neglect involving preferentially the personal rather than the extrapersonal space.

4. General discussion and conclusion

The studies summarised here illustrate the necessity to use a quantitative and validated test battery for

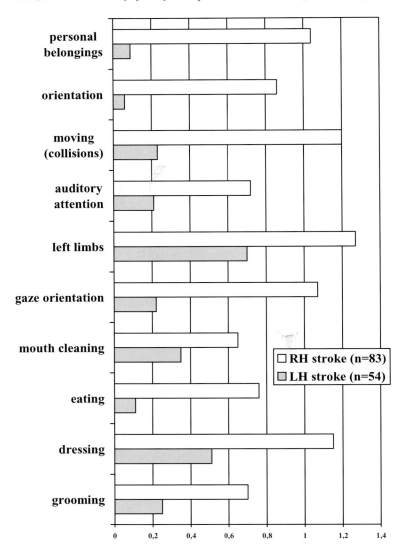

Fig. 2. Mean score (/3) on each item of the Catherine Bergego Scale obtained by patients with right and left hemisphere (RH and LH respectively) stroke.

assessment of UN. It is necessary to compare performance of patients with that of matched healthy controls. A significant effect of age and/or education was found for several tests in healthy controls, suggesting that these factors should be taken into account. Moreover, it is clear that clinical tasks for UN are of variable sensitivity. Tasks including a strong visual component were the most sensitive in our battery, and the automatic rightward orientation bias appeared to be the best indicator of unilateral neglect. In addition, several tests were more likely to uncover evidence of neglect than a single test. The BEN also addresses disorders such as personal neglect, anosognosia and extinction, that are not addressed in other widely used batteries.

Surprisingly, although UN in the extrapersonal space was more frequent and severe after right than left hemisphere stroke, personal neglect was of quite similar frequency in the two groups of patients.

An important finding, replicated across several studies with different groups of patients, was that behavioural assessment of neglect in daily life was more sensitive than any other single measure of neglect. As recently suggested [21], such behavioural measures should be included in any therapeutic trial of UN. The CBS is a reliable, valid and sensitive measure of behavioural neglect, that can easily be used in a rehabilitation setting. It also permits an assessment of anosognosia for neglect in everyday life, that can be dissociated from anosognosia for hemiplegia or hemianopia. Finally, it should be reminded that neglect is not an all-or-nothing phenomenon. Apparently recovered neglect patients may demonstrate signs of spatial bias when confronted to a novel situation [8]. Non specific factors, such as motivation, fatigue, emotional state, may also be of influence and should be taken into consideration in the assessment of neglect patients.

Aknowledgements

We are mostly grateful to E Bisiach, G Gainotti, L Gauthier, Y Joanette, J Ogden, and P van Eeckhout, for authorizing us to include their tests in the battery.

We thank the members of the coordination team of the French Collaborative Study Group on Assessment of Unilateral Neglect (GEREN/GRECO): T Bernati, S Chokron, C Keller, M Leclercq, A Louis-Dreyfus, F Marchal, Y Martin, G de Montety-Bensmail, N Morin, S Olivier, C Prairial, G Rode, C Samuel, E Sieroff, L Wiart, and many students and colleagues who participated in data collection.

We thank also Dr. Luigi Tesio (Milano, Italy) for running the Rasch analysis on data from the CBS.

References

[1] M. Albert, A simple test of visual neglect, *Neurology* **23** (1973), 658–664.

[2] P. Appelros, G.M. Karlsson, A. Seiger and I. Nydevik, Neglect and anosognosia after first-ever stroke: incidence and relationship to disability, *J Rehabil Med* **34**(5) (2002), 215–220.

[3] P. Appelros, G.M. Karlsson, A. Seiger and I. Nydevik, Prognosis for patients with neglect and anosognosia with special reference to cognitive impairment, *J Rehabil Med* **35**(6) (2003), 254–258.

[4] P. Azouvi, F. Marchal, C. Samuel, L. Morin, C. Renard, A. Louis-Dreyfus, C. Jokic, L. Wiart, P. Pradat-Diehl, G. Deloche and C. Bergego, Functional consequences and awareness of unilateral neglect: Study of an evaluation scale, *Neuropsychological Rehabilitation* **6** (1996), 133–150.

[5] P. Azouvi, S. Olivier, G. de Montety, C. Samuel, A. Louis-Dreyfus and L. Tesio, Behavioral assessment of unilateral neglect: Study of the psychometric properties of the Catherine Bergego Scale. *Archives of Physical Medicine and Rehabilitation* **84** (2003), 51–57.

[6] P. Azouvi, C. Samuel, A. Louis-Dreyfus, T. Bernati, P. Bartolomeo, J. Beis, S. Chokron, M. Leclercq, F. Marchal, Y. Martin, G. de Montety, S. Olivier, D. Perennou, P. Pradat-Diehl, C. Prairial, G. Rode, E. Sieroff, L. Wiart and M. Rousseaux, Sensitivity of clinical and behavioural tests of spatial neglect after right hemisphere stroke, *Journal of Neurology, Neurosurgery and Psychiatry* **73** (2002), 160–166.

[7] M.J. Bailey, M.J. Riddoch and P. Crome, Evaluation of a test battery for hemineglect in elderly stroke patients for use by therapists in clinical practice, *NeuroRehabilitation* **14** (2000), 139–150.

[8] P. Bartolomeo, The novelty effect in recovered hemineglect, *Cortex* **33** (1997), 323–332.

[9] P. Bartolomeo and S. Chokron, Levels of impairment in unilateral neglect, in: *Handbook of Neuropsychology, 2nd ed., vol4: Disorders of Visual Behavior*, M. Behrmann, F. Boller and J. Grafman, eds, Elsevier Science Publishers, Amsterdam, 2001, pp. 67–98.

[10] P. Bartolomeo and S. Chokron, Orienting of attention in left unilateral neglect, *Neuroscience and Biobehavioral Review* **26**(2) (2002), 217–234.

[11] J. Beis, C. Keller, N. Morin, P. Bartolomeo, T. Bernati, S. Chokron, M. Leclercq, A. Louis-Dreyfus, F. Marchal, Y. Martin, D. Perennou, P. Pradat-Diehl, C. Prairial, G. Rode, M. Rousseaux, C. Samuel, E. Sieroff, L. Wiart and P. Azouvi, Right spatial neglect after left hemisphere stroke: Qualitative and quantitative study, *Neurology* **63** (2004), 1600–1605.

[12] C. Benaim, D.A. Perennou, J. Villy, M. Rousseaux and J.Y. Pelissier, Validation of a standardized assessment of postural control in stroke patients: the Postural Assessment Scale for Stroke Patients (PASS), *Stroke* **30**(9) (1999), 1862–1868.

[13] C. Bergego, P. Azouvi, C. Samuel, F. Marchal, A. Louis-Dreyfus, C. Jokic, L. Morin, C. Renard, P. Pradat-Diehl and G. Deloche, Validation d'une échelle d'évaluation fonctionnelle de l'héminégligence dans la vie quotidienne: l'échelle CB, *Annales de Réadaptation et de Médecine Physique* **38** (1995), 183–189.

[14] A. Berti and G. Rizzolatti, Is neglect a theoretically coherent unit? *Neuropsychological Rehabilitation* **4** (1994), 111–114.

[15] N. Beschin and I.H. Robertson, Personal versus extrapersonal neglect: A group study of their dissociation using a reliable clinical test, *Cortex* **33** (1997), 378–384.

[16] E. Bisiach, C. Bulgarelli, C. Sterzi and G. Vallar, Line bisection and cognitive plasticity of unilateral neglect of space, *Brain and Cognition* **2** (1983), 32–38.

[17] E. Bisiach, C. Luzzatti and D. Perani, Unilateral neglect, representational schema and consciousness, *Brain* **102** (1979), 609–618.

[18] E. Bisiach, D. Perani, G. Vallar and A. Berti, Unilateral neglect: personal and extrapersonal, *Neuropsychologia* **24** (1986), 759–767.

[19] E. Bisiach, G. Vallar, D. Perani, C. Papagno and A. Berti, Unawareness of disease following lesions of the right hemisphere: anosognosia for hemiplegia and anosognosia for hemianopia, *Neuropsychologia* **24** (1986), 471–482.

[20] A. Bowen, N.B. Lincoln and M. Dewey, Cognitive rehabilitation for spatial neglect following stroke, *Cochrane Database Systematic Review* (2) (2002), CD003586.

[21] A. Bowen, N.B. Lincoln and M.E. Dewey, Spatial neglect: is rehabilitation effective? *Stroke* **33**(11) (2002), 2728–2729.

[22] A. Bowen, K. McKenna and R.C. Tallis, Reasons for the variability in the reported rate of occurrence of unilateral neglect after stroke, *Stroke* **30** (1999), 1196–1202.

[23] D. Bowers and K.M. Heilman, Pseudoneglect: effect of hemispace on a tactile line bisection task, *Neuropsychologia* **18** (1980), 491–498.

[24] J.L. Bradshaw, J.A. Bradshaw, G. Nathan, N.C. Nettleton and L.E. Wilson, Leftwards error in bisecting the gap between two points: stimulus quality and hand effects, *Neuropsychologia* **24** (1986), 849–855.

[25] L.J. Buxbaum, M.K. Ferraro, T. Veramonti, A. Farne, J. Whyte, E. Ladavas, F. Frassinetti and H.B. Coslett, Hemispatial neglect: Subtypes, neuroanatomy, and disability *Neurology* **62**(5) (2004), 749–756.

[26] D.C. Campbell and J.M. Oxbury, Recovery from unilateral visuo-spatial neglect? *Cortex* **12** (1976), 303–312.

[27] G. Cocchini, N. Beschin and M. Jehkonen, The Fluff Test: A simple task to assess body representation neglect, *Neuropsychological Rehabilitation* **11** (2001), 17–31.

[28] V. Dauriac-Le Masson, L. Mailhan, A. Louis-Dreyfus, G. de Montety, P. Denys, B. Bussel and P. Azouvi, Double dissociation entre négligence unilatérale gauche et anosognosie, *Revue Neurologique* **158** (2002), 427–430.

[29] E. De Renzi, M. Gentilini, P. Faglioni and C. Barbieri, Attentional shift towards the rightmost stimuli in patients with left visual neglect, *Cortex* **25** (1989), 231–237.

[30] G. Denes, C. Semenza, E. Stoppa and A. Lis, Unilateral spatial neglect and recovery from hemiplegia, *Brain* **105** (1982), 543–552.

[31] J. Edmans and N.B. Lincoln, The frequency of perceptual deficits after stroke, *Clinical Rehabilitation* **1** (1987), 273–281.

[32] G. Gainotti, P. D'Erme and P. Bartolomeo, Early orientation of attention toward the half space ipsilateral to the lesion in patients with unilateral brain damage, *Journal of Neurology, Neurosurgery and Psychiatry* **54** (1991), 1082–1089.

[33] G. Gainotti, P. Messerli and R. Tissot, Qualitative analysis of unilateral spatial neglect in relation to laterality of cerebral lesions, *Journal of Neurology, Neurosurgery and Psychiatry* **35** (1972) 545–550.

[34] L. Gauthier, F. Dehaut and Y. Joanette, The Bells test: A quantitative and qualitative test for visual neglect, *International Journal of Clinical Neuropsychology* **11** (1989), 49–54.

[35] B. Gialanella and F. Mattioli, Anosognosia and extrapersonal neglect as predictors of functional recovery following right hemisphere stroke, *Neuropsychological Rehabilitation* **2** (1992), 169–178.

[36] C.V. Granger and B.B. Hamilton, UDS report; the uniform data system for medical rehabilitation report of first admission for 1990, *Am J Med Rehabil* **72** (1992), 108–113.

[37] P.W. Halligan, J. Cockburn and B. Wilson, The behavioural assessment of visual neglect, *Neuropsychological Rehabilitation* **1** (1991), 5–32.

[38] P.W. Halligan, G.R. Fink, J.C. Marshall and G. Vallar, Spatial cognition: evidence from visual neglect, *Trends in Cognitive Science* **7**(3) (2003), 125–133.

[39] P.W. Halligan and J.C. Marshall, How long is a piece of string? A study of line bisection in a case of visual neglect, *Cortex* **24** (1988), 321–328.

[40] P.W. Halligan and J.C. Marshall, Left neglect for near but not for far space in man, *Nature* **350** (1991), 498–500.

[41] P.W. Halligan, J.C. Marshall and D.T. Wade, Visuospatial neglect: Underlying factors and test sensitivity, *The Lancet* **2**(908–910) (1989).

[42] P.W. Halligan and I.H. Robertson. The assessment of unilateral neglect, in: *A Handbook of Neuropsychological Assessment,* J.R. Crawford, D.M. Parker and W.W. McKinlay, eds, Lawrence Erlbaum Associates, Hove, 1992, pp. 151–175.

[43] K.M. Heilman, R.T. Watson and E. Valenstein, Neglect and related disorders, in: *Clinical Neuropsychology,* K.M. Heilman and E. Valenstein, eds, Oxford University Press, New York, 1993, pp. 279–336.

[44] G. Jewell and M.E. Mc Court, Pseudoneglect: A review and meta-analysis of performance factors in line bisection tasks, *Neuropsychologia* **38** (2000), 93–110.

[45] L. Kalra, I. Perez, S. Gupta and M. Wittink, The influence of visual neglect on stroke rehabilitation, *Stroke* **28** (1997), 1386–1391.

[46] G. Kinsella and B. Ford, Acute recovery patterns in stroke patients, *Medical Journal of Australia* **2** (1980), 663–666.

[47] J. Linacre and B. Wright, *BIGSTEPS: Rasch model computer program,* Chicago: Mesa Press, 1994.

[48] J.C. Marshall and P.W. Halligan, Line bisection in a case of visual neglect; Psychophysical studies with implications for theory, *Cognitive Neuropsychology* **7** (1990), 107–130.

[49] J.B. Mattingley, J.L. Bradshaw, J.A. Brashaw and N.C. Nettleton, Residual rightward attentional bias after apparent recovery from right hemisphere damage: Implications for a multicomponent model of neglect, *Journal of Neurology, Neurosurgery and Psychiatry* **57** (1994), 597–604.

[50] R.D. McIntosh, E.E. Brodie, N. Beschin and I.H. Robertson, Improving the clinical diagnosis of personal neglect: a reformulated comb and razor test, *Cortex* **36**(2) (2000), 289–292.

[51] A. Menon and N. Korner-Bitensky, Evaluating unilateral spatial neglect post stroke: working your way through the maze of assessment choices, *Top Stroke Rehabil* **11**(3) (2004), 41–66.

[52] J.A. Ogden, Anterior-posterior interhemispheric differences in the loci of lesions producing visual hemineglect, *Brain and Cognition* **4** (1985), 59–75.

[53] S. Paolucci, G. Antonucci, C. Guariglia, L. Magnotti, L. Pizzamiglio and P. Zoccolotti, Facilitatory effect of neglect rehabilitation on the recovery of left hemiplegic stroke patients: A cross-over study, *Journal of Neurology* **243** (1996), 308–314.

[54] P.M. Pedersen, H.S. Jorgensen, H. Nakayama, H.O. Raaschou and T.S. Olsen, Hemineglect in acute stroke. Incidence and prognostic implications. The Copenhagen stroke study, *American Journal of Physical Medicine and Rehabilitation* **76** (1997), 122–127.

[55] A. Peskine and P. Azouvi, Anosognosia and denial after right hemisphere stroke, in: *The Behavioural and Cognitive Neurology of Stroke,* O. Godefroy and J. Bogousslavsky, eds, Cambridge University Press, Cambridge, UK, in press, pp.

[56] L. Pizzamiglio, A. Judica, C. Razzano and P. Zoccolotti, Toward a comprehensive diagnosis of visuo-spatial disorders in unilateral brain damaged patients, *Psychological Assessment* **5** (1989), 199–218.

[57] G. Rasch, *Probabilistic models for some intelligence and attainment tests,* Chicago: Mesa Press, 1992.

[58] I.H. Robertson, Cognitive rehabilitation: attention and neglect, *Trends Cogn Sci* **3**(10) (1999), 385–393.

[59] I.H. Robertson and P.W. Halligan, *Spatial Neglect: A Clinical Handbook for Diagnosis and Treatment,* Hove, UK: Psychology Press, 1999.

[60] G. Rode, F. Mauguière, C. Fischer and D. Boisson, Lésions hémisphériques droites et négligence unilatérale; La part de la déafférentation, *Annales de Réadaptation et de Médecine Physique* **38** (1995), 324.

[61] G. Rode, M.T. Perenin and D. Boisson, Negligence de l'espace représenté: Mise en évidence par l'évocation mentale de la carte de France, *Revue Neurologique* **151** (1995), 161–164.

[62] M. Rousseaux, J.M. Beis, P. Pradat-Diehl, Y. Martin, P. Bartolomeo, T. Bernati, S. Chokron, M. Leclercq, A. Louis-Dreyfus, F. Marchal, D. Perennou, C. Prairial, G. Rode, C. Samuel, E. Sieroff, L. Wiart and P. Azouvi, Présentation d'une batterie de dépistage de la négligence spatiale. Normes et effet

de l'âge, du niveau d'éducation, du sexe, de la main et de la latéralité, *Revue Neurologique* **157** (2001), 1385–1400.

[63] C. Samuel, A. Louis-Dreyfus, R. Kaschel, E. Makiela, M. Troubat, N. Anselmi, V. Cannizzo and P. Azouvi, Rehabilitation of very severe unilateral neglect by visuo-spatio-motor cueing: Two single-case studies, *Neuropsychological Rehabilitation* **10** (2000), 385–399.

[64] T. Schenkenberg, D.C. Bradford and E.T. Ajax, Line bisection and unilateral visual neglect in patients with neurological impairment, *Neurology* **30** (1980), 509–517.

[65] X. Seron, G. Deloche and F. Coyette, A retrospective analysis of a single case neglect therapy: a point of theory, in: *Cognitive approaches in neuropsychological rehabilitation*, X. Seron and G. Deloche, eds, Lawrence Erlbaum Associates, Hillsdale, 1989, pp. 289–316.

[66] S.P. Stone, B. Wilson, A. Wroot, P.W. Halligan, L.S. Lange, J.C. Marshall and R.J. Greenwood, The assessment of visuospatial neglect after acute stroke, *Journal of Neurology, Neurosurgery and Psychiatry* **54** (1991), 345–350.

[67] L. Tesio, Measuring behaviours and perceptions: Rasch analysis as a tool for rehabilitation research, *J Rehabil Med* **35**(3) (2003), 105–115.

[68] K. Tham and R. Tegner, The baking tray task: A test of spatial neglect, *Neuropsychological Rehabilitation* **6** (1996), 19–25.

[69] D. Towle and N.B. Lincoln, Development of a questionnaire for detecting everyday problems in stroke patients with unilateral visual neglect, *Clinical Rehabilitation* **5** (1991), 135–140.

[70] P. Van Eeckhout, J. Sabadel, J.L. Signoret and B. Pillon, *Histoires insolites pour faire parler*, Paris: MEDSI, 1982.

[71] B. Wilson, J. Cockburn and P. Halligan, Development of a behavioral test of visuospatial neglect, *Archives of Physical Medicine and Rehabilitation* **68** (1987), 98–102.

[72] P. Zoccolotti, G. Antonucci and A. Judica, Psychometric characteristics of two semi-structured scales for the functional evaluation of hemi-inattention in extrapersonal and personal space, *Neuropsychological Rehabilitation* **2** (1992), 179–191.

[73] P. Zoccolotti and A. Judica, Functional evaluation of hemineglect by means of a semistructured scale: Personal extrapersonal differentiation, *Neuropsychological Rehabilitation* **1** (1991), 33–44.

Spatial and non-spatial attention deficits in neurodegenerative diseases: Assessment based on Bundesen's theory of visual attention (TVA)

Peter Bublak[a,c,*], Petra Redel[b] and Kathrin Finke[b,c]
[a]*Neuropsychology Unit, Neurology Clinic, Friedrich Schiller University, Jena, Germany*
[b]*General and Experimental Psychology, Ludwig Maximilian University, Munich, Germany*
[c]*Neuro-cognitive Psychology, Ludwig Maximilian University, Munich, Germany*

Received 1 April 2006
Revised 2 June 2006
Accepted 22 June 2006

Abstract. *Purpose*: The aim was to present evidence that, similarly as in neglect, a combined pattern of spatial and non-spatial deficits of visual attention can also be typically observed in patients suffering from neurodegenerative disorders.
Method: Whole and partial report of brief letter arrays, based on Bundesen's 'theory of visual attention' (TVA), was applied in patients suffering from Huntington's disease (HD), mild cognitive impairment (MCI), or Alzheimer's disease (AD). TVA-based parameter estimates were derived reflecting (a) perceptual processing speed and visual working memory storage capacity as non-spatial aspects of visual attention (determined by whole report performance), and (b) spatial attentional weighting (determined by partial report performance).
Results: Processing speed was severely slowed in HD, and also reduced, although to a lesser degree, in MCI and AD patients. In HD and AD patients, but not in MCI patients, a strong leftward bias of spatial attention was observed.
Conclusion: Neglect and neurodegenerative diseases both involve a similar constellation of non-spatial and spatial deficits of visual attention. Therefore, by using TVA-based measurement, results from both fields of research may fruitfully inform each other in future studies, thus improving our understanding of the interaction of spatial and non-spatial attention deficits and its behavioral consequences.

Keywords: Perceptual disorders, hemispatial neglect, neuropsychology, neuropsychological tests, Huntington's disease, Alzheimer's disease

1. Introduction

In this article we will present evidence that, quite similar as in visual hemi-neglect, a combined pattern of spatial and non-spatial deficits of visual attention can also be typically observed in patients suffering from neurodegenerative disorders. Our focus will be on Huntington's disease and Alzheimer's disease. We will not survey the attention literature on these illnesses, as excellent reviews already exist [54,79]. Instead, we show data obtained from a method based on a theory of normal attention functions, that has already been applied successfully in neglect patients [18]: the 'the-

*Corresponding author: Peter Bublak, Neuropsychology Unit, Neurology Clinic, Friedrich Schiller University Jena, Erlanger Allee 101, D-07747 Jena, Germany. Tel.: +49 3641 9323475; Fax: +49 3641 9323472; E-mail: peter.bublak@med.uni-jena.de.

ory of visual attention', TVA [8–10]. By providing directly comparable measures, therefore, we hope to make a convincing case that attentional deficits in neglect and dementia have more in common than previously thought. In Section 2, we will explain the theoretical and methodological issues. Then, some of our results will be presented in Section 3. First, however, we shortly point out how investigation of impaired attention in neurodegenerative diseases builds upon the progress made in neglect research.

1.1. From spatial to non-spatial aspects of attention and back

In neglect research, a major progression in understanding impaired attention in this complex syndrome has been made by shifting perspective from a pure spatial view to the recognition of spatially non-lateralised aspects of attention to be at least equally important. Traditionally, neglect had been assumed to result from an impairment in orienting spatial attention to the contra-lesional hemi-field [56]. The higher frequency of left-sided neglect was attributed to a right-hemispheric dominance in governing spatial attention functions [49], and the region of the right temporo-parietal junction (TPJ) has been considered as especially important in this regard [27,73]. This line of research has made important contributions, for instance, in developing a number of tests like line bisection, cancellation and drawing tasks that have become something like a gold standard for assessing neglect patients [51,77]. Also, procedures manipulating spatial attention were identified which were able to modulate the ipsi-lesional bias in patients and seemed to be appropriate also for treatment purposes [35,58] (for a review, see [45]; for a critical evaluation of neglect rehabilitation studies, see [43]).

While the presence of additional attention deficits like low arousal, reduced speed of stimulus processing, or lapses of sustaining attention was clearly recognised from the beginning, such non-spatial impairments were not considered as directly contributing to the hemi-spatial nature of the neglect syndrome. Starting with the seminal work of Robertson and colleagues, however, who were able to demonstrate that modulations of the level of alertness in patients actually had an influence on the degree of the spatial bias [59], the significance of spatially non-lateralised attentional components has been increasingly acknowledged. They are now presumed to be involved both in the evocation and severity of neglect symptoms [33,78] and in their alleviation [45,59,71]. The fact that left-sided neglect occurs more frequently than right-sided neglect may even be more related to the dominant role of the right TPJ region in non-lateralised aspects than to its dominant role in spatially lateralised aspects of attention [34].

Thus, the current view on neglect embraces the knowledge gained by both the "spatial" and the "non-spatial" lines of research. It assumes that neglect patients suffer from a combined deficit of an ipsi-lesional bias of spatial attention together with a profound limitation of processing resources, the latter giving rise to non-spatial deficiencies like a reduction of perceptual speed and visual working memory storage capacity [14, 34]. While these deficits could be observed in isolation under a variety of states of brain dysfunction and are not specifically related to neglect, they interact in neglect patients in a unique way to provoke the specific picture observed. That is, although a spatial attentional bias to the ipsi-lesional side may be equally pronounced after left- and right-hemispheric lesions (see, e.g. [47]), a right-hemispheric dominance of spatially non-lateralised functions may be responsible for the greater severity of the lateralised deficit in patients with left hemi-neglect.

Such a multi-componential view on neglect seems to be better suited than the classical 'pure spatial' position to account for the complex nature of the neglect syndrome which becomes manifest in a large, inter- as well as intra-individual, variability of the clinical picture. It is also in line with the evidence that anatomically, neglect can emerge after damage to a large variety of brain areas, cortical as well as subcortical, with each presumably making a specific contribution to lateralised as well as to non-lateralised deficits of attention.

A challenge for neuropsychological assessment arising from such conceptual progress is how distinct spatially lateralised and non-lateralised deficits of visual attention can be specifically measured [21]. This problem is not easily solved by using classical tasks, because many of them involve more than one attentional component. For example, performance in a cancellation task is at least affected by both spatial bias and spatial working memory storage capacity (e.g. [44]). Of course, some tasks may be sufficiently independent to be applied for assessing distinct attentional components. For instance, Malhotra et al. [44] found a spatial working memory task not to be associated with a measure of lateral bias, i.e. line bisection. However, these tasks also differ considerably with respect to stimulus and response conditions and thus may also be unrelated due to other reasons. Moreover, their application is primarily driven by convention and practicability reasons than by conceptual considerations. As a result, it is difficult to reduce them to a common theoretical basis which would enable unambiguous explanations and predictions. Obviously, then, for the conceptual progress in neglect research to proliferate, more specific and sensitive assessment tools for grasping spatial and non-spatial aspects of attention would definitely be advantageous.

Such a method could also be usefully applied to other kinds of neuropsychological disorders different from neglect. If impaired attention in neglect would only reflect an idiosyncratic combination of impaired, spatial and non-spatial, components, they may be detectable in other states of brain dysfunction, too, albeit with a different phenomenological result. Neurodegenerative diseases like, for example, Huntington's disease, Parkinson's disease or Alzheimer's disease, are a candidate field for closer scrutiny in this regard. Although these disorders are primarily characterised by non-spatial deficits, i.e. general capacity reductions and global cognitive decline, deficits of spatial attention are suggestive, for example, due to anatomical asymmetries during the degenerative progress. In fact, Vecera and Rizzo [74] recently made a case for a more intensive investigation of spatial attentional deficits in neurodegenerative diseases. Thus, a development complementary to neglect research seems to proceed in studying neurodegenerative diseases, with a shift in focus from non-spatial towards spatial attentional deficits.

2. The theory of visual attention and whole and partial report of brief letter arrays

2.1. The theory

The "theory of visual attention" (TVA) developed by Bundesen [8–10] is a mathematically explicit framework which characterises the process of visual selection in terms of four independent parameters representing separate attentional components:[1] perceptual processing speed (parameter C), visual working memory storage capacity (K), top-down control (α), and spatial attentional weighting across the visual field (w_λ). On this account, selective visual attention results from the coordinated interaction of both spatially lateralised (w_λ) and non-lateralised (C, K, α) attentional components. As a detailed description together with the equations of TVA is given by Kyllingsbæk [41]; see also [18, 29], we here give only a short sketch of its main ideas. For a detailed neural interpretation of mathematically specified TVA concepts, considering attentional effects at the single-cell level, the interested reader is referred to Bundesen et al. [11].

TVA is closely related to the 'biased competition" approach, the currently dominating view of visual attention in cognitive neuroscience [15,16,20,38,57,64]. On this view, objects (perceptual units) in the visual field are processed in parallel and compete for representation within the information processing system ("selection"). The resulting race among objects can be biased in such a way that some objects are favored for selection, based either on stimulus-driven, "bottom-up" factors (e.g., a single black circle among white ones) or on intentional, "top-down" factors (e.g., a search for a face in a crowd).

According to TVA, selection of an object is synonymous with its encoding into a visual working memory store. It has a limited capacity and the few visual objects it 'contains' represent what can be perceived consciously at any given moment (e.g. [65,67]). TVA assumes that encoding is a result of a speed competition between objects where only the fastest objects racing towards the working memory store are selected. That is, the probability of an object x to be encoded into visual working memory is determined by its processing rate v_x, with v_x denoting the speed of object x within the race. The object's processing rate v_x depends on the relative attentional weight (w_x) it receives, which reflects a fraction of the total weight distributed across all objects within the visual field. Thus, increasing the relative weight of a given object x decreases the relative weights of the other objects, biasing the race in favour of object x. Hence, it has a higher probability of being selected. The result of this parallel and capacity-limited processing is that only a subset of the non-consciously processed objects is consciously represented within the visual working memory store. Selected objects are available for further processing and goal-directed actions, such as verbal report.

In summary, the probability of selection of an object is determined by (i) an object's processing rate which is a function of the attentional weight it receives, and (ii) the capacity of the working memory store (if the store is filled, the race for selection terminates). TVA provides quantitative estimates for characterizing both the general processing efficiency of the information process-

---

[1] It should be noted that, in some studies [29,30], a fifth TVA parameter, the perception threshold t_0, has also received considerable interest.

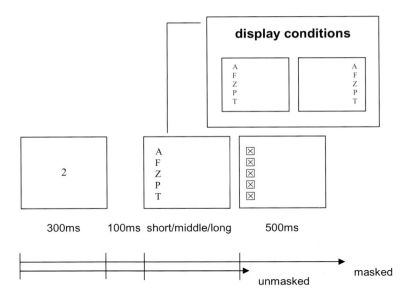

Fig. 1. Schematic representation of the whole report procedure and the possible display conditions. First, a digit is presented that has to be fixated by the subject. After a short ISI, the letter display is briefly presented with one of three different exposure durations (e.g. 86, 157, or 300 ms), either in the left or the right visual hemi-field (randomly determined). In masked trials, square masks are presented immediately at each previous letter position, constraining letter processing to their presentation time. In unmasked trials, due to visual persistence, letter processing is prolonged beyond their presentation time, by several hundred milliseconds. In this way, by using three exposure durations in either masked or unmasked trials, six effective exposure durations result. The subject's task is to report as many letters as possible.

ing system (processing rate and storage capacity), and specific aspects of attentional weighting. Two weighting aspects are considered: first, the ability to process objects from both visual hemi-fields equivalently (spatial attentional weighting); and second, the ability to confer a competitive advantage to target objects at the expense of the processing of distractor objects (task-related weighting). As a result, four attentional parameters emerge, which can be assessed within two simple psychophysical tasks, whole and partial report, that will be explained in the next section.

2.2. The method[2]

Processing rate and working memory storage capacity, the two general efficiency aspects of the visual processing system, are assessed in a whole report experiment (see e.g. [66,68,69]). In this task, aspects of spatial or task-related weighting are irrelevant. Five letters are briefly presented (see Fig. 1), for variable exposure durations, in a column either within the left or the right hemi-field, and subjects have to verbally report as many items as possible. In this task, performance accuracy as a function of presentation time is represented by an exponential growth function (see Fig. 2). It is fitted (based on a maximum-likelihood procedure) by the TVA computational model (see [41]). Thereafter, estimates can be derived for the growth parameter of the exponential curve (parameter C, derived from the rate parameters v for each single object) and for the asymptote of the curve (parameter K). Parameter C (estimated separately for each hemi-field, C_L, C_R), reflects processing speed (the number of elements that can be processed per second). It is represented by the initial slope of the growth function (Fig. 2). Parameter K (also estimated separately for each hemi-field, K_L, K_R), reflects the capacity of the working memory store (the number of elements that can be maintained in parallel). It is represented by the asymptote of the growth function (dashed line in Fig. 2).

In a similar way, by combining TVA with a partial-report paradigm, attentional weighting of an object can be estimated. In partial report (see Fig. 3), one or two letters are presented at one or two out of four possible locations (one in each display quadrant), and subjects have to verbally report only those (target) stimuli

---

[2]The method described here is closely related to the design used by Duncan et al. [18] and is distinguished by a large norm data base and a ready-to-use software package [6,24,41]. However, there are several possible variations of whole/partial report designs that can be applied [30,53].

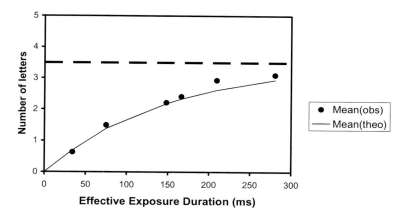

Fig. 2. Whole report performance for a typical healthy subject ($K = 3.5$ elements; $C = 22.3$ elements/s). The mean number of correctly reported letters is shown as a function of effective exposure duration. Solid lines represent the best fits from the Theory of Visual Attention to the observations. The estimate of the visual working memory storage capacity K is marked by a dashed horizontal line. For this subject, exposure durations were 43, 86, and 157 ms, the estimated visual detection threshold, t_0, was 9 ms, the prolongation of visual stimulus persistence in unmasked conditions, estimated as parameter μ, was 132 ms. Thus, the six resulting effective exposure durations were 34, 77, and 148 ms in the three masked and 166, 209, and 280 ms in the three unmasked conditions (more comprehensive explanations are given in [18,24]. *Note:* Mean(obs): observed mean; Mean(theo): predicted mean.

that belong to a pre-specified category (e.g., color: red items), whilst ignoring distractors (e.g., green items). Each subject's accuracy in performing this task is fitted by the TVA computational model (see [41], for mathematical details), using a maximum-likelihood procedure. This produces estimates of the attentional weight (w) assigned to a target or, respectively, distractor at each of the four locations. From these eight weight estimates (four targets and four distractors), it is possible to derive parameters reflecting spatial distribution of attention (parameter w_λ), and efficiency of top-down control (parameter α).

Parameter w_λ indicates whether attentional weighting of objects – averaged across targets and distractors – is equal in the left and the right visual hemifield. If objects in the left visual field receive the same amount of attentional weighting as those in the right field (i.e., $w_L = w_R$), the spatial lateralization parameter $w_\lambda = w_L/(w_L + w_R)$ equals 0.5. By contrast, greater weighting of objects within the right hemi-field, as in visual neglect, is reflected by values of $w_\lambda < 0.5$, denoting a rightward bias of spatial attention. Conversely, a bias to the left visual field is indicated by values of $w_\lambda > 0.5$.

Parameter α indicates whether – averaged across locations – attentional weighting of targets is greater than that of distractors. If so, the ratio between distractor and target weights (w_D/w_T), expressed by α, would be less than 1, with lower α-values indicating more efficient top-down control. Impaired control functions, by contrast, would give rise to equally weighted target and distractor processing, increasing α to approach 1.

Taken together, TVA-based modelling of whole- and partial-report performance in terms of the independent parameters described above permits selective-attention functions to be "fractionated" into four separable, theoretically integrated sub-components.

2.3. Usability for neuropsychological assessment

TVA based parameter estimates have proven to account for a wide range of findings in the cognitive psychological literature on normal attentional processes [8]. Moreover, they can even account for a large part of the findings on attentional effects assessed at the single-cell level in monkeys [11]. As regards neuropsychological assessment, the TVA-based measurement also bears a number of important methodological advantages for clinical purposes:

First, since TVA integrates the distinct attentional components within a unifying theoretical framework, the observed raw data can be transformed into parameter estimates that are directly related to the underlying theoretical constructs and to their assumed, recently specified [11], neural basis. A subject's visual-attentional performance can be characterized in terms of four numerical, easily interpretable values: the number of visual elements she/he can process per second; the number of elements she/he can maintain in parallel in "conscious" visual working memory; the degree to which she/he can preferentially process targets as com-

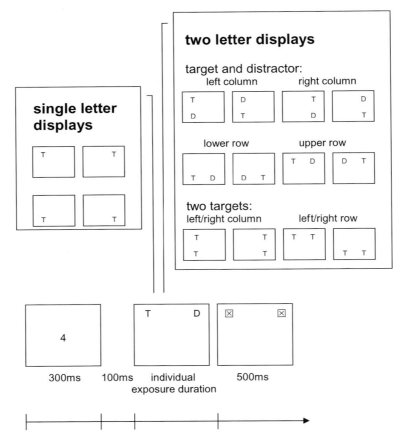

Fig. 3. Schematic representation of the partial report procedure and the possible display conditions. First, a digit is presented that has to be fixated by the subject. After a short ISI, either a single letter or a two letter display is briefly presented with an exposure duration individually determined for each subject (e.g. 100 ms). In single letter displays, a red target letter (depicted as "T") appears at one of four possible positions (the corners of an imaginary square). In displays with two letters, a red target letter appears either in combination with a green distractor letter (depicted as "D"), or together with a second target letter. The second letter (target or distractor) appears within either the same or the opposite hemi-field. Letters are always presented in either columns or rows, never diagonally. In each trial, a square mask is presented immediately at each previous letter position. The subject's task is to report only red (target) letters, whilst ignoring green (distractor) letters.

pared to distractors; and the degree of her/his spatial bias towards one visual hemi-field.

Second, as a reasonable approximation, the estimates of the four attentional components are delivered by mathematically independent fitting algorithms. So, the assessment tool bears the possibility to measure distinctive attentional components with unconfounded measurement.

Third, in contrast to the heterogeneity of conventional clinical attentional tests, all attentional components are measured using tasks that are highly similar in terms of stimulus material and response modality. They therefore impose comparable demands on the subjects' cognitive as well as motor skills.

Fourth, the attentional components, especially processing speed, are not measured in terms of response latency, but rather in terms of accuracy at certain exposure durations. The measurement of perceptual, rather than response, speed in patients has critical advantages. Whereas a motor deficit may slow responses in any attentional task that requires speeded motor (e.g. manual) responses, it should not influence perceptual processing speed. Moreover, the individual processing speed does not affect the other parameters: While the measurement of processing speed relies on the performance at certain exposure durations, that of the three other components does not include a time-critical component. They are either measured as asymptotes of performance increases indicating the individually achievable maxima or assessed based on *relative*, within-subject performance differences across conditions.

Finally, the simplicity of the tasks, the individual adjustment of experimental parameters (exposure durations), and the verbal, non-speeded response modus permit the testing to be adapted to the basic performance levels of subjects with a broad range of motor, attentional and general cognitive abilities.

In their path-breaking study proving the high value of TVA for clinical purposes, Duncan et al. [18] used this method to obtain estimates of the four above mentioned attentional components in a group of neglect patients. Subsequent studies extended this approach to a fine-grained analysis of attention deficits at the single case level. They were able to demonstrate a high sensitivity of a TVA based procedure for even subtle attentional deficits [29], and the possibility to disentangle basic attentional deficits underlying complex disorders like simultanagnosia [19]. More recently, studies in larger groups of patients differing with respect to lesion location have begun to analyse the cerebral correlates of the different TVA based attentional parameters [30, 53].

Based on the preceding clinical studies, it was tempting to hypothesise that a TVA based approach could also be of considerable value to enhance the assessment of attentional impairments within a standard clinical setting. However, the tasks applied had been rather time consuming, requiring more than two hours in some cases, and thus were hardly feasible for a more widespread clinical use. To that end, an important pre-requisite was to demonstrate that sufficiently reliable measures could be obtained with a procedure short enough to be applicable for clinical purposes.

Therefore, Finke et al. [24] developed shorter experimental test versions and assessed their reliability and validity. Both whole and partial report proved to have sufficient internal consistency to be shortened substantially to test durations of about 30 minutes each, still delivering robust and accurate parameter estimates with satisfactory reliability. In addition, the independence assumption of TVA, that is, the specificity of the independently modeled parameters was empirically confirmed. By and large, non-significant correlations were found between the different parameters, apart from a modest correlation between the whole report parameters processing speed and visual working memory storage capacity. Therefore, all parameters seem to have high functional independence. Finally, since the parameters showed higher correspondence with theoretically related than with unrelated neuropsychological standard test procedures, it was shown that TVA based assessment provides valid and clinically useful information.

In a first clinical validation study of these shortened paradigms, a double dissociation in two patients with right-hemispheric brain damage was demonstrated [6]. A patient with a right-sided parietal lesion encroaching the angular gyrus suffered from a pathological (rightward) spatial bias of attentional weighting but had preserved efficiency of top-down control. In contrast, a patient with a right-sided superior fronto-medial lesion, in the presence of equally balanced attentional weighting of the two visual hemi-fields, was severely impaired with regard to top-down control.

3. Application to neurodegenerative diseases

3.1. Huntington's disease

After the successful demonstration that even substantially shortened versions of the TVA based assessment tools provide reliable and meaningful results on attentional deficits in patients with acquired brain damage, we directed our focus to the assessment to neurodegenerative diseases. Several reasons prompted us to move into this direction. Many studies have been conducted investigating the question of impaired selective attention in disorders like Huntington's disease or Alzheimer's disease (see e.g. [23,54]). However, despite the wealth of data acquired, and although progress in neuroimaging has significantly improved our understanding of the structural changes occurring in degenerating brains in characteristic ways, a consistent and clear-cut pattern did not emerge. It still remains unclear whether basic attentional deficits are a core feature of these disorders, occur already at early disease stages, or how they develop during progression. Thus, they are more or less considered as part of the global pattern of decline without any specific pathognomonic value.

One possible circumstance contributing to this inconsistent pattern of results may be different characteristics of the taks applied in patients (task difficulty, stimulus complexity, response features etc). After all, a critical problem for assessing patients with dementing illnesses is how well they are able to understand task instructions. Another one is related to the necessity to use response buttons for acquiring speed measures. While this may not be a major problem at early disease stages, difficulties are inevitable at later stages when intellectual decline procedes and motor symptoms are present (in fact, in some types of dementia these represent core and even diagnostic features). Therefore, we thought that the TVA based approach, with its clear and repetitory trial structure and its lack of a manual response requirement, would be well suited to be applied in patients with global cognitive decline and severe motor problems, and would possibly provide new clues for qualifying as well as quantifying attentional impairments in patients with dementia.

Assessment of non-spatial as well as spatial attentional deficits in Huntington's disease [23] appeared to be an especially promising starting point into this area. In Huntington's disease (HD), a progressive atrophy of the caudate nucleus and the putamen occurs, giving rise to a progressive disruption of functionally segregated fronto-striatal loops [3,12]. Recently, neuroanatomical studies have indicated that this striatal degeneration is asymmetrical. While there is a bilateral volume reduction of the striatum that seems to be related to the severity of the genetic pathology, it seems to be more pronounced on the left-side in both presymptomatic and symptomatic patients [39,52,60,70]. The striatum is closely involved in the control of visuomotor behaviour and attention [32]. The anterior portion of the caudate nucleus receives input from the posterior parietal cortex [1,32] and is among the first striatal regions affected by HD. In monkeys, unilateral lesions of the caudate nucleus have been shown to induce deficits in oculomotor and attentional orienting to the contralateral hemifield [32]. In humans, deficits of spatial attention after unilateral striatal lesions have also been described [13,22,29,37,63]. These lines of evidence suggested the hypothesis, given the stronger left-sided atrophy in HD, that a leftward bias of spatial attentional weighting would be observable in a TVA based partial report task.

In addition, by using whole report, we also expected to find a reduction of processing capacity in HD patients. After all, Habekost and Bundesen [29] found non-spatial attention deficits of bilaterally reduced processing speed and working memory storage capacity in a patient with a unilateral, right-sided lesion involving basal ganglia structures (see also [30]). Moreover, in their neural interpretation of TVA, Bundesen and colleagues [11] have proposed speed of visual stimulus processing to be proportionally related to the number of cortical neurons representing a visual object. In HD, increasing cortical atrophy, especially in posterior areas, and consequently increasing neuronal loss occurs during disease progression [4,61,62].

In fact, in our study of 18 HD patients [23], the most obvious visual attentional change was a severe reduction of processing speed to an extent, that HD patients were unable to even process a quarter of the objects processed by the control group. None of the patients reached the speed of the slowest healthy control subject. Data from a representative HD patient are shown in Fig. 4. The working memory storage capacity or the number of objects that could consciously be maintained and identified was also significantly reduced in the group of HD patients. The extent of the reduction of both parameters was significantly related to disease duration since onset. Thus, the reduction of speed and storage capacity might represent possible state markers for the state of disease progression.

In addition to these prominent non-spatial impairments, however, we also found a consistent change of the spatial distribution of attentional weighting across the left and the right visual hemi-field. Nearly all patients (94%) showed a lateral bias towards the left side, resulting in a highly significant difference from the control group who showed a balanced attentional weighting across both sides. This result could neither be explained by unilateral sensory loss or by an inability to keep fixation since performance in unilateral displays was absolutely comparable. The lateralised deficit exclusively occured in conditions with stimuli presented bilaterally, one in each hemi-field. Here, performance for left-sided targets was much better than that for the right-sided targets (a typical example is shown in Fig. 5). Therefore, the pathological leftward bias found in HD seems to represent an extinction phenomenon – an inability to report a right-sided stimulus when a second stimulus is presented simultaneously on the left – not from neglect with a complete unawareness of one hemi-field [17,46,50]. The TVA parameter reflecting spatial distribution of attentional weighting was highly significantly correlated with the severity of the genetic defect in HD patients. Thus, the leftward bias might have the potential to serve as a valid trait marker reflecting the intensity of the underlying pathogenic mechanisms in HD.

3.2. Alzheimer's disease

Recently, we continued our attempt to assess spatial and non-spatial attention deficits in neurodegenerative diseases by investigating subjects suffering from mild cognitive impairment (MCI), and Alzheimer's disease (AD). As in HD, accumulating evidence suggests that also in AD the neural degeneration, although generally affecting both sides of the brain, may be asymmetric, again with a more pronounced involvement of left compared to right brain structures. This has been suggested by lateralised glucose metabolism [75], volume reductions [72], post-mortem anatomical abnormalities [42], and bioelectrical brain activity [2].

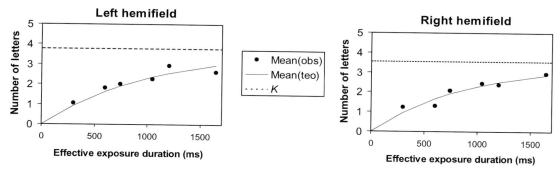

Fig. 4. Whole report performance for both visual hemi-fields in a representative, 39 year old, female Huntington's disease patient (patient MS). Her first symptoms had appeared at the age of 37. Solid lines represent the best fits from the Theory of Visual Attention to the observations (dark spots). The estimate of the visual working memory storage capacity K is marked by a dashed horizontal line. Processing speed was estimated as parameter $C = 3.7$ elements/s (averaged across hemi-fields). Nevertheless, in her case, working memory storage capacity was quite high, $K = 3.7$ elements (also averaged across hemi-fields), and comparable to healthy control subjects. Note that performance differences between hemi-fields are only minimal. *Note:* Mean(obs): observed mean; Mean(theo): predicted mean; K: working memory storage capacity.

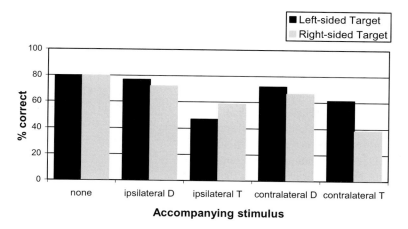

Fig. 5. Partial report results from the same patient (MS) also presented in Fig. 4. Mean proportion of correctly reported letters is shown as a function of trial type, separately for left- (black bars) and right-sided targets (grey bars). Trial type is indicated as follows: "none" = no accompanying stimulus (single letter display); "ipsilateral D" = target is accompanied by a distractor letter presented within the same hemi-field; "ipsilateral T" = target is accompanied by a second target letter presented within the same hemi-field; "contralateral D" = target is accompanied by a distractor letter presented within the opposite hemi-field; "contralateral T" = target is accompanied by a second target letter presented within the opposite hemi-field. Probability of correct target report is equal in both hemi-fields for single target conditions. In contrast, accuracy of report decreases significantly for a right sided target when it is accompanied by a stimulus (especially a target) in the left hemi-field, indicative of right-sided extinction. This is reflected by the TVA based parameter estimate of $w_\lambda = 0.66$, indicating a leftward spatial bias of attention.

The brain region typically undergoing the most accentuated glucose metabolism reductions in the case of AD is not a subcortical but a cortical region, that is the parietotemporal cortex [25,31,36,40,75], the key region in visual hemi-neglect [37]. Given the bilateral cortical degeneration in AD that may be more pronounced in the left hemisphere, Bartolomeo et al. [5] have suggested that, on the behavioural level, signs of right-sided neglect might emerge relatively often and therefore should be assessed systematically in AD. Indeed, in a number of AD patients symptoms of right-sided neglect have been found in paper-and-pencil neglect batteries [5,26,48] and, in a single case, also a progression of the spatial inattention during the course of the disease [5]. However, also patients with left-sided neglect have been documented, partly within the same studies [26,48].

In our study, we again assumed that, based on the TVA methodology, a more homogeneous pattern of results might be obtained. Preliminary data, from 19 patients with MCI and 9 patients with a diagnosis of probable AD so far, suggest a slowing of visual perceptual processing speed, in both MCI and in AD patients [55], even though the speed reduction is not as striking as in HD. Figure 6 shows typical examples of one patient with MCI, one with probable AD, together with data from a control subject. Like in HD patients, and to a comparable degree, we also found a leftward bias of spatial attentional weighting [7]. Whereas in the MCI group the distribution of attentional weights assigned to left- and right-sided objects was more or less equally balanced, in AD patients a systematic deviation towards the left side of visual space was found.

Figure 7 shows separately the mean proportion of target letters correctly identified by two representative patients, one with MCI and one with mild AD, and by a control subject, in each hemi-field for the five experimental conditions known from Fig. 5. Visual field differences are present in the patient with mild AD, only. Whereas this subject achieved similar values for both hemi-fields when reporting single targets, performance was clearly asymmetrical when two stimuli were presented bilaterally. In these cases, accuracy was much higher for left- compared to right-sided targets, regardless of whether the opposite stimulus was a distractor or a target stimulus. In contrast, the MCI patient (like the normal control subject) performed comparably across both hemi-fields in all conditions. These results indicate that, like in HD, right-sided inattention resulting in extinction of stimuli presented in the right hemi-field may also accompany AD. As the spatial bias was not observed in MCI patients, the hypothesis emerges that the leftward deviation may develop during the course of neurodegenerative progression. It will be interesting to see whether spatial weighting, as well as processing speed, are related to other clinical variables, like e.g. intellectual decline.

4. Discussion

Using TVA based assessment of components of selective attention, we observed the same pattern of spatial and non-spatial attentional deficits in two different types of neurodegenerative diseases, one of primarily subcortical (HD) the other one of primarily cortical (AD) origin. Both patients with HD and those with AD showed fundamental modifications of non-spatial aspects of attention. Speed of visual stimulus processing was consistently reduced. In some cases, this was true also for visual working memory storage capacity, although to a lesser degree. In addition, in both HD and AD, a marked leftward spatial bias of attention was identified.

An interesting result was the observation that the speed reduction was already present in MCI, a probable precursor stage of AD. In contrast, the leftward spatial bias was observed only in AD, but not in MCI. Based on the assumption that cortical degeneration (predominantly in posterior regions) occurs relatively early in AD (and thus may already be present at the MCI stage), these results suggest that speed reductions could mainly reflect the degree of cortical atrophy. In line with this assumption, speed (TVA parameter C), like storage capacity (TVA parameter K), was significantly associated with disease duration in HD, where substantial cortical degeneration (in particular at posterior sites) seems to be a prominent feature not until later stages of the disease [60]. The beginning of HD is primarily characterized by striatal atrophy, instead, which appears to be closely linked to the spatial attentional bias. The fact that a leftward spatial bias was also found in AD, but not in MCI, may thus reflect the increasing involvement of subcortical (striatal) structures at more advanced stages of AD.

Thus, based on our preliminary data, it appears tempting to speculate that, although every dementing illness is a result of both cortical and subcortical pathology, the course of degeneration may start from different "centers of gravity" that may be detected by sensitive assessment of spatial and non-spatial aspects, respectively, of attentional impairment. While this interesting possibility deserves attention, future studies are definitley required, with testing of patients at different disease stages, to test this hypothesis. Results of other studies clearly underline this point. TVA parameters seem to be affected by damage to several different structures [30], and a main factor for lateral attentional bias may even be cortical lesion volume [53]. Thus, a consistent relationship between TVA parameters and possible cerebral correlates has yet to be established.

Our results clearly show that, in a similar manner as for hemi-spatial neglect, the presence of both spatial and non-spatial deficits of attention also characterizes neurodegenerative diseases. Despite this commonality, an important difference should certainly not be ignored. Neither the patients with AD nor those with HD tested in our study showed any obvious neglect signs at the behavioural level. The TVA results also suggested a pattern of stimulus extinction during bilateral stimulation, rather than complete neglect of one hemifield. However, as Bartolomeo et al. [5] had already mentioned, spatial deficits have traditionally not been a focus of research in dementia, and more thorough investigations may indeed find more clear-cut signs of

Healthy subject

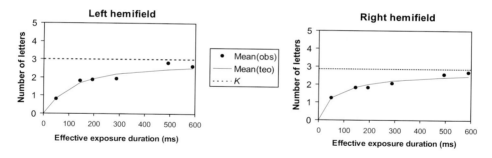

MCI patient

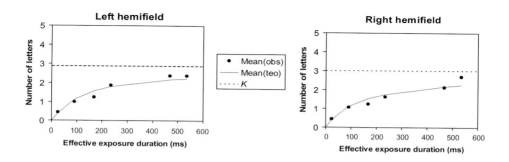

AD patient

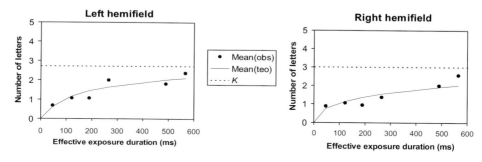

Fig. 6. Whole report results from three representative subjects: a 79-years old male control subject (upper panel), a 64-years old male MCI patient (middle panel), and a 60-years old female AD patient. Solid lines represent the best fits from the Theory of Visual Attention to the observations (dark spots). The estimate of the visual working memory storage capacity K is marked by a dashed horizontal line. For both the MCI and the AD subject (and more notedly for the latter), the curve shows a less steep initial slope compared to the control subject, indicating reduced perceptual speed. TVA parameter estimates were $C = 22.93$ for the control, $C = 19.14$ for the MCI, and $C = 14.73$ for the AD subject, respectively. Nevertheless, working memory storage capacity was quite comparable for all three subjects, with parameter estimates $K = 2.93$ (control), $K = 2.94$ (MCI), and $K = 2.86$ (AD).

hemi-inattention comparable to neglect patients (see also [74]). On the other hand, the severity of non-spatial deficits may be greater in dementia than in neglect patients, and behavioural effects are perhaps mainly dominated by these aspects. In fact, the speed reduction found in HD patients was extremely severe. In preceding studies, comparable reductions of visual speed and storage capacity have only been documented in two patients with simultanagnosia so far [19]. A possible hypothesis, therefore, derived from this fact could be

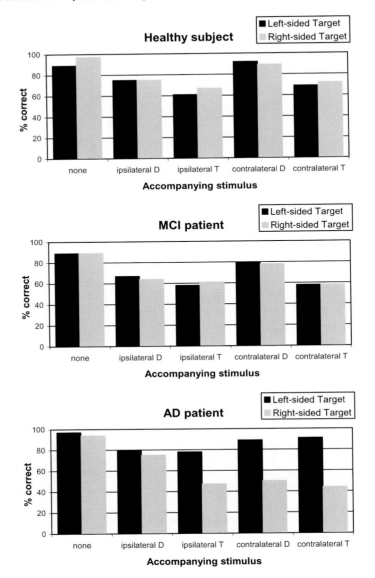

Fig. 7. Partial report results from three representative subjects: a 79-years old male control subject (upper panel), a 64-years old male MCI patient (middle panel), and a 60-years old female AD patient. Mean proportion of correctly reported letters is shown as a function of trial type, separately for left- (black bars) and right-sided targets (grey bars). Trial types are the same as in Fig. 5. Hemi-field differences are absent in both the control and the MCI subject, whereas the AD subject shows extinction of right-sided targets in the presence of left-sided stimuli. TVA parameter estimates for spatial attentional weighting indicate balanced weighting in the control subject ($w_\lambda = 0.48$) and the MCI patient ($w_\lambda = 0.52$), but a large leftward spatial bias in the AD patient ($w_\lambda = 0.74$). None of the control subjects tested so far ($N = 25$) had a comparably large deviation.

that symptoms of simultanagnosia might be expected to occur regularly in dementia. In sum, the search for behavioural correlates of the attention deficits detected by TVA based assessment in HD and AD, respectively, appears to be another urgent issue for future investigations.

Another difference refers to the hemi-field that obtains weaker attentional weight. It is the left hemi-field in neglect, but the right side in neurodegenerative diseases. In neglect the ipsi-lesional bias is clearly related to a right-hemispheric lesion. The matter appears to be less clear with HD or AD. A leftward spatial bias has been found after bilateral posterior lesions [76], and bilateral degeneration is without any doubt occurring in neurodegenerative diseases. However, modern neuroimaging has now consistently revealed stronger degeneration within the left, i.e. domiant hemisphere (in dextrals). Thus, leftward spatial bias in HD and AD may also be an expression of a unilateral effect, i.e. more pronounced left-hemispheric pathology.

Notwithstanding these clear differences, we would like to stress at the end of this article, that, as regards visual attentional deficits, hemi-spatial neglect and states of dementia, assessed cross-sectionally at a given point in time, may not be as different from each other as they were considered to be hitherto. The combination of spatial and non-spatial attentional deficits prevailing in both neglect on the one hand and in diseases like HD and AD on the other is so striking, that it may be justifiable to say that each of theses disorders involves a highly similar syndrome of impaired visual attention, with emphasis of the non-dominant hemisphere in the case of the neglect patient, and of the dominant hemisphere in the case of the patient with dementia.

Of course, this similarity should not be driven too far. Visual attention certainly is an important cognitive domain affected in all three kinds of disorder, but each one also includes deficits in other domains, like memory, spatial cognition, language, motor function etc (for the role of body representation in neglect, see [28]). Instead of simplifying things, our aim is to point to an important potential for clinical research in identifying these parallels. Recognizing them may open the possibility for both fields of research to inform each other. For example, understanding the interaction between spatial and non-spatial deficits of attention and the resulting behavioural consequences is a main issue in studying neglect as well as neurodegenerative diseases. TVA based assessment can be a powerful tool for that purpose, because it allows measurement of distinct components of attention not only in neglect but can be appropriately applied also in patients with severe intellectual decline.

Acknowledgements

We wish to thank Christian Sorg, Alexander Kurz and Hans Foerstl from the Psychiatry Hospital, Technical University of Munich, Germany, for their support in assessing MCI and AD patients, Matthias Dose from the Huntington Center South, Taufkirchen/Vils, Germany, for his support in assessing HD patients. We also thank Joseph Krummenacher for programming the experiments, as well as Hermann J. Müller and Werner X. Schneider, Department of Psychology, University of Munich, Germany, for their support in realising the project. We also thank Tanja Sonnfeld and Irmgard Maurer for their help in data acquisition. Finally, we are very grateful to Thomas Habekost for helpful comments on an earlier draft of this paper. This work was funded by the Deutsche Forschungsgemeinschaft (DFG; projects Mu 773/6-1, Mu FOR 480-Bu 1327/2-1).

References

[1] G.E. Alexander, M.R. De Long and P.L. Strick, Parallel organization of functionally segregated circuits linking basal ganglia and cortex, *Annual Review of Neuroscience* **9** (1986), 357–381.

[2] X.A. Alvarez, R. Mouzo, V. Pichel, P. Perez, M. Laredo, E. Fernandez-Novoa, L. Corzo, R. Zas, M. Alcarez, J.J. Secades, R. Lozano and R. Cacabelos, Double-blind placebo-controlled study with citicoline in APOE genotyped Alzheimer's disease patients. Effects on cognitive performance, brain bioelectrical activity and cerebral perfusion, *Methods and Findings in Experimental and Clinical Pharmacology* **21** (1999), 633–644.

[3] T.C. Andrews and D.J. Brooks, Advances in the understanding of early Huntington's disease using the functional imaging techniques of PET and SPET, *Molecular Medicine Today* **4** (1998), 532–539.

[4] E.H. Aylward, N.B. Anderson, F.W. Bylsma, M.V. Wagster, P.E. Barta, M. Sherr, J. Feeney, A. Davis, A. Rosenblatt, G.D. Pearlson and C.A. Ross, Frontal lobe volume in patients with Huntington's disease, *Neurology* **50** (1998), 252–258.

[5] P. Bartolomeo, G. Dalla Barba, M.F. Boisse, A.C. Bachoud-Levi, J.D. Degos and F. Boller, Right-side neglect in Alzheimer's disease, *Neurology* **51** (1998), 1207–1209.

[6] P. Bublak, K. Finke, J. Krummenacher, R. Preger, S. Kyllingsbæk, H.J. Müller and W.X. Schneider, Usability of a theory of visual attention (TVA) for parameter-based measurement of attention II: evidence from two patients with frontal or parietal damage, *Journal of the International Neuropsychological Society* **11** (2005), 843–854.

[7] P. Bublak, P. Redel, C. Sorg and K. Finke, Top-down-control and spatial attention in mild cognitive impairment and Alzheimer's disease: parametric assessment based on a theory of visual attention (TVA), Joint Meeting of the German Society of Neuropsychology and the International Neuropsychological Society, Zurich, Switzerland, 2006.

[8] C. Bundesen, A theory of visual attention, *Psychological Review* **97** (1990), 523–547.

[9] C. Bundesen, A computational theory of visual attention, *Philosophical Transactions of the Royal Society London B* **353** (1998), 1271–1281.

[10] C. Bundesen, A general theory of visual attention, in: *Psychology at the turn of the millennium: Vol. 1. Cognitive, biological, and health perspectives*, L. Bäckman and C. von Hofsten, eds, Psychology Press, Hove, 2002, pp. 179–200.

[11] C. Bundesen, T. Habekost and S. Kyllingsbæk, A neural theory of visual attention: bridging cognition and neurophysiology, *Psychological Review* **112** (2005), 291–328.

[12] T.W. Chow and J.L. Cummings, Frontal-subcortical circuits, in: *The human frontal lobes*, B.L. Miller and J.L. Cummings, eds, Guilford Press, New York, 1999, pp. 3–26.

[13] A.R. Damasio, H. Damasio and H.C. Chui, Neglect following damage to frontal lobe or basal ganglia, *Neuropsychologia* **18** (1980), 123–132.

[14] J. Danckert and S. Ferber, Revisiting unilateral neglect, *Neuropsychologia* **44** (2006), 987–1006.

[15] R. Desimone, Visual attention mediated by biased competition in extrastriate visual cortex, *Philosophical Transactions of the Royal Society London B* **353** (1998), 1245–1255.

[16] R. Desimone and J. Duncan, Neural mechanisms of selective visual attention, *Annual Review of Psychology* **18** (1995), 193–222.

[17] J. Driver and P. Vuilleumier, Perceptual awareness and its loss in unilateral neglect and extinction, *Cognition* **79** (2001), 39–88.

[18] J. Duncan, C. Bundesen, A. Olson, G. Humphreys, S. Chavda and H. Shibuya, Systematic analysis of deficits in visual attention, *Journal of Experimental Psychology: General* **128** (1999), 450–478.

[19] J. Duncan, C. Bundesen, A. Olson, G. Humphreys, R. Ward, S. Kyllingsbæk, M. Van Raamsdonk, C. Rorden and S. Chavda, Attentional functions in dorsal and ventral simultanagnosia, *Cognitive Neuropsychology* **20** (2003), 675–702.

[20] J. Duncan, G. Humphreys and R. Ward, Competitive brain activity in visual attention, *Current Opinion in Neurobiology* **7** (1997), 255–261.

[21] J. Fan, B.D. McCandliss, T. Sommer, A. Raz and M.I. Posner, Testing the efficiency and independence of attentional networks, *Journal of Cognitive Neuroscience* **14** (2002), 340–347.

[22] B. Fimm, R. Zahn, M. Mull, S. Kemeny, F. Buchwald, F. Block and M. Schwarz, Asymmetries of visual attention after circumscribed subcortical vascular lesions, *Journal of Neurology Neurosurgery, and Psychiatry* **71** (2001), 652–657.

[23] K. Finke, P. Bublak, M. Dose, H.J. Müller and W.X. Schneider, Parameter-based assessment of spatial and non-spatial attentional deficits in Huntington's disease, *Brain* **129** (2006), 1137–1151.

[24] K. Finke, P. Bublak, J. Krummenacher, S. Kyllingsbæk, H.J. Müller and W.X. Schneider, Usability of a theory of visual attention (TVA) for parameter-based measurement of attention I: evidence from normal subjects, *Journal of the International Neuropsychological Society* **11** (2005), 832–842.

[25] N.L. Foster, T.N. Chase, L. Mansi, R. Brooks, P. Fedio, N.J. Patronas and G. Di Chiro, Cortical abnormalities in Alzheimer's disease, *Brain Research* **691** (1984), 83–91.

[26] I. Freedman and L.E. Dexter, Visuospatial ability in cortical dementia, *Journal of Clinical and Experimental Neuropsychology* **13** (1991), 677–690.

[27] R.J. Friedrich, R. Egly, R.D. Rafal and D. Beck, Spatial attention deficits in humans: a comparison of superior parietal and temporal-parietal junction lesions, *Neuropsychology* **12** (1998), 193–207.

[28] D. Glocker, P. Bittl and G. Kerkhoff, Construction and psychometric properties of a novel test for body representational neglect (Vest Test), *Restorative Neurology and Neuroscience* this issue, (2006).

[29] T. Habekost and C. Bundesen, Patient assessment based on a theory of visual attention (TVA): subtle deficits after a right frontal-subcortical lesion, *Neuropsychologia* **41** (2003), 1171–1188.

[30] T. Habekost and E. Rostrup, Persisting asymmetries of vision after right side lesions, *Neuropsychologia* **44** (2006), 876–895.

[31] K. Herholz, FDG PET and differential diagnosis of dementia, *Alzheimer Disease and Associated Disorders* **9** (1995), 6–16.

[32] O. Hikosaka, Y. Takikawa and R. Kawagoe, Role of the basal ganglia in the control of purposive saccadic eye movements, *Physiological Reviews* **80** (2000), 953–978.

[33] M. Husain, S. Mannan, T. Hodgson, E. Wojciulik, J. Driver and C. Kennard, Impaired spatial working memory across saccades contributes to abnormal search in parietal neglect, *Brain* **124** (2001), 941–952.

[34] M. Husain and C. Rorden, Non-spatially lateralized mechanisms in hemispatial neglect, *Nature Reviews Neuroscience* **4** (2003), 26–36.

[35] S. Ishiai, K. Seki, Y. Koyama and R. Okiyama, Effects of cueing on visuospatial processing in unilateral spatial neglect, *Journal of Neurology* **242** (1995), 367–373.

[36] W.J. Jagust, J.L. Eberling, B.R. Reed, C.A. Mathis and T.F. Budinger, Clinical studies of cerebral blood flow in Alzheimer's disease, *Neurology* **50** (1997), 1585–1593.

[37] H.-O. Karnath, A.D. Milner and G. Vallar, *The cognitive and neural bases of spatial neglect*, Oxford University Press, Oxford, 2002.

[38] S. Kastner and L. Ungerleider, Mechanisms of visual attention in the human cortex, *Annual Review of Neuroscience* **23** (2000), 315–341.

[39] C.M. Kipps, A.J. Duggins, N. Mahant, L. Gomes, J. Ashburner and E.A. McCusker, Progression of structural neuropathology in preclinical Huntington's disease: a tensor based morphometry study, *Journal of Neurology Neurosurgery, and Psychiatry* **75** (2005), 650–655.

[40] D. Kogure, H. Matsuda, T. Ohnishi, T. Asada, M. Uno, T. Kunihiro, S. Nakano and M. Takasaki, Longitudinal evaluation of early Alzheimer's disease using brain perfusion SPECT, *Journal of Nuclear Medicine* **41** (2000), 1155–1162.

[41] S. Kyllingsbæk, Modeling visual attention, *Behavior Research Methods* **38** (2006), 123–133.

[42] F. Li, E. Iseki, M. Kato, Y. Adachi, M. Akagi and K. Kosaka, An autopsy case of Alzheimer's disease presenting with primary progressive aphasia: a clinicopathological and immunohistochemial study, *Neuropathology* **20** (2000), 239–245.

[43] N.B. Lincoln and A. Bowen, The need for randomised treatment studies in neglect research, *Restorative Neurology and Neuroscience*, this issue, (2006).

[44] P. Malhotra, H.R. Jäger, A. Parton, R. Greenwood, E.D. Playford, M.M. Brown, J. Driver and M. Husain, Spatial working memory capacity in unilateral neglect, *Brain* **128** (2005), 424–435.

[45] T. Manly, Cognitive rehabilitation for unilateral neglect: review, *Neuropsychological Rehabilitation* **12** (2002), 289–310.

[46] C.A. Marzi, M. Girelli, E. Natale and C. Miniussi, What exactly is extinguished in unilateral visual extinction? Neurophysiological evidence, *Neuropsychologia* **39** (2001), 1354–1366.

[47] J.B. Mattingley, N. Berberovic, L. Corben, M.J. Slavin, M.E.R. Nicholls and J.L. Bradshaw, The greyscales task: a perceptual measure of attentional bias following unilateral hemispheric damage, *Neuropsychologia* **42** (2004), 387–394.

[48] M.F. Mendez, M.M. Cherrier and J.S. Cymerman, Hemispatial neglect on visual search tasks in Alzheimer's disease, *Neuropsychiatric, Neuropsychological, and Behavioural Neurology* **10** (1997), 203–208.

[49] M.-M. Mesulam, Spatial attention and neglect: parietal, frontal, and cingulate contributions to the mental representation and attentional targeting of salient extrapersonal events, *Philosophical Transactions of the Royal Society London B* **354** (1999), 1325–1346.

[50] A.D. Milner, Neglect, extinction, and the cortical streams of visual processing, in: *Parietal lobe contributions to orientation in 3D space*, H.-O. Karnath and P. Thier, eds, Springer, Berlin, 1997, pp. 3–22.

[51] A. Parton, P. Malhotra and M. Husain, Hemispatial neglect, *Journal of Neurology, Neurosurgery, and Psychiatry* **75** (2004), 13–21.

[52] J.S. Paulsen, J.L. Zimbelman, S.C. Hinton, D.R. Langbehn, C.L. Leveroni, M.L. Benjamin, N.C. Reynolds and S.M. Rao, fMRI biomarker of early neuronal dysfunction in presymptomatic Huntington's disease, *American Journal of Neuroradiology* **25** (2004), 1715–1721.

[53] P.V. Peers, C.J.H. Ludwig, C. Rorden, R. Cusack, C. Bonfiglioli, C. Bundesen, J. Driver, N. Antoun and J. Duncan, Attentional functions of parietal and frontal cortex, *Cerebral Cortex* **15** (2005), 1469–1484.

[54] R.J. Perry and J.R. Hodges, Attention and executive deficits in Alzheimer's disease: a critical review, *Brain* **122** (1999), 383–404.

[55] P. Redel, P. Bublak, C. Sorg and K. Finke, Perceptual processing speed and visual working memory storage capacity in mild cognitive impairment and Alzheimer's disease: parametric assessment based on a theory of visual attention (TVA), Joint Meeting of the German Society of Neuropsychology and the International Neuropsychological Society, Zurich, Switzerland, 2006.

[56] P.A. Reuter-Lorenz and M.I. Posner, Components of neglect from right-hemisphere damage: an analysis of line bisection, *Neuropsychologia* **28** (1990), 327–333.

[57] J.H. Reynolds and R. Desimone, Interacting roles of attention and visual salience in V4, *Neuron* **37** (2003), 853–863.

[58] M.J. Riddoch and G.W. Humphreys, The effect of cueing on unilateral neglect, *Neuropsychologia* **21** (1983), 589–599.

[59] I.H. Robertson, J.B. Mattingley, C. Rorden and J. Driver, Phasic alerting of neglect patients overcomes their spatial deficit in visual awareness, *Nature* **395** (1998), 169–172.

[60] H.D. Rosas, J. Goodman, Y.I. Chen, B.G. Jenkins, D.N. Kennedy, N. Makris, M. Patti, L.J. Seidman, M.F. Beal and W.J. Koroshetz, Striatal volume loss in HD as measured by MRI and the influence of CAG repeat, *Neurology* **57** (2001), 1025–1028.

[61] H.D. Rosas, N.D. Hevelone, A.K. Zaleta, D.N. Greve, D.H. Salat and B. Fischl, Regional cortical thinning in preclinical Huntington disease and its relationship to cognition, *Neurology* **65** (2005), 745–747.

[62] H.D. Rosas, A.K. Liu, S. Hersch, M. Glessner, R.J. Ferrante, D.H. Salat, A. Van der Kouwe, B.G. Jenkins, A.M. Dale and B. Fischl, Regional and progressive thinning of the cortical ribbon in Huntington's disease, *Neurology* **58** (2002), 695–701.

[63] Y. Sakashita, Visual attentional disturbance with unilateral lesions in the basal ganglia and deep white matter, *Annals of Neurology* **30** (1991), 673–677.

[64] W.X. Schneider, VAM: a neuro-cognitive model for visual attention control of segmentation, object recognition, and space based-motor action, *Visual Cognition* **2** (1995), 331–375.

[65] W.X. Schneider, Visual-spatial working memory, attention, and scene representation: a neuro-cognitive theory, *Psychological Research* **62** (1999), 220–236.

[66] H. Shibuya and C. Bundesen, Visual selection from multi-element displays: measuring and modeling effects of exposure duration, *Journal of Experimental Psychology: Human Perception and Performance* **14** (1988), 591–600.

[67] D.J. Simons and D.T. Levin, Change blindness, *Trends in Cognitive Sciences* **1** (1997), 261–267.

[68] G. Sperling, The information available in brief visual presentations, *Psychological Monographs* **74** (1960), 11.

[69] G. Sperling, A model for visual memory tasks, *Human Factors* **5** (1963), 19–31.

[70] M.J. Thieben, A.J. Duggins, C.D. Good, L. Gomes, N. Mahant, F. Richards, E. McCusker and R.S.J. Frackowiack, The distribution of structural neuropathology in pre-clinical Huntington's disease, *Brain* **125** (2002), 1815–1828.

[71] M. Thimm, G.R. Fink, J. Küst, H. Karbe and W. Sturm, Impact of alertness training on spatial neglect: a behavioural and fMRI study, *Neuropsychologia* **44** (2006), 1230–1246.

[72] K. Ueyama, H. Fukuzako, T. Fukuzako, Y. Hokazono, K. Takeuchi, T. Hashiguchi, M. Takigawa, T. Yamanaka and K. Matsumoto, CT study in senile dementia of Alzheimer type, *International Journal of Geriatric Psychiatry* **9** (1994), 919–924.

[73] G. Vallar, Spatial hemineglect in humans, *Trends in Cognitive Sciences* **2** (1998), 87–97.

[74] S.P. Vecera and M. Rizzo, Spatial attention: normal processes and their breakdown, *Neurologic Clinics of North America* **21** (2003), 575–607.

[75] N.D. Volkow, W. Zhu, C.A. Felder, K. Mueller, T.F. Welsh, G.-J. Wang and M.J. de Leon, Changes in brain functional homogeneity in subjects with Alzheimer's disease, *Psychiatry Research Neuroimaging* **114** (2002), 39–50.

[76] S. Weintraub, K.R. Daffner, G.L. Ahern, B.H. Price and M.-M. Mesulam, Right sided hemispatial neglect and bilateral cerebral lesions, *Journal Of Neurology, Neurosurgery, and Psychiatry* **60** (1996), 342–344.

[77] B. Wilson, J.J. Cockburn and P. Halligan, Development of a behavioral test of visuospatial neglect, *Archives of Physical Medicine and Rehabilitation* **68** (1987), 98–102.

[78] E. Wojciulik, M. Husain, K. Clarke and J. Driver, Spatial working memory deficit in unilateral neglect, *Neuropsychologia* **39** (2001), 390–396.

[79] K.K. Zakzanis, The subcortical dementia of Huntington's disease, *Journal of Clinical and Experimental Neuropsychology* **20** (1998), 565–578.

Construction and psychometric properties of a novel test for body representational neglect (Vest Test)

D. Glocker[a], P. Bittl[a] and G. Kerkhoff[a,b,*]
[a]*Department of Biological, Clinical and Neuropsychology, Catholic University Eichstätt-Ingolstadt, Germany*
[b]*Clinical Neuropsychology Unit, Saarland University, Saarbrücken, Germany*

Received 1 January 2006
Revised 4 July 2006
Accepted 5 July 2006

Abstract. *Purpose*: Multimodal spatial neglect manifests itself also in nonvisual modalities such as audition, touch and body representation. Yet, quantitative tests for the diagnosis of nonvisual neglect are still quite rare. The purpose of the present paper was to develop and evaluate a novel, simple and sensitive test for the assessment of body representational neglect (BRN) in patients with left or right cerebral hemispheric lesions.
Methods: The vest test covers the front part of the trunk. The blindfolded subject wears the vest and is instructed to pick up all objects from the 24 pockets of the vest (12 on each side) as quickly as possible using the ipsilesional, nonparetic hand. Two samples of healthy control subjects (each $N = 25$) using either their left or their right hand performed the test in identical way to obtain normative data for patients searching with their left hand (i.e. left hemisphere stroke patients) versus their right hand (i.e. right hemisphere stroke patients). The test can be performed within 5 minutes, even with aphasic or apractic stroke patients.
Results: Psychometric evaluations in a sample of 50 patients with unilateral stroke (25 leftsided, 25 rightsided) show high objectivity, high internal consistency (Cronbach's alpha = 0.96), good retest-reliability (0.79 after 1 week in neglect patients) and good validity as compared with two other measures of BRN or multimodal neglect. Patient examples show that BRN as assessed with the vest test allows the detection of qualitatively and quantitatively different patterns of BRN, and shows double dissociations from visual neglect and from apraxia in left hemisphere stroke patients. Details of the test including instructions and cut-off values are given for users in the appendix of this article.
Conclusions: In conclusion, the vest test is a sensitive, quick and reliable test for BRN which complements the assessment of visuo- and audiospatial neglect and allows to measure recovery (spontaneous or treatment-induced) in patients with BRN. Furthermore, it can help to improve our knowledge about the multisensory coding of our body and the surrounding space in the human brain.

Keywords: Stroke, neglect, test, body, human, space

1. Introduction

Spatial neglect commonly refers to a complex neurological disorder where patients fail to attend, process and respond appropriately towards stimuli in the contralesional, usually the left hemispace [15]. The most obvious behavior in patients with this disorder is their failure to attend to even the most conspicuous and rele-

*Corresponding author: Prof. Dr. Georg Kerkhoff, Clinical Neuropsychology Unit, Faculty of Social Sciences, Saarland University, Postbox 151150, D-66041 Saarbrücken, Germany. E-mail: Kerkhoff@ mx.uni-saarland.de.

vant *visual* stimuli such as persons or obstacles on their contralesionial side, food on their contralesional side of the plate or copy a daisy or a house on a sheet of paper. As omissions of contralateral visual stimuli are the most obvious behaviour of patients with spatial neglect it is not surprising that numerous studies have focused on *visual* neglect after unilateral brain lesions [23]. Consequently, there exists a number of quantitative tests for the diagnosis of visual neglect (cf. BIT [24]; line cancellation tests Bells Test [11]; visual cancellation tests, cf [10]. Recent studies on the nature of neglect in other modalities have shown that the majority of patients with visual neglect also shows auditory neglect [18], tactile neglect [22], or representational neglect [8]. Unfortunately, only few standardized clinical tests are available for the diagnosis of *nonvisual* neglect. As a result of this, the relationship between visual and nonvisual neglect is far from clear and is difficult to assess in the clinical setting.

In this paper we report the construction and psychometric evaluation of a novel and clinical sensitive test for the assessment of body representational neglect (further abbreviated as BRN) in stroke patients. The paper is split into five parts: after a short survey of existing tests for BRN, the basic idea of the novel test, its purpose and differences to other tests are outlined. In the third part results of 50 healthy control subjects are reported. Part four describes results of patient studies, and in the fifth part psychometric properties (objectivity, reliability, validity, practicability) are outlined. In the Appendix of the paper the potential user finds more detailed informations for the self-construction as well as a scoring sheet and normative data for the test.

2. Existing tests for the assessment of body representational neglect

So far, only a few tests have been reported for the measurement of BRN. Three tests will be shortly described: Bisiach's test [7], the comb and razor/compact-test developed by Beschin and Robertson [6] and the Fluff test developed by Cocchini et al. [9].

Bisiach's test: Bisiach and coworkers [7] operationalized BRN (personal neglect in their terminology) as an inability to touch the contralesional arm with the ipsilesional arm. The patient is asked to reach out for the left hand using his/her right arm with eyes closed. The performance is rated on a four-point-scale (*0 points: the patient reaches his contralesional arm immediately; 3 points: no movement towards the contralesional arm*). This test allows a simple and quick (bedside) screening of BRN and could well differentiate between personal and extrapersonal neglect [7]. A possible drawback may reside in the few number of "items" (only one). Furthermore, the patient may be "cued" by the *explicit* instruction to search for the *contralesional* (left) arm. Such cueing effects are well known [19] and may overcome the neglect deficit transiently.

– *Comb- and- razor/ compact-test*: this test by Beschin and Robertson [6] was developed on the basic of Zoccolotti's and Judica's semi-quantitative rating scale [25]. First, patients are asked to comb their hair for 30 seconds. Second, men are instructed to shave and women to make up their face for 30 s. The number of strokes is recorded for each side of the head or the face. A marked difference in the number of strokes on the two sides of the head indicates BRN (with fewer strokes on the contralesional side).

While Bisiach's test and the Comb-and-razor/compact-test require the subject to search for specific, personal body-parts the Fluff-test is desined as a body-scanning test in the representational modality where the subjects has to search the front part of his/her body.

– *Fluff-test*: Because the comb-and-razor/compact-test focuses exclusively on the subject's face and head Cocchini et al. [9] developed a test involving almost the entire body. The so-called Fluff test requires patients to remove all targets ("fluffs") which are placed on the front of their clothes using their ipsilesional arm. 24 identical circular patches (6 on the contralesional arm, 6 on each leg and 6 on the upper part on the body) are placed by the examiner on the patient's clothes after blindfolding the patient. In order to reduce the tactile information and stimulation (hence "cueing") the patients were diverted by a conversation. 27 patients with right brain damage, 11 patients with left sided lesions and 38 normal subjects were investigated in the original study [9]. According to the cut-off score (*13 targets on the contralesional side*) 10 right brain damaged patients with extrapersonal, visual neglect, two patients without extrapersonal neglect and two patients with left sided lesion showed a BRN in the Fluff test. Furthermore, a double dissociation between the performance in the Fluff Test and the comb-and-razor/compact-test was reported. Psychometric evaluations showed that the

Fluff test is highly reliable und sensitive for BRN. Possible drawbacks may reside in the asymmetrical distribution of targets (15 contralesional, 9 ipsilesional) on the two body sides which may reduce test sensitivity and implies that an asymmetrical cortical representation of the body surface is searched by the patient. Furthermore, it can not be excluded that implicit cueing processes occur when the experimenter places the targets on the patient's body – this could improve performance.

3. Description of the vest test

With the above specific aspects and possible limitations in mind we tried to construct a simple, quick, symmetric, sensitive and reliable test of BRN which can be performed in acute as well as chronic patients with left or right hemisphere lesions *and* despite frequently associated deficits such as apraxia or aphasia. The vest test aims at evaluating the pattern of performance and differential hemispheric contributions in the manual exploration and spatial representation of the two trunk halves. As the front part of the vest is firmly attached to the body surface (see instructions for use in the Appencix) it can be conceived as a veridical test of BRN. It might be objected that searching a vest filled with common but not personal objects can not be considered a test of BRN. However, as the vest is attached firmly to the patient's body surface we believe that it is very likely that vest and body surface are merged together, just as when you attach fluffs or other targets on the subject's pullover or trouser for search. Neurophysiologically, we believe that it is very likely that objects firmly attached to the skin are *merged* into personal space, just as grasping a tool immediately leads to the merging of personal and peripersonal space [5].

Practically, 24 everyday objects (i.e. battery, text marker, lipstick) are hidden in 24 pockets of the vest (one object per pocket, 12 targets per body-half of the vest; see Appendix A). After blindfolding the subjects are instructed to search for all objects and give them to the experimenter (detailed instruction, see Appendix). Patients with right sided lesions perform the vest test with their right hand and left brain damaged patients search with their left hand. Before running the test one practice trial is run with a "practice" vest that contains only one target which is hidden in a pocket on the ipsilesionale side. To minimize the stimulation on the body surface, this practice vest and a "test vest" (with all 24 targets) are used sequentially and put on passively with the help of the experimenter. Hence, the subject never views the vest and its spatial layout. The test is finished when the subject indicates that he/she has found all objects. Otherwise, the examiner stops the test after 5 minutes. Test performance was videotaped in all subjects and analyzed offline. After 150 seconds the original instruction was repeated once again to remind subjects of the task.

4. Normative data

4.1. Samples and procedures

To obtain normative data for the vest test 50 healthy control subjects without neurological or psychiatric disease were examined. All subjects were matched in terms of age and sex to the patient group (Section 5, below). 25 normal subjects (all righthanded) performed the vest test with their right hand (termed N-RH; corresponding to the 25 patients with right sided lesions). The remaining 25 normal subjects (21 righthanded, 4 ambidextrous) searched with their left hand (termed N-LH; corresponding to the 25 left brain damaged patients). Table 1 summarizes the demographic data of all normal subjects. Although the N-LH group was slightly younger than the N-RH group (*t-test*: $t = 2.57$; $d.f. = 48$; $p = 0.013$) we will show that neither age nor performing hand per se have a significant effect on task performance. The number of targets detected was rated cumulatively in 30 second intervals (bins) for each trunk halve separately. Furthermore, the individual performance time to complete the vest test was also evaluated.

4.2. Time and number of targets

The N-RH performed the vest test in 171.52 seconds ($sd = 39.34$), the N-LH group in 153.32 seconds ($sd = 27.66$). The difference is not significant ($t = -1.89$; $d.f. = 48$; $p > 0.05$). N-RH found on their maximum 9.96 objects on the right vest side and 10.84 targets on the left trunk side. N-LH detected at maximum 10.08 objects on the right and 10.96 targets on the left side of the vest. Neither the difference between both groups nor between both halves of the vest in each group were significant ($p > 0.05$ in all comparisons).These data also indicate the equivalence of the two halves of the vest test.

Table 1
Descriptive data of the normal subjects: sd = standard deviation, N-RH = normals using the right hand, N-H = normals using the left hand

variable / group		N-RH	N-LH
age	arithmetic mean	63,20	55,56
	(sd)	(9,87)	(11,14)
	minimum	36	32
	maximum	77	75
sex	male	12	15
	female	13	10
handedness	right	25	21
	left	0	0
	ambivalent	0	4

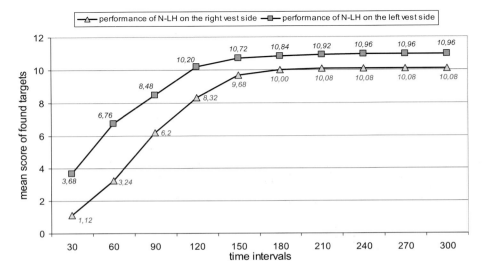

Fig. 1. Cumulative increase of the mean number of targets per time interval (in seconds) in the vest test for 25 normal control subjects using their left hand (N-LH).

4.3. Cut-off scores

To define conservative cutoff-scores the mean scores of detected targets in each time interval and trunk halve were compared for both control groups separately by paired sample t-tests. Figure 1 shows the cumulative increase of mean scores for both sides of the vest side in the N-LH group, and Fig. 2 shows the equivalent data for the H-RH group. As values in successive time intervals are dependent we used paired t-test to determine up to which time period significant increases in performance (targets detected) between adjacent were observed. For N-LH the significant increase in the number of targets detected on the right trunk side declined after 180 seconds ($t = -1$; $d.f. = 24$, $p > 0.05$; Fig. 1). T-tests for paired samples showed in the N-RH-group that after 210 seconds no significant further increase in the number of targets detected occurred ($t = -1.00$; $d.f. = 24$, $p = 0.32$; see Fig. 2). To establish a homogeneous cut-off criterion we set the cut-off score for the performance time at 210 seconds for both halves of the vest.

In a second step we calculated how many targets the majority of normal subjects (at least 90%) had detected after 210 seconds on the vest side contralateral to their searching hand. Only one subject in the N-RH found less than 9 objects on the left side of the vest. Hence, 96% (24 out of 25 N-RH) detected at least nine targets or more within 210 seconds on the left vest side. The distribution of targets detected on the ipsilateral side of the vest is somewhat different. 5 out of 25 N-RH found less than 9 targets after 210 seconds (20%).

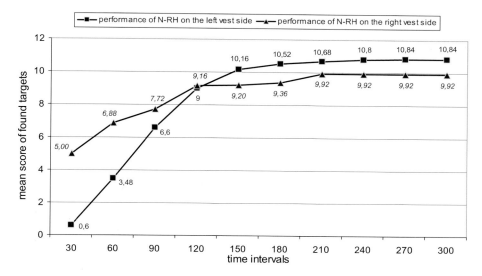

Fig. 2. Cumulative increase of the mean number of targets per time interval (in seconds) in the vest test for 25 normal control subjects using their right hand (N-RH).

Comparably 92% (23 out of 25 N-LH) of the N-LH group found at least 9 objects on the right side of the vest test after 210 seconds. On the ipsilateral, left side of the vest 96% (24 out of 25 N-LH) detected at least 9 targets within 210 seconds.

From these results the following, conservative cutoff-criteria were derived: BRN in the vest test is defined:

- when a patient detects less than 9 objects on the *contralesional* side of the vest within 210 seconds.
- The corresponding cut-off score for the *ipsilesional* side is also 9 targets within 210 seconds (see Table 2).

Although ipsilesional omissions are not viewed as a key deficit in patients with spatial neglect, such deficits have recently received much attention [14]. We therefore also calculated cutoff scores for the ipsilesional side of the vest. In Section 5.2 (patient studies) we will show that both contralateral and ipsilateral deficits may be found in some patients with multimodal neglect.

We considered the idea whether a left-right-ratio would be more specific to identify BRN in the vest test. However, apart from the left-right-distribution our percentile ranges (see below) indicate additionally whether a patient shows impaired target detection on both sides of the trunk. As is shown below in some representative cases poor performance on both sides of the vest was observed in several patients with unilateral right-sided lesions, but not in patients with unilateral left-sided lesions. Such a result might constitute an important information which would be lost with the calculation of a left-right-ratio of targets detected.

4.4. Effects of age on test performance

Age was not correlated (Pearson coefficients) significantly ($r = -0.11$) with test performance on the left vest side, nor on the right side of the vest ($r = -0.24$) at 210 seconds in the collapsed two normal samples. Furthermore, we entered the number of detected targets after 210 seconds for both sides of the vest and all groups in a one-way ANOVA. The ANOVA showed no significant effect of age (*left vest side:* $F = 0.36$; $d.f. = 25$; $p = 0.99$; *right vest side:* $F = 1.21$; $d.f. = 25$; $p = 0.32$). Consequently, age was no crucial variable for the performance in the vest test in healthy subjects.

5. Patient studies

5.1. Total patient sample

We consecutively tested 50 patients with unilateral stroke (25 left sided, 25 rightsided) in two neurological hospitals with acute stroke patients (Bad Aibling, Kipfenberg, Germany). Exclusion criteria were: multiple vascular lesions, dementia, additional neurological diseases like Parkinson's disease or brain tumours; infratentorial lesions). The leftsided lesioned patient group (14 male, 11 female) had a mean age of 55 years

Table 2
Percentile range of the number of targets detected in the vest test for both sides of the vest after 210 seconds in the two groups of normal subjects (N-RH = subjects using their right for search; N-LH = subjects using their left hand for search)

percentile range of		number of targets detected	6	8	9	10	11	12
	N-RH	left side of the vest	< 4	4	28	40	60	100
		right side of the vest	< 20	20	28	72	88	100
	N-LH	left side of the vest	< 4	4	12	28	56	100
		right side of the vest	< 8	8	20	68	96	100

(range: 30–73). Mean time since lesion was 10 weeks (range: 1–24). The rightsided lesioned patient group (13 male, 12 female) had a mean age of 64 years (range: 36–79). Their mean time since lesion was 10 weeks (range: 3–21). Age was significantly lower in the left-hemisphere lesioned patients as in the right hemisphere lesioned patients ($T = 2.795; p < 0.007$). However, age did not correlate significantly with performance in the vest test at 210 seconds (all patients together: Pearson correlation coefficient, left vest side: $r = -0.11$, $p > 0.05$; right vest side: $r = -0.24, p > 0.05$). Thus, age does not seem to contribute significantly to test performance – neither in normal subjects nor in stroke patients.

Contralateral BRN in the vest test, according to the above defined cutoff-criteria, was found in 48% of stroke patients with left hemisphere lesions and 80% of patients with right hemisphere lesions, the difference is highly significant (Mann-Whitney-test, $U = 0.00$; $z = -4.71; p < 0.01$). These results identify contralesional BRN as a frequent deficit in patients with unilateral stroke, and shows that it is not a rare phenomenon in patients with left hemisphere lesioned patients. This finding confirms also recent findings on right visuospatial neglect after left hemisphere stroke [.[3]]. The results of our ongoing patient studies will be published in detail in a separate paper.

However, in order to show the diagnostic usefulness of the vest test, we present here five representative single cases from the total patient sample (3 with right brain damage, 2 with left brain damage) who demonstrate different patterns of results and reveal dissociations between BRN and visual neglect as well as to other neuropsychological disorders (see complete patient data in Table 3).

5.2. Patient examples

5.2.1. Patient PR

PR was a 73 old man who had suffered from a right sided intracerebral hemorrhage 13 weeks before our investigation, lesioning the temporo-occipital cortex. Visual neglect tests (line bisection, number cancellation task, copying and reading) showed a severe leftsided visual neglect. Furthermore, patient PR showed a leftsided homonymous hemianopia. In the vest test PR found only 5 objects on the left and 4 objects on the right side (PR <4 for both sides). According to our cutoff-criteria this patient showed a clear leftsided BRN in the vest test. Unexpectedly, he also showed clear *rightsided* BRN but no rightsided visual neglect. This striking pattern was found in a significant number of right brain damaged patients (to be published in a separate paper). Possible explanations are alluded to in the discussion of this paper.

5.2.2. Patient MP

MP was a 71 year old lady who had suffered from a rightsided, hypertensive thalamo-striatal hemorrhage 17 weeks before. In analogy to patient PR this woman also showed severe leftsided visual neglect and leftsided, homonymous hemianopia. However, in clear contrast to PR she showed a more lateralized pattern of BRN in the vest test (7 objects on the right and 0 objects on the left side; PR < 4 for both sides).

5.2.3. Patient ER

ER had sustained a right sided thalamic hemorrhage and was examind 13 weeks post onset. The 74 year old man showed no signs of left visual neglect, but a moderate BRN on both sides of the vest test (7 objects on the left and 8 objects on the right side, PR <4 for both sides). Hence, ER shows the same bilateral deficit as patient PR, but in a milder form. Furthermore, ER demonstrates that mild BRN can occur in isolation, hence in the absence of any signs of visual neglect.

5.2.4. BRN versus apraxia

As many patients with left hemisphere lesions are often aphasic and apractic and may show contralateral neglect to a significant degree [3,15] it is of considerable clinical interest whether the vest test can also be performed reliably with such patients. To this purpose we have chosen one left brain damaged patient with severe apraxia but without BRN and one patient with severe unilateral BRN but without apraxia. Apraxia was tested conventionally with a pantomime and a hand movement test [12]. For testing pantomime the patient was shown 10 pictures of everyday objects and asked to demonstrate the use of the objects by pantomime. Performance was rated as impaired if the patient made more than 2 mistakes [12]. The second test required the imitation of 10 meaningless hand movements [12]. The patient is allowed 2 trials per hand movement (hence $10 \times 2 =$ maximum 20 correct points). Performance was rated as pathological if the total score was <16 points in the hand movment test.

5.2.5. Patients example for BRN versus apraxia: JO versus EB

JO was a 64 year old man with a leftsided, subarachnoid hemorrhage. He was examined 7 weeks post onset. He showed neither signs of visual neglect nor any apractic deficits, but in the vest test he demonstrated a clear BRN, with 0 detected objects on the right side but 9 objects on the left (hence PR < 4 for the right side and PR = 20 for the left side). Put differently, JO showed isolated rightsided BRN in the vest test without visual neglect.

In contrast to JO patient EB, a 50 year old man with a left sided middle cerebral artery infarction 10 weeks before examination, showed no BRN in the vest test (12 targets detected on the left vest side, PR = 100; 11 targets detected on the right vest side; PR = 96), but severe apraxia in both tests of apraxia (0 points in pantomime, 6 points in hand movements). This case indicates a clear double dissociation between BRN and another neuropsychological disorder involving body knowledge and representation, namely apraxia. Furthermore, this example indicates that apraxia per se has no influence on the test performance in the vest test so that left hemisphere lesioned subjects with or without apraxia can perform the vest test properly with their left hand.

6. Psychometric evaluations

We evaluated the typical psychometric criteria [13] such as objectivity, internal consistency, retest reliability and validity in all 50 stroke patients (patients described in Section 5.2).

6.1. Objectivity

Objectivity indicates how (in)dependent a test result is from the person who examines the patient, scores or interprets the test results [13]. As the instructions, test protocol, scoring and interpretation of the results are standardized the vest test can be viewed as highly objective. The cutoff-criteria and the normative data guarantee the correct interpretation of the test performance.

6.2. Internal consistency and retest-reliability

Internal consistency

We evaluated reliability using Cronbach's alpha, which is a measure for internal consistency. The average inter-item-correlation was $r = 0.35$, hence Cronbach's alpha was $\alpha = \mathbf{0.96}$. This indicates a high internal consistency of the vest test.

Retest-reliability

The two patient groups described above (5.2.) were retested 5 to 14 days (mean: 7.2) after the first investigation with the vest test in the same clinic. For the computation of retest-reliability we compared the number of targets (left and right side separately) at the critical cutoff time (210 seconds) for the first test and the retest with the vest test (see Table 4). The average item-intercorrelation was $r = 0.49$, resulting in a Cronbach's alpha of $\alpha = \mathbf{0.79}$. Hence, the vest test is a reliable instrument also for retest evaluations which is important when studying spontaneous or treatment-induced recovery from BRN.

Although retest-reliability of the vest test was high, there might be systematic differences in test performance between test and retest, due to familiarity with the test on the second occasion, fatigue, learning or recovery. We therefore verified by paired t-tests whether the patients did show any improvements in the retest condition of the vest test (performance cutoff was after 210sec). Neither patients with nor patients without BRN showed any significant improvements in the vest test (right brain damaged patients with BRN: $t_{\text{left vest side 210sec test-retest}} = 1.03$; $p = 0.32$; right brain damaged patients

Table 3
Descriptive and test data of the patient examples. N: normal; pathological performances are printed in bold

	Patients	PR	MP	ER	JO	EB
descriptive data	Age	73	71	74	64	50
	Sex	male	female	male	male	male
	Time after lesion in weeks	13	17	13	7	10
	Etiology and Lesion	right sided intracerebral hemorrhage in the temporo-occipital cortex	right sided hypertensive thalamo-striatal hemorrhage	right sided thalamic hemorrhage	left sided subarachnoid hemorrhage	left sided middle cerebral artery infarction
	Handedness	right	right	right	right	right
visual neglect tests	Line Bisection with deviation in mm	**40**	**69**	2	4	**-60**
	Cancelation task - missings on the left side	**10**	**10**	2	1	0
	Cancelation task - missings on the right side	**6**	**9**	3	1	0
	Reading (Neglect dyslexia)	**impaired**	**impaired**	N	N	Aphasia
	Copy - left side	**impaired**	**impaired**	N	N	N
	Copy - right side	N	**impaired**	N	N	N
	visual field defects	left sided hemianopia	left sided hemianopia	N	N	N
vest test	targets detected on the left side	**5**	**0**	7	9	12
	targets detected on the right side	**4**	**7**	8	**0**	11
Apraxia	Score in pantomime	**6**	**8**	10	10	**0**
	Score in hand movements	**8**	**6**	18	20	**6**
CBS - Items for body representational neglect	missing of body care of the head and face, like razor and make up	**mildly impaired**	**mildly impaired**	N	N	**moderately impaired**
	difficulties to put the cloth on	**severely impaired**	**severely impaired**	**mildly impaired**	N	**moderately impaired**
	forget to clean the left/ right side of the mouth after eating	**mildly impaired**	**moderately impaired**	N	N	**moderately impaired**
	don t pay attention for the left/ right part of the body, like don t use the left/ right arm for activities	**mildly impaired**	**mildly impaired**	**moderately impaired**	N	**mildly impaired**
digit span	forward	7	4	7	6	Not tested
	backward	5	2	5	3	Not tested
Test battery for attentional performance TAP	T- Score for the trials without a warning tone	**20**	---	**26**	34	34
	T- Score for the trials with a warning tone	**24**	---	**25**	37	35

without BRN: $t_{\text{left vest side 210sec test-retest}} = -0.61$; $p = 0.53$; left brain damaged patients with BRN: $t_{\text{right vest side 210sec test-retest}} = -1.58$; $p = 0.14$; left brain damaged patients without BRN: $t_{\text{right vest side 210sec test-retest}} = -0.32$; $p = 0.75$). Hence, comparable values are found when two investigations are performed within 7 days in acute stroke patients. Nevertheless, this does not rule out small, though insignificant learning effects due to familiarity with the vest on retesting. We therefore calculated the averaged number of targets on the left and right side of the vest during the first test and the retest for comparison (Table 5). The mean improvement (over both sides and both measurements) shows an improvement of 0.35 targets. This effect must be considered as very small when we take into account that patients were familiar with the vest on the second occasions, and when we consider that some, although very limited recovery can have taken

Table 4
Intercorrelations (Pearson Product-Moment-Correlations) of different variables in the first test and the re-test with the vest test. Abbreviations: vest-210sec-r = number of detected targets after 210 seconds on the right vest side; re-vest-210sec-r = number of detected targets after 210 seconds on the right vest side on the second measure point; vest-210sec-l = number of detected targets after 210 seconds on the left vest side; re-vest-210sec-l = number of detected targets after 210 seconds on the left vest side on the second measure point; x = arithmetic mean; sd = standard devision

Variables	vest-210sec-r ($x = 7,44; sd = 2,96$)	re-vest-210sec-r ($x = 8,16; sd = 2,78$)	vest-210sec-l ($x = 8,50; sd = 2,26$)	re-vest-210sec-l ($x = 8,48; sd = 2,82$)
vest-210sec-r	*1.00*			
re-vest-210sec-r	**.66**	*1.00*		
vest-210sec-l	.34	.37	*1.00*	
re-vest-210sec-l	.44	.39	**.77**	*1.00*

place within one week. Finally, it should be kept in mind that all patients received treatment (behavioural and pharmacological) within the retest period. Given all these possible influence factors the retest reliability of the vest test quite high.

6.3. Validity

6.3.1. Relations to the fluff test

In a first analysis we compared the results of the vest test with those obtained from a slightly modified version of the Fluff test. For a better comparison with the vest test we did not place the 24 targets on the patient's body surface (as is done in the standard Fluff test). Instead the targets were attached to a jacket and the front side of a trouser before examination. Both jacket and trouser were dressed on in the same way as we put the vest on. By this procedure we tried to eliminate the tactile stimulation of the body which is inevitable when placing targets on the patient's clothes. Thus, both tests were made more comparable by this modification.

The same 50 patients with unilateral stroke were examined with both tests on separate occasions (maximal 1–2 days apart). The results were transformed into z-scores and correlated. The Pearson correlation coefficients between the test performance of both tests after the critical time Cut-off (for the Fluff test 180 sec and for the vest test 210 sec) were between $r = 0.31$ and $r = 0.60$ (see Table 6). All correlations were significant at least at the 5%- level.

6.3.2. Relation to the Catherine Bergego Scale (CBS)

Furthermore we compared the results of the vest test with those of a semiquantitative rating (CBS-scale) concerning the patient's neglect deficits obtained from the nursing staff. The Catherine Bergego Scale (CBS) was developed by Azouvi et al. [1,2]. This well constructed scale is highly reliable and valid for the detection of unilateral neglect. The quality and severity of the neglect syndrome is first rated by the person who suffers from neglect and then compared to the ratings of a relative or staff. The difference between both ratings results in the anosognosia score. The Scale contains 10 questions about relevant activities of daily living. The four items related to BRN are printed in bold.

- **lack of body care on the contralesional side on the head and face**
- **difficulties to put the clothes on**
- forgetting the food on the left/right side of the plate
- **forget to clean the left/right side of the mouth after eating**
- difficulties to look leftwards/rightwards
- **nonuse of the left/right arm for activities**
- ignoring sounds coming from the left/right side
- collision with persons or objects on the left/right side
- difficulties to find the way to the left/right side for well known places in the clinic
- difficulties to find personal things in the own room or in the bathroom if they are on the left/right side

The person has to rate on a three-point-scale whether the patient has no, mild or severe problems with the activity. Patients showing no evidence of unilateral neglect received the score 0 in the CBS scale. Mild behavioural unilateral neglect is scored with values between 1 and 10. A score between 11 to 20 reflects moderate neglect, and patients with a severe behavioural neglect receive scores of more than 20 points [1].

Four of the 10 questions are related directly to BRN and were therefore used for our validity measurements.

Table 5

Averaged number of targets detected on the left and right side of the vest test during the first examination and the retest (7 days later) in 25 patients with left hemispheric stroke (LBD) and 25 patients with right hemispheric stroke (RBD). Abbreviations: vest-210sec-r = number of detected targets after 210 seconds on the right vest side on the first measurement; re-vest-210sec-r = number of detected targets after 210 seconds on the right vest side on the retest; vest-210sec-l = number of detected targets after 210 seconds on the left vest side on the first measurement; re-vest-210sec-l = number of detected targets after 210 seconds on the left vest side on the retest

group \ variable	vest-210sec-r	re-vest-210sec-r	vest-210sec-l	re-vest-210sec-l
RBD	7,12	7,76	7,08	6,84
LBD	7,76	8,56	9,92	10,12

Table 6

Intercorrelations (Person Product-Moment-Correlations) of the modified Fluff test and the vest test. Abbreviations: vest-210sec-r = number of detected targets after 210 seconds on the right vest side; vest-210sec-l = number of detected targets after 210 seconds on the left vest side; Fluff-180sec-ipsi = number if detected targets after 180 seconds on the ipsilesional body side; Fluff-180sec-con = number if detected targets after 180 seconds on the contralesional body side; * = significant at the 5%- level; ** = significant at the 1%- level

Variables	vest-210sec-r	vest-210sec-l	Fluff-180sec-ipsi	Fluff-180sec-con
vest-210sec-r	--			
vest-210sec-l	.34*	--		
Fluff-180sec-ipsi	.61**	.50**	--	
Fluff-180sec-con	.31*	.49**	.42**	--

In analogy to the scoring of the total CBS, the following scoring procedure was adapted. The 4 items could have a maximum score of 12, which indicates a very severe deficit (9 to 12 points). A moderate form of BRN in the CBS was considered when the patient reached 5 to 8 points. A score between 1 to 4 was considered as mild BRN. Accordingly, we calculated Spearman rank correlations between the ratings in these four questions of the CBS and the performance in the vest test over all time intervals (Fig. 3). Highly significant correlations ($p < 0.05$ in all cases) were obtained, ranging up to 0.6 or even 0.8. The negative values are due to the different polarity of scores in both tests (CBS: high scores indicate severe deficit; Vest: high score indicate better performance).

6.4. Sensitivity and specificity of the vest test

6.4.1. Vest test versus other tests of BRN

We were interested in a test which measures BRN separately from other neglect modalities and which measures BRN more sensitively. 80% of the patients

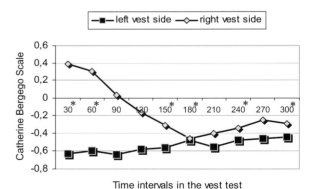

Fig. 3. Spearman's rank correlations between the scores of the Catherine Bergego Scale (four items related to BRN) and the number of detected targets in the two halves of the vest test over all time intervals (in seconds): * = significant correlation with $p < 0.05$. For details see text.

having right sided lesions showed a pathological performance in the vest test, whereas the Fluff test registered only 68% of BRN within this group (see Table 6). 60% of the patients with right brain damages showed a BRN in both tests. In addition 20% demonstrated

BRN only in the vest test, whereas the Fluff test detected only 8% of BRN separately. Within the patient group with left sided lesions 24% showed a BRN in both tests. Furthermore 24% of all left brain damaged patients showed a pathological performance only in the vest test, and another 24% showed a BRN selectively in the Fluff test. This discrepancy might result from the fact that different body parts are searched in the two tests.

Assessment tools with a very high sensitivity run the risk of showing lower specificity. Two aspects indicate satisfactory specificity of the vest test: first, nearly all healthy control subjects (>92%) showed nearly perfect performance in the vest test, and second we encountered dissociations between BRN and visual neglect (see below).

As is obvious from Table 7, 52% of the left-hemisphere lesioned patients showed pathological results in the four BRN items of the CBS (this percentage is achieved when the numbers for the four BRN-items of the CBS-scale are added). This indicates that the CBS is also sensitive for left brain damaged patients with BRN. However, four of the patients with leftsided lesions scored normally in these four items of the CBS, but showed moderate to severe BRN in the vest. Hence, although the CBS is a highly sensitive behavioural measure of neglect, it may miss patients with rightsided BRN. Obviously the ideal diagnostic strategy for identifying patients with BRN might be a battery of differnt tests, including the CBS, the vest test and the Fluff test. This battery approach has yielded the highest sensitivity in the assessment of *visual* neglect (see last row in Table 7).

6.4.2. BRN in the vest test versus visual neglect

Many of the right brain damaged patients showed visual neglect (84%). Three patients (12%) with right brain lesions were unimpaired in the visual neglect tests but showed a clear BRN in the vest test. Four right brain damaged patients (16%) showed the opposite pattern (visual neglect but no BRN). For the left brain damaged patients 36% showed visual neglect. 40% of the left brain lesioned patients showed no visual neglect, but a BRN in the vest test (see also patient JO, Table 3). In contrast 28% of the patients with left sided lesions showed visual neglect but no BRN. This shows clearly that the vest test can detect BRN separately from other modalities of the neglect syndrome.

7. Summary and conclusions

7.1. Psychometric criteria and practical aspects of the vest test

In this study we showed that the vest test is a simple and sensitive test for the assessment of BRN. Performance takes only 5–10 minutes and patients with hemiparesis, apraxia or aphasia can also be assessed with this test as these deficits do not prevent proper execution of the test. Furthermore, it avoids the tactile stimulation of the patient's body surface and contains a *symmetrical* number of targets on both trunk halves – thus making it more comparable to visual scanning tasks frequently used to assess visual neglect [5].

In comparison to Bisiach's test of personal neglect and the Comb-and-razor-compact-test the vest test assesses body representational neglect via a manual body scanning procedure which requires knowledge about the shape, spatial layout and left-right-configuration of the front part of the patient's trunk. Furthermore, it is likely that an efficient manual search of the own body surface is facilitated by mechanisms subserving spatial memory for body locations (in the sense of distinguishing old from new locations). If this hypothesis is correct, deficits in body spatial working memory should covary with the degree of BRN.

The psychometric analyses show good to excellent results for reliability and validity when taking into account that we tested patients with *recent* brain damage and manifold associated neuropsychological deficits such as apraxia, aphasia, and attentional impairments. Furthermore, spontaneous recovery and medications are likely to affect especially retest-reliability and validity estimates in acute stroke patients due to fluctuations in performance. In sum, our results demonstrate the usefulness of this simple test for the measurement of BRN after brain damage which hopefully contributes to a better understanding of BRN and its relation to sensory and motor neglect. For the clinician it enables a better diagnosis and treatment of those patients suffering from spatial neglect. We suggest, that – as in visual neglect – the combination of a rating procedure (CBS) and one or two tests of BRN (vest test, fluff test) to form a battery might be the best strategy to detect and follow up BRN.

7.2. Patterns of dissociation

The five case examples show that BRN and visual neglect can be associated or dissociated. Furthermore, we

Table 7
Incidence (%) of contralateral neglect in different neglect tests in two patient samples: patients with unilateral leftsided stroke ($n = 25$) and patients with unilateral rightsided stroke ($n = 25$). As cut-off scores we adopted those described in Figs 1 and 2 for the vest test. Other cut-off scores were taken from the literature

Test variable	% BEYOND CUT-OFF or/and mean scores	
	Leftsided lesion	Rightsided lesion
Vest Test	48	80
Fluff Test (modified)	48	68
CBS – mild unilateral neglect	48	36
CBS – moderate unilateral neglect	4	56
CBS – severe unilateral neglect	4	8
CBS - (items for BRN- mild BRN)	28	20
CBS - (items for BRN- moderate BRN)	20	64
CBS - (items for BRN- severe BRN)	4	12
Line bisection, 20cm (visual)	33,3	68
Line bisection, 6 lines with 10cm	68	96
Cancellation (visual)	12	68
Reading	8	56
Copy	8	72
Visual neglect (all tests concluded)	36	84

found – surprisingly – that many right brain damaged patients typically show a *bilateral* deficit in the vest test, whereas left brain damaged patients seem to display either no neglect or a strictly rightsided, lateralized BRN. The reasons for this interesting finding are currently under intensive investigation in our group (for example differences in the search strategies between patients with or without BRN and between patients and normals; revisiting patterns etc.). First, the lesions could simply be larger or differently located in those patients with bilateral versus unilateral BRN. Second, a general arousal deficit [20,21] or spatially nonlateralized attentional impairments [14] could be responsible for such a pattern of results in the vest test. Third, deficient *manual* scan paths could be responsible – in analogy to the disordered *visual* scan paths [17] found in patients with neglect. Fourth, impaired spatial working memory for *body* positions (misjudging already searched pockets as new ones) in analogy to deficient *visuospatial* working memory in neglect patients might cause such a pattern of results [16]. Finally, a combination of these factors might be present in some patients with BRN.

7.3. Multiple mechanisms of body representation

Another interesting finging of our investigations is that BRN seems to be dissociable from apraxia. For the clinician, this means that apractic patients can properly perform the vest test with their ipsilesional hand despite the presence of limb apraxia. Furthermore, although preliminary, this result may indicate dissociable mechanisms of body representation: one mechanism is crucial for the imitation of hand movements and pantomime [12] whereas the other is probably involved in the cortical representation of the own trunk surface [4] and its spatial updating during manual search.

Acknowledgements

We are grateful to Prof. Preger, head of the Neurological Clinic Kipfenberg, Germany and Prof. König, head of the Neurological Clinic Bad Aibling, Germany for patient access and PD Dr. Ingo Keller, Bad Aibling, and DP Christiane Zeller for excellent organization and providing test facilities.

References

[1] P. Azouvi, P. Bartolomeo, J.-M. Beis, D. Perennou, P. Pradat-Diehl and M. Rousseaux. A battery of tests for the quantitative assessment of unilateral neglect, *Restor Neurol Neurosci* in press, (2006).

[2] P. Azouvi, F. Marchal, C. Samuel, L. Morin, C. Renard, A. Louis-Dreyfus, C. Jokic, L. Wiart, P. Pradat-Diehl, G. Deloche and C. Bergego, Functional consequences and awareness of unilateral neglect: Study of an evaluation scale, *Neuropsychological Rehabilitation* **6** (1996), 133–150.

[3] J.M. Beis, C. Keller, N. Morin, P. Bartolomeo, T. Bernati, S. Chokron, M. Leclercq, A. Louis-Dreyfus, F. Marchal, Y. Martin, D. Perennou, P. Pradat-Diehl, C. Prairial, G. Rode, M. Rousseaux, C. Samuel, E. Sieroff, L. Wiart and P. Azouvi, Right spatial neglect after left hemisphere stroke: qualitative and quantitative study, *Neurology* **63** (2004), 1600–1605.

[4] G. Berlucchi and S. Aglioti, The body in the brain: neural bases of corporeal awareness, *Trends Neurosci* **20** (1997), 560–564.

[5] A. Berti and F. Frassinetti, When far becomes near: remapping of space by tool use, *Journal of Cognitive Neuroscience* **12** (2000), 415–420.

[6] N. Beschin and I.H. Robertson, Personal versus extrapersonal neglect: a group study of their dissociation using a reliable clinical test, *Cortex* **33** (1997), 379–384.

[7] E. Bisiach, G. Vallar, D. Perani, C. Papagno and A. Berti, Unawareness of disease following lesions of the right hemispherre: anosognosia for hemiplegia and anosognosia for hemianopia, *Neuropsychologia* **24** (1986), 471–482.

[8] E. Bisiach and C. Luzzatti, Unilateral neglect of representational space, *Cortex* **14** (1978), 129–133.

[9] G. Cocchini, N. Beschin and M. Jehkonen, The Fluff test: a simple task to assess body representation neglect, *Neuropsychological Rehabilitation* **11** (2001), 17–31.

[10] S. Ferber and H.-O. Karnath, How to assess spatial neglect – line bisection or cancellation tasks? *J Clin Exp Neuropsychol* **23** (2001), 599–607.

[11] L. Gauthier, F. Dehaut and Y. Joanette, The bells test: a quantitative and qualitative test for visual neglect, *Int J of Clin Neuropsychol* **11** (1989), 49–54.

[12] G. Goldenberg, Defective imitation of gestures in patients with damage in the left or right hemispheres, *Journal of Neurology, Neurosurgery, and Psychiatry* **61** (1996), 176–180.

[13] W.L. Hays, *Statistics for the social sciences*, Holt, Rinehart and Winston, London, 1973.

[14] M. Husain and C. Rorden, Non-spatially lateralized mechanisms in hemispatial neglect, *Nature Neuroscience* **4** (2003), 26–36.

[15] H.-O. Karnath, A.D. Milner and G. Vallar, *The cognitive and neural bases of spatial neglect*, Oxford University Press, Oxford, 2002, pp. 1–401.

[16] P. Malhotra, H.R. Jager, A. Parton, R. Greenwood, E.D. Playlinebreak ford, M.M. Brown, J. Driver and M. Husain, Spatial working memory capacity in unilateral neglect, *Brain* **128** (2005), 424–435.

[17] S.K. Mannan, D.J. Mort, T.L. Hodgson, J. Driver, C. Kennard and M. Husain, Revisiting previously searched locations in visual neglect: role of right parietal and frontal lesions in misjudging old locations as new, *Journal of Cognitive Neuroscience* **17** (2005), 340–354.

[18] F. Pavani, M. Husain, E. Ladavas and J. Driver, Auditory deficits in visuospatial neglect patients, *Cortex* **40** (2004), 347–365.

[19] M.J. Riddoch and G.W. Humphreys, The effect of cueing on unilateral neglect, *Neuropsychologia* **21** (1983), 589–599.

[20] I.H. Robertson, Do we need the lateral in unilateral neglect? Spatially nonselective attention deficits in unilateral neglect and their implications for rehabilitation, *Neuroimage* **14** (2001), S85–S90.

[21] I.H. Robertson, J.B. Mattingley, C. Rorden and J. Driver, Phasic alerting of neglect patients overcomes their spatial deficit in visual awareness, *Nature* **395** (1998), 169–172.

[22] R. Sterzi, G. Bottini, M.G. Celani, E. Righetti, M. Lamassa, S. Ricci and G. Vallar, Hemianopia, hemianaestesia, and hemiplegia after right and left hemisphere damage. A hemispheric difference, *Journal of Neurology Neurosurgery and Psychiatry* **56** (1993), 308–310.

[23] S.P. Stone, B. Wilson, A. Wroot, P.W. Halligan, L.S. Lange and J.C. Marshall, The assessment of visuo-spatial neglect after acute stroke, *Journal of Neurology Neurosurgery and Psychiatry* **54** (1991), 345–350.

[24] B. Wilson, J. Cockburn and P. Halligan, Development of a behavioral test of visuospatial neglect, *Arch Phys Med Rehabil* **68** (1987), 98–102.

[25] P. Zoccolotti and A. Judica, Functional evaluation of hemineglect by means of a semistructured scale: personal extrapersonal differentiation, *Neuropsychological Rehabilitation* **1** (1991), 33–44.

Appendix

A Picture, protocol and figure of the vest test

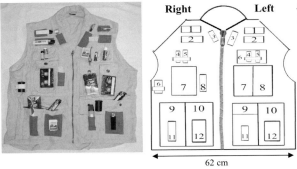

PROTOCOL

Time interval	30s	60s	90s	120s	150s	180s	210s	240s	270s	300s	330s	360s
left												
1. key												
2. bookmark												
3. Pen												
4. battery												
5. lipstick												
6. matchbox												
7. handkerchiefs												
8. cassette												
9. filmcan												
10. chocolatebar												
11. marker												
12. lighter												
right												
1. lighter												
2. marker												
3. key												
4. battery												
5. lipstick												
6. filmcan												
7. cassette												
8. bookmark												
9. handkerchiefs												
10. chocolatebar												
11. pen												
12. matchbox												

Sum	30s	60s	90s	120s	150s	180s	210s	240s	270s	300s	330s	360s
Left												
right												

Verbal instruction for nonaphasic patients:

"Now we put you a vest on. The vest has many pockets. In these pockets are objects. Please search all objects (blindfolded) *and place them into my hand. You do not have to name the objects, just find them! You do not have to search on the backside of your body. Use only the right hand* (for right brain damaged patients) */left hand* (for left brain damaged patients) *and give me a sign, when you believe that you are ready with your search."*

Instruction for aphasic patients

For aphasic patients we explained a little bit more in the practice trial before the test performance by learning by doing. The patient was instructed like the nonaphasic patients to search for an object, which was hidden in one pocket. If the patient did not understand the verbal instruction, the examiner put his hand to the relevant pocket and opened it with his hand. Then the object was put out of the pocket by guiding the patient's hand. After this procedure the trial was repeated. In our sample all aphasic patients understood the purpose of the test at the latest after the second practice trial.

Additional instructions for the user

Ensure that the front part of the vest is firmly attached to the subject's body. If the vest is too large for an individual, use one or several clips to tighten the cloth on the patient's back side.

Postural disorders and spatial neglect in stroke patients: A strong association

Dominic Pérennou
*Service de Rééducation Neurologique, CHU, INSERM ERM207 Motricité et plasticité, Centre de Médecine Physique & Réadaptation, 23 rue Gaffarel, BP 77908 F, 21079 Dijon cedex, France
Tel.: +33 380 293 371; Fax: +33 380 293 643; E-mail: dominic.perennou@chu-dijon.fr*

Received 10 January 2006
Revised 6 March 2006
Accepted 22 June 2006

Abstract. *Purpose*: In this paper we analyse the arguments for a strong association between spatial neglect and postural disorders and attempt to better understand the mechanisms which underlie that.
Methods: We first provide a general overview of the available tools for a rational assessment of postural control in a clinical context. We then analyse the arguments in favour of a close relationship, although not necessarily causal, between spatial neglect and: 1) body orientation with respect to gravity (including verticality perception i.e. the visual vertical, the haptic vertical, and the postural vertical); 2) body stabilisation with respect to the base of support; 3) posturographic features of stroke patients; 4) and finally their postural disability in daily life. This second part of the paper is based both on the literature review and on results of our current research.
Results: Neglect patients show a dramatic postural disability, due both to problems in body orientation with respect to gravity and to problems in body stabilisation. It might be that these problems are partly caused by a neglect phenomenon bearing on graviceptive (somaesthetic > vestibular) and visual information serving postural control. This could correspond to a kind of postural neglect involving both the bodily and nonbodily domains of spatial neglect. The existence of distorsion(s) in the body scheme are also probably involved, especially to explain the weight-bearing asymmetry in standing, and probably an impaired multisegmental postural coordination leading to an impaired body stabilisation.
Conclusion: The present paper explains why neglect patients show longer/worse recovery of postural-walking autonomy than other stroke patients.

Keywords: Spatial cognition, body scheme, subjective vertical, verticality perception, stabilisation, postural control, balance

1. Introduction

Three main functions can be attributed to postural control: regulate posture to counter gravity (orientation), provide a stable base for a subsequent action (stabilisation), and contribute to the construction of the different systems of spatial co-ordinates (spatial cognition). The interplay between body posture and spatial cognition has first been emphasised by Paillard [76], who postulated that the postural space co-ordinate system has the advantage of being physically anchored to the invariant direction of gravity which provides, at least on Earth, the unique absolute frame of reference. There is now much evidence that body posture influences the degree of spatial neglect [24,59,72,92,106]. Conversely much less is known about the influence of neglect on postural control in terms of balance. In order to better understand the association between postural disorders and spatial neglect after stroke, the present paper analyses the interplay between spatial cognition tackled in terms of spatial neglect, and postural control tackled both in terms of orientation with respect to gravity and stabilisation of the centre of mass.

2. Postural disorders after stroke: some landmarks

Since postural control involves most brain areas [51], many brain lesions may cause a perturbation of postural control, and postural disorders represent one of the most frequent disabilities after stroke. Their nature and their severity depend on the ability of undamaged brain areas to compensate, therefore on age [85] and premorbid status, as well as on lesion size [85,87] and location [19,34,54,57,73,77,87,118]. After a stroke, the ability to maintain or to change a position can be altered in the three basic postures : the lying, the sitting, and the standing posture. Consequently assessment of these critical postures is often standardised for clinical follow-up. One week after stroke, about 40% of patients *are not able to roll from supine to side lateral* [78]. On day-30 after stroke, only 60–70% of patients can perform this change of posture without any help [9], 20–25% with help [9], and the other 10–15% are still not able to roll from supine to side lateral, always more difficult toward the non affect side [9,78]. *The restoration of an independent sitting posture* being a key point for the patient autonomy, the sitting posture has long been one of the most frequently postures analysed after stroke. Up to 75–80% of patients keep or recover the ability to maintain an independent sitting posture for several minutes within the first month [9,91,105]. The Median time to recover the ability to sit independently one minute covaries with the size and site of the lesion: from 0 days for a lacunar or a posterior circulation infarct to 11 days (25th–75th percentile = 7–19.3 days) for a total anterior circulation infarct [108]. In stroke patients undergoing rehabilitation, the mean time to achieve independent sitting from admission is approximately 11 days [71]. This recovery is better or/shorter in patients with a left lesion than in those with a right lesion [16,85,119,120], especially those displaying spatial neglect [14,85,112]. We will further discuss this point later. One month after stroke onset, 40% of patients undergoing rehabilitation are able to stand independently for one minute, 40% are not able to stand at all, and the other 20% can stand with help [9]. The median time to recover the ability *to stand* 10 seconds covaries with the size and site of the lesion: 0 days for a lacunar infarct, 4 days for a posterior circulation infarct, and 44 days (25th–75th percentile = 38–57 days) for a total anterior circulation infarct [108].

These landmarks show how postural disorders constitute a primary disability in stroke patients, leading to a loss of autonomy and exposing patients to a risk of falling. The risk of falling is so high in the first weeks after stroke onset, that it must be considered as a significant problem in stroke rehabilitation. The incidence rate is about 1–2 falls per 100 patient-day of hospitalisation [38,75,116]. Falls occur mainly while transfers (active changes of posture) [53,75], and their number increases with age and depression [117]. Their risk is not linearly related to the number of impairments, individuals with heavy deficits being less mobile and therefore less exposed to hazardous activities than more independent patients [123]. After discharge in non-institutionalised individuals with long-standing stroke, the risk of falling is more than twice as high for patients with stroke than for elderly controls [41,55]. Although the detrimental role of spatial neglect and overall anosodiaphoria is suspected, it remains to show that spatial neglect and/or anosodiaphoria are independent factors increasing the risk of falling after a stroke.

3. Assessing postural disorders in neglect and no-neglect patients

Postural assessment of stroke patients has evolved in the last few years. Postural disability per se is now assessed, and distinguished from the assessment of other functions such as walking and the assessment of basic impairments such as range of motion, muscle power and sensory loss. This evolution in the assessment of stroke patients is associated to an improvement of the practical, quantitative properties of functional scales, including balance scales. By practical properties we mean good feasibility and specific meaning for the clinical team. Quantitative or metric properties include validity, reliability, internal consistency, lack of ceiling or floor effects, and ability to discriminate changes.

3.1. Ordinal scales

Generic balance scales such as the Berg Balance Scale (BBS) or the Functional Reach Test (FRT) are gradually making way for categorical scales whose psychometric characteristics are better in terms of validity, reproducibility, reliability, internal consistency, absence of threshold effect (floor or ceiling), and thus in their capacity to distinguish between or detect changes. Most of the scales put forward in recent years have benefited from a complete statistical validation procedure, which was not the case 15 years ago. We suggest that the scales may be classified as *"Rapid postural evalu-*

ation" done in around a minute at the patient's bedside and as *"complete postural evaluation"* carried out in 10–20 min in a rehabilitation room.

Rapid postural evaluations only investigate one aspect of postural impairment in order to describe and/or quantify a given behaviour, such as the inability to remain seated [105] or standing [15], to analyse a crucial point such as trunk control [27] or to detect lateropulsion and or pushing [56,64]. Balance in a sitting position or control of the trunk can also be assessed by using the corresponding items of more complete scales [40, 52]. These quick tests are perfectly suitable for an initial evaluation performed as soon as the patient arrives in the unit, and is medically stable enough to be tested. Most of them can be considered bedside tests. They provide a first impression about the prognosis and the severity of the impairment. For example, trunk control can easily be evaluated by asking the patient to roll over from dorsal decubitus to lateral decubitus and then to sit up. By using this type of scale it has been shown for example that evaluation of trunk control gives a relatively good indication of a patient's independence at discharge from the rehabilitation unit [36,42]. Although there is a growing interest in the understanding of the pushing behaviour, one of the most puzzling motor behaviour after stroke, it is noticeable than the *ad hoc* ordinal scales proposed to detect pushing [56,64] are subjective since the item "*resistance to passive correction*" which differentiate lateropulsion with pushing from lateropulsion without pushing is not objectively measured but just scored yes or no depending on a clinical impression. It is far to be certain that these scales have satisfactory psychometric properties, that could explain huge differences in the pushing prevalence between studies [28,58,64,80]. This subjectivity is a major drawback for the diagnosis and the quantification of such a complex trouble. Instead of these scales, the likely link between pushing and a tilt of the biological vertical used to organise postural control in these patients [56,86] argues for a more systematic assessment of verticality perception after stroke, based the three subjective verticals available in clinical practice: the visual vertical, the haptic or tactile vertical, and above all the postural vertical (see below).

Complete postural evaluation scales specifically devoted to stroke examine the patient in all of the principal postural situations in everyday life, by testing both the ability to maintain and change a given posture. The *postural assessment scale for stroke patients* or PASS [9] was the first complete evaluation score for balance specifically devoted to stroke patients. The PASS was designed to be useful for any stroke patient, whatever the severity of the handicap. It contains 12 items on 4 levels (from 0 to 3) which assess the postural abilities in increasingly difficult tasks with the patient lying, sitting and standing for a total score ranging from 0 to 36 (Table 1). As it comprises a protocol guide and a clearly defined scoring system, the PASS is an easy and relatively quick postural evaluation test; it takes less than 12 min. Compared to the measurement characteristics of the BBS or the balance section of the Fugl-Meyer, those of the PASS are satisfactory, in particular during the 3 months following the stroke [9,68]. The internal consistency and reproducibility are excellent. Postural impairment as measured by the PASS takes into account both postural orientation and stabilisation [9]. The PASS is particularly suitable for distinguishing between groups of patients [85], detecting change [9,68], and predicting recovery [52]. These qualities make the PASS an excellent tool in both clinical practice and research. Another tool, which is very similar to the PASS, has recently been proposed. The Postural Control and Balance for Stroke or PCBS [95] differs from the PASS in that there are more items, and that scores are not based on independence as in the (PASS), but on the assistance required. The first psychometric characteristics of the PCBS to be analysed have proved to be satisfactory. It has been suggested that the two intermediate levels of the PASS be combined [121]. The resulting loss of information would not diminish the reproducibility or the predictive validity of the scale. In terms of validation, the PASS, in its original form, has the merit of being advantageously compared to other scales by others than those who designed and validated it.

3.2. Chronometric assessment

Many ordinal balance scales check if a given patient is able to maintain a given posture during a given time. The results are then converted into item levels. Chronometric measurements of postural abilities can be also used, especially for assessing the ability to maintain standing posture, possibly with increasing difficulties according to the variation of the base of support (feet apart or together, sharpened Romberg also termed tandem stance because feet are placed in a heel-to-toe position, eventually single limb stance) and the sensory availability (at least eyes open and closed). Although often used as predictor of falls in elderly, these tests are often too difficult for hemiparetics, and in the end are not used for routine assessment of their balance

Table 1
Items of the postural assessment scale for stroke (PASS) and criteria for scoring [9]

Maintaining a posture
1. Sitting without support (*sitting on the edge of an 50 cm height examination table – a Bobath plane for instance – with the feet touching the floor*)
    0 = cannot sit
    1 = can sit with slight support, for example by one hand
    2 = can sit for more than 10 seconds without support
    3 = can sit for 5 minutes without support
2. Standing with support (*feet position free, no other constraints*)
    0 = cannot stand even with support
    1 = can stand with strong support of two persons
    2 = can stand with moderate support of one person
    3 = can stand with only one support of one hand
3. Standing without support (*feet position free, no other constraints*)
    0 = cannot stand without support
    1 = can stand without support for 10 seconds or leans heavily on one leg
    2 = can stand without support for 1 minute or stands slightly asymmetrically
    3 = can stand without support for more than 1 minute and at the same time perform arm movements above the shoulder level
4. Standing on non-paretic leg (*no other constraints*)
    0 = cannot stand on non-paretic leg
    1 = can stand on non-paretic leg for a few seconds
    2 = can stand on non-paretic leg for more than 5 seconds
    3 = can stand on non-paretic leg for more than 10 seconds
5. Standing on paretic leg (*no other constraints*)
    Same scoring as item 4

Changing posture
Scoring items 6–12 (*items 6 to 11 are to perform with a 50 cm height examination table, like a Bobath plane; items 10–12 are to perform without any support. No other constraints*). 0 = cannot perform the activity, 1 = can perform the activity with much help, 2 = can perform the activity with little help, 3 = can perform the activity without help.
6. Supine to affected side lateral
7. Supine to non-affected side lateral
8. Supine to sitting up on the edge of the bed
9. Sitting on the edge of the bed to supine
10. Sitting to standing up
11. Standing up to sitting down
12. Standing, picking up a pencil from the floor

disorders. However, they can be useful to detect impairments in patients who appear clinically to have adequate postural control [26]. As already mentioned, timed balance tests support the analysis of the sensory contribution to postural control, especially in erect stance. The sensory organisation balance test (SOT) is a posturography based test which evaluates somatosensory, visual and vestibular contribution to the maintaining of the upright posture [32,107]. Using a clinical variant of the SOT (the 'foam and dome' test; see Fig. 7 and below under 'Other assessment tools'), Di Fabio and Badke [33] analysed stance duration of hemiplegics required to stand with eyes open, eyes closed, or wearing a visual dome to produce inaccurate visual information, either on a hard flat floor or on a compliant foam surface. They found that visual deprivation or visual conflict conditions did not decrease the duration of the task when stance was performed on a stable surface, whereas stance duration was lower when patients stood on a compliant surface. Visual compensation was evident during the compliant-surface condition because stance duration showed the greatest reductions with eyes closed and with the visual dome. Di Fabio and Badke [33] concluded that the ability of stroke patients to integrate somatosensory information from the lower extremities is compromised. Such a paradigm could be very interesting to further analyse the postural imbalance of neglect patients.

3.3. *The subjective verticals*

To know if the postural imbalance of certain patients is in part due to an orientation problem with respect to gravity, one simply has to measure their perception of the vertical. Though research laboratories have been measuring perception of the vertical for a long time [67], clinical interest in these measurements is much more recent, dating back to the 1990s for vestibular [5,13,17,111] and neurological diseases [19,35,56, 60,83,84,103,125].

Several sources of information about verticality can be distinguished. Firstly the direction of gravity, which constitutes the physical vertical and is the only absolute co-ordinate. Most living organisms exert responses against this force. The nature of these responses characterises the antigravitational behaviour of species. The orientation of the body relative to the ambient gravito-inertial force constitutes the *behavioural vertical* [89] that is the expression of an implicit representation of verticality used to control balance. In upright humans, the *behavioural vertical* usually corresponds to the direction of the longitudinal body axis. It can be measured by movement analysis systems. It is also possible to estimate the direction of the longitudinal body axis by means of a force platform, allowing an indirect assessment of body orientation in a standing subject [50, 126]. However, body orientation with respect to gravity can be estimated by the projection of the centre of mass onto the ground only when the body is aligned along the gravitational force. It is far from being the case when subjects must ensure a dynamic balance, or when there is an obvious asymmetry of weight-bearing as in hemiplegics. This is why it has been proposed to estimate the behavioural vertical (active postural vertical) using a rocking chair paradigm (Fig. 1). With this paradigm, it is possible to measure the mean orientation of the supporting surface and so to estimate the direction of the trunk in the roll plane [83,84]. The relevance of this type of measurement is however limited by the possible covariation between postural orientation and stability (that it is only possible to dissociate in microgravity conditions), and also by the fact that the most severely impaired patients are not able to perform the task. The *behavioural vertical* must be distinguished from the explicit perceptions of verticality, namely the *visual vertical*, the *haptic (tactile) vertical* and the *postural vertical*. These modality-related perceptions of verticality usually provide convenient and complementary ways of drawing inferences about the sense of verticality in a given individual. To assess the *visual vertical*, the subject in darkness is asked to visually adjust a luminous rod to the estimated vertical direction (Fig. 2a). This assessment is normally very precise with errors of less than one degree [67]. To assess the *haptic vertical*, the subject in darkness is asked to set a rotating bar to vertical using his tactile sense (Fig. 2b). Again this adjustment is precise, although subject to a possible directional hand-side effect [8]. For the assessment of the *postural vertical* [122], the subject seated on a tilting chair in darkness is asked to set himself to vertical (Fig. 2c). Normally with practice this *body adjustment* is remarkably accurate [25,67,109,122]. The subjective visual vertical has widely been assessed in stroke patients [3,10,12,19,22,31,35,61,113,114,125]. Although more recently applied in stroke patients, the measurement of the subjective haptic vertical [21,43, 60] and that of the subjective postural vertical [2,56, 84,89] are promising. Indeed, correlation between VV and postural abilities in daily life are not so strong as expected [60,89]. Since VV is a poorer predictor of postural abilities than HV or PV [89], and because dissociation can occur between VV and PV or HV [13, 21,56,90], VV cannot be used in isolation as a guide to rehabilitation in stroke patients [89]. Therefore, there is an increasing demand for routine measurement of the postural vertical in neurorehabilitation context. Fly simulators or motorised gimbal used in research laboratories are not suitable for stroke patients so Gresty, Pérennou, and Bronstein designed a device suited for the measurement of the postural vertical in stroke patients [89,90]. Patients are strapped into a sitting position to a framework within a wheel (Fig. 3), with the head, trunk and lower limbs aligned in an upright position. In order to determine the postural vertical, the subject is tilted to a given position to either side of the vertical. The wheel is then rolled towards the other side until the patient reports to have reached an upright position. The wheel is manually turned as gently and steadily as possible at a relatively low velocity. Ten unpredictable trials are performed, 5 from left to right, and 5 from right to left, the mean value yielding the postural vertical. Only patients who display a supramodal bias in the perception of vertical (tilt in VV, HV and also PV) are suspected to have a high order disruption in the construction of the vertical, i.e. a tilted representation of the vertical [89,90]. One can assume that they actively adjust their erect sitting or standing posture to this tilted subjective vertical. According to this view, disorders of balance encountered by stroke patients should be partly due to a bias in the representation of the verticality, severe bias being incompatible with the maintenance of an autonomous erect posture. Most often these patients have a hemisphere lesion, patients with brain stem lesion having a net VV tilt, with PV and HV normal or slightly tilted. There are very often dissociation between VV, HV and PV [4,21,56]. The metrological characteristics for these should be specified and compared as soon as possible, particularly in terms of reproducibility and clinical relevance [81].

3.4. Posturography

Posturography (also termed stabilometry) is the measurement of postural body sway (Fig. 4). It is usually

Rocking platform paradigm

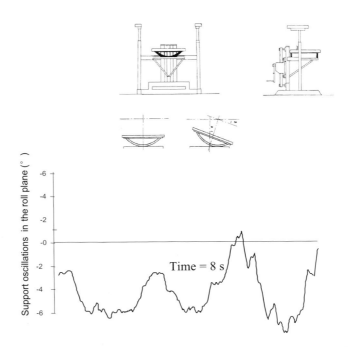

Fig. 1. Rocking platform (chair) paradigm adapted for analysing dynamic lateral balance of neurological patients in a sitting posture. Patients seat on a rigid plane support mounted on a seesaw allowing lateral oscillations. They are asked to maintain an upright sitting posture as still as possible while looking straight ahead and fixing a target for 8 seconds. During the trials their hands were crossed, resting on the thighs. Safety armrests are disposed at the sides to prevent falls. The height of the sitting support is adjustable so that the subject's legs hang freely. To perform the task, patients typically execute continual corrective movements with an overall oscillatory characteristic. Most of stroke patients become able to perform this dynamic postural task within the two or three months after the stroke onset. In stroke patients this model has at least four advantages. Firstly, because the sitting posture is the first posture to be restored, paradigms based upon sitting posture are those which are the most suited to an early analysis of balance after a stroke. Secondly, because this task is a dynamic balance task, it increases the sensory contribution to body balance, and subsequently is helpful in revealing troubles in the integration of sensory inputs. Moreover, since the axis of rotation did not pass through the supporting surface, the movements of the rocking platform combined rotations around an anterior-posterior axis and lateral translations. Consequently, no absolute stable reference frame is available that might increase the contribution of internal models to succeeding in performing the task. Thirdly, balancing on a rocking platform is a self-perturbed and self-regulated dynamic task, the subject himself being responsible both for his imbalance and active correction. While the subject keeps the same location inside the room, this ecological model allows the analysis of natural strategies of equilibrium, by simultaneously measuring segmental orientation and stability. Fourthly, challenging (stressing) balance laterally is interesting given that many stroke patients show an attentional/representational spatial gradient in the frontal plane. Kinematics of body movements in roll can be analysed by means of an automatic optical TV image processor [83]. More simply the support oscillations with respect to the horizontal plane may be recorded using an accelerometer used as an inclinometer [84,88]. The control of body tilt is termed 'orientation'. The control of the oscillations is termed 'stabilisation'. The raw data show both a left tilt and large oscillations.

recorded by force platform(s), measuring the successive positions of the centre of foot pressure inside the base of support during a given period of time. The centre of pressure is also the application point of the resultant upward force exerted by the support surface on the feet in reaction to gravity. Although many postures can be quantified using posturography (in particular the ability to maintain a short single limb stance), clinical posturography usually serves to characterise and quantify bipedal erect stance. In standing still, the body is normally kept upright and the centre of mass projects over the base of support provided by the two feet. In the sagittal axis the base of support is determined by foot length. In the lateral axis the base of support is defined by the distance between the outside edges of the feet. Posturographic assessment can be made by one or two force platforms. The use of a single force platform yields information about positions and displacements of the centre of pressure (metric data) together with information about rhythmic aspects of postural sways. To evaluate postural instability, one can compute either the length of the sway path (mm), the

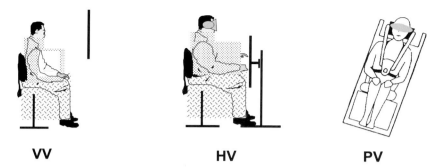

Fig. 2. Three modalities to measure verticality perception: the visual vertical (VV), the haptic vertical (HV) and the postural vertical (PV).

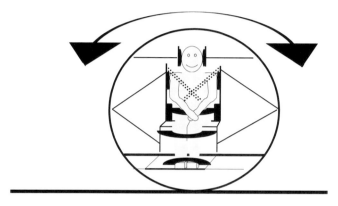

Fig. 3. Schematic view of the apparatus (wheel) designed by Gresty, Pérennou and Bronstein for measuring the subjective postural vertical in a clinical context.

stabilogram area (mm^2), or the dispersion of the centre of pressure co-ordinates on the lateral and sagittal axes during a given time. If the instruction is to stand still, one assumes that the more the body sways, the less stable the person is. In addition to this, the use of two force platforms yields direct information about the symmetry of weight-bearing, expressed in percentage of body weight loaded on each foot. This is especially relevant in hemiplegics. The term "static posturography" refers to the ability to maintain balance on a fixed platform whereas "dynamic posturography" measures postural reactions in response to a translation/rotation of the support. This latter technique being may be of value for analysing postural reflexes [74], dizzy patients or for specific retraining purposes, but only static posturography will be considered in this section.

Static posturography is now often used in stroke patients. Three main patterns may be observed (Fig. 5): – 1) A weight-bearing asymmetry, with more weight on the non paretic leg. With a single platform, a lateral shift of the centre of pressure toward the non paretic leg is observed. This behaviour is due to biomechanical and cognitive impairments, and is partly the result of a compensatory strategy. – 2) An increase of the centre of pressure displacements, both in sagittal and lateral axes. These large body sways reflect postural instability which may result from orthopaedic, sensory-motor and cognitive impairments. 3) A small limit of stability beyond which the centre of pressure cannot move further without exposing the person to a loss of balance. This represents the inability to control a stressed equilibrium system or an impaired co-ordination between posture and movement [70]. In stroke patients posturography seems especially interesting to monitor the postural recovery [29].

4. Postural disorders and spatial neglect: A strong association

It has long been known that the postural recovery is worse after right hemispheric strokes than after left hemispheric strokes, especially in patients displaying spatial neglect. This disadvantage concerns the standing posture [49,65,85,97,102], the sitting posture [16, 85,88,119], and the lying posture as well [85]. It leads

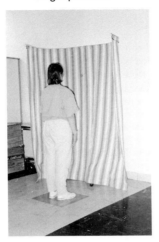
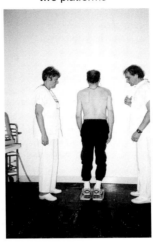

Fig. 4. Posturographic assessment can be made by one or two force platforms. The use of a single force platform (here integrated in the ground to facilitate assessments in disabled people) yields information about positions and displacements of the centre of pressure (metric data) together with information about rhythmic aspects of postural sways. In addition to these indices, the use of two force platforms yields direct information about the symmetry of weight-bearing, expressed in percentage of body weight loaded on each foot. This is especially relevant in neglect patients who underuse the paretic leg as compared to no-neglect patients.

to a longer/worse recovery of the autonomous gait in left hemiplegics [23,48] and more generally of many other motor tasks involving postural control [11,30]. We will successively consider the clues for an association between spatial neglect and troubles in body orientation with respect to gravity (the subjective verticals), between spatial neglect and troubles in body stabilisation, between spatial neglect and some posturographic features of patients, and overall between spatial neglect and the more general postural disability in daily life.

4.1. Association between a tilted biological vertical and spatial neglect

4.1.1. What are the evidences?

The relative contribution of each cerebral hemisphere to actively orientate the body against gravity cannot be analysed by brain imaging. Indeed, this technique imposes restraints on head movements that is not easily compatible with a balance task. Therefore, behavioural studies of postural controlling are still the best way of analysing the possible association between spatial neglect and a tilt in the behavioural vertical (*or active postural vertical*). We have unpublished data showing a similar body orientation with respect to gravity for left and right stroke patients submitted to the rocking platform paradigm in sitting (Fig. 6). This absence of difference between the active body orientation of LBD and RBD with respect to gravity confirms our previous study which revealed for the first time the existence of a contralesional bias in the active postural vertical (behavioural postural) of some patients with a hemisphere stroke, specially those showing spatial neglect [84]. These findings are congruent with studies concerning verticality perception after stroke. Indeed, no significant difference has been found between left and right hemisphere strokes for the subjective visual vertical [19,22,60] or the subjective haptic vertical [60]. However, among studies having analysed the possible relationship between spatial neglect and one of the three modalities of the subjective vertical, all [43,60,61,83,84,104,125] but two [56,63] found that spatial neglect magnified the contralesional tilt of subjective vertical. This finding has been reported for the subjective visual vertical [61,104,125], the subjective haptic vertical [43,60] and also for the behavioural vertical [83,84] and postural vertical [90].

4.1.2. How to interpret these findings?

Spatial neglect is a behaviour which refers to a lateral axis whereas body orientation with respect to gravity refers to a vertical axis: how could a deficit expressed on a vertical axis could be linked to a deficit expressed on a lateral axis? We put forward three interpretations. *In the first*, a given lesion perturbs two distinct but close one from the other neural networks,

CP mean position and oscillations

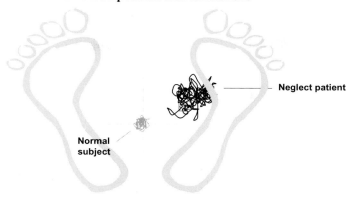

Fig. 5. Static posturography in a neglect patient showing a rightward shift of the centre of pressure, and big postural oscillations.

which code, one for spatial information referring to a lateral axis, the other for spatial information referring to a vertical axis. In that case, a same lesion induces two specific deficits which are merely associated due to the anatomical extension of the lesion. This interpretation is plausible since most neglect patients have a quite large lesion whereas the evidence from monkey physiology shows that even closely neighbouring areas of the parietal lobe are involved in subtly different functions, albeit according to similar computational principles [94]. *The second interpretation* implies that some networks might have the competency to process spatial information in three dimensions. If a lesion overlaps the area of this neural network, it may disrupt the processing of the multidimensional spatial information and thus may induce both lateral neglect and biased verticality. These two scenarios suggested by Kerkhoff and Zoelch [60] can be described as *associative*. *The third interpretation* which only concerns verticality construction from vestibular and/or somaesthetic information is rather *causative*. As already mentioned, an intact somaesthetic information is crucial for the construction of the *postural vertical* [2,20] and also for the construction of the *behavioural vertical* [83, 84]. This means that the brain compares the graviceptive information originated in the left hemibody to that originated in the right hemibody with a view to computing a resulting idiotropic vector which determines the subjective direction of verticality. In the case of spatial neglect, it might be that the graviceptive information normally provided by the left hemibody is not correctly integrated, thus inducing a systematic error in the co-ordinate system coding with respect to the vertical. It has been shown that the error made by neglect patients when bisecting a line in supine position (which decreases the gravitational information from the otolith organs) or when sitting up a visuo-tactile vertical was smaller as that made in erect position [92,104]. This suggests that, in patients with neglect, gravitational information is processed in a non-symmetrical fashion, with a rightward bias towards the side of the lesion. These studies also argue in favour of a strong association between the processing of lateral and vertical spatial information. In Fig. 7, the pelvis and not the head was found misoriented. This reflects an asymmetric integration of the somaesthetic graviceptive information originated in the pelvis, and a more symmetric integration of the otolithic cues. This confirms a previous study [83] and argues for a disruption at a high order level in the processing of somaesthetic gravitational information, which may be *graviceptive neglect* [83].

4.2. Impaired postural stabilisation and spatial neglect

4.2.1. What are the evidences?

The rocking platform paradigm allows to analyse simultaneously body orientation and body stabilisation. We used this paradigm to analyse both postural orientation [83,84] and stabilisation [88] in normal subjects and stroke patients with or without spatial neglect. Regarding postural stabilisation we hypothesised that neglect patients had a worse postural stability as compared to non-neglect patients and normals, and also latent postural capacities which could be unmasked by an appropriate somatosensory manipulation. We used TENS applied on the contralesional side of the neck during the postural task. Subjects were informed that we compared two intensities of stimulation and that they may or may not feel any sensation. An effec-

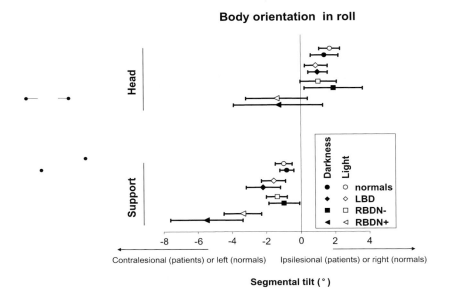

Fig. 6. Head and pelvic orientation with respect to horizontal of 35 subjects performing the rocking platform paradigm in sitting: 8 healthy subjects, 12 patients with a right stroke without neglect, 8 patients with a left stroke without neglect (LBD), and 7 patients with a left stroke with neglect. (LBD N+). With a view to comparing postural orientation with respect to the side of the lesion, data signs were transformed so that a negative angle indicated a contralesional tilt whereas a positive angle indicated an ipsilesional tilt. In controls, a negative angle corresponded to a leftward tilt. Data are in the form mean ± standard error. Vision did not contributed to body orientation with respect to gravity. The head and pelvic orientations were opposite to one another, presumably to facilitate an active maintenance of upright posture. Head orientation did not differ between groups and remained close to the horizontal plane. This meant that, in spite of a hemispheric lesion, vestibular information is able to orient the head correctly. Regardless of the visual condition, pelvic orientation was biased in RBDN+ that might reflect an underintegration of the somaesthetic graviception originated in the left hemibody (graviceptive neglect). RBDN- and LBD behaved similarly, which indicated that both hemispheres are competent to orient the body against gravity.

tive stimulation (intensity corresponding to the threshold of perception, TENS+) was compared to a placebo stimulation (0.01 × threshold of perception, TENS−). Postural performance in each trial was monitored using two criteria: the number of aborted trials due to loss of balance and the angular dispersion of the support oscillations in roll. This latter, which increased with body instability, was defined as 2 standard deviations of the angular distribution. Patients showing neglect displayed pronounced postural instability as compared to other patients and normals. While their dramatic postural instability was spectacularly and systematically reduced with TENS, no effect was observed in patients without neglect (Fig. 7).

It has long been known that vision is a major determinant in balance control [37,99]. Any movement of the body gives rise to an optic flow field at the eye, which affords information about the oscillations of the body relative to the environment [66]. This optic flow is used in postural stabilisation which consists in minimising body oscillations around a given orientation. Interestingly, a recent paper by Yelnik et al. [124] reported that 2 patients with spatial neglect submitted to an optokinetic stimulation during a postural task were resistant to this perturbation. This finding suggest that visual information subserving postural stabilisation could be neglected in patients with spatial neglect. To quantify the use of the optic flow in reducing the amount of sway of normals and stroke patients performing a dynamic postural task on a rocking platform with or without vision, we computed their visual gain using the formula proposed by Lacour et al. [62]. The visual gain was 25% in normals meaning that they were 25% more stable with eyes open in daylight than with eyes closed in darkness. As for patients, the visual gain in stability was lower in those with hemianopia than in others that corroborated several experimental and clinical studies [1,6,79,100,110]. We found an interaction between hemianopia and visual neglect factors. In fact, neglect patients without hemianopia did not use visual information for stabilising the body as well as they should have. To the best of our knowledge, this is the first demonstration that visual information can be neglected in the control of postural stability, exposing patients to postural impairment.

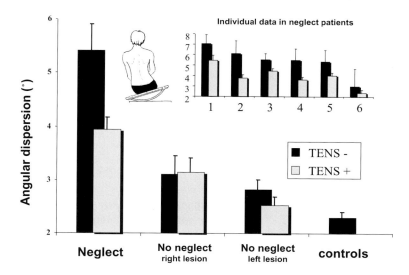

Fig. 7. Body stabilisation in controls, neglect patients, and patients without neglect performing the rocking platform paradigm in sitting. The data represent the mean value ± s.e.m of the support angular dispersions. Firstly can be noted, a greater postural imbalance in patients showing neglect than in others. Secondly, patients showing neglect were spectacularly improved by TENS (27% on average) whereas no significant change was induced in other patients. Thirdly, individual behaviour in response to TENS attests that improvement in body stability was systematic in neglect patients.

4.2.2. How to interpret these findings

The "postural body scheme" plays a crucial role in postural stabilisation [47]. This concept incorporates body geometry and orientation as well the interface between bodily and non-bodily spaces and body dynamics [69]. Spatial neglect, often associated with a disruption of, or failure to attend to, the body scheme represents an interesting way to analyse cognitive aspects of postural control. Currently, rather than a concept of a unitary representation of egocentric space, the concept of multiple representations of space appears more convenient to account for numerous disorders involving spatial cognition. Stabilising the body consists of regulating the position of body segments, either with respect to each other, or to external support or to absolute space. One may assume that this function relies on multisegmental body representations (for instance eye-head, head-shoulders, shoulders-pelvis, pelvis-lower legs, feet-supporting surface). The transformation of the co-ordinates of these multisegmental body representations could be vulnerable in patients with neglect [93]. The postural instability of neglect patients could partly result from difficulty in the multisegmental postural co-ordination process [88]. This concept could explain why neglect patients display postural instability whatever the postural task considered [85].

TENS activates afferent nerve fibers, which convey stimuli to the contralateral hemisphere. The study by Pérennou et al. [88] suggests that TENS applied to the neck facilitates the reorganisation and/or improves the functioning of the neural network including the polymodal sensory area. This leads to an improvement in the regulation of positions of head and trunk, either with respect to each other, or to external support, or absolute space.

The sustained artificial TENS stimulation delivered somatotopically at the neck level could thus be active through a transient mechanism of somatosensory substitution, based on the activation of undamaged parts of the neural network underlying multisensory integration. Due to the technical advantages of TENS including its portability and prolonged duration of stimulation, we have suggested that this technique could perhaps be used as a sensory prosthesis [88]. However, as in most studies analysing the effects induced by sensory manipulations in brain-damaged patients, the number of patients with neglect was quite small in that study, and the possible clinical interest of TENS for restoring body balance in neglect patients will need to be confirmed by studies carried out on larger groups of patients.

The underuse of the visual information to stabilise the body in neglect patients does not necessarily mean that optic flow is itself neglected. In the paradigm used, subjects had to look straight ahead at a fixation point placed at gaze level on a visual pattern. This procedure was aimed at optimising the capture of visual information from surroundings, the contribution

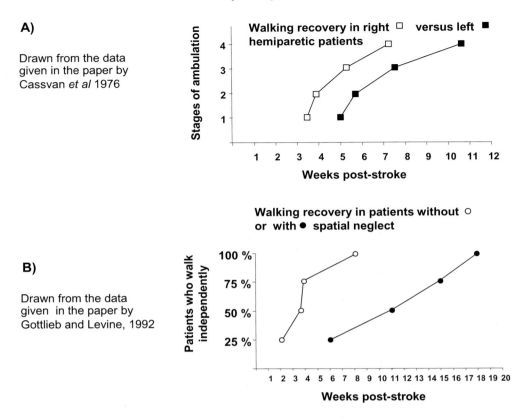

Fig. 8. Comparison of the walking recovery between left and right stroke (A, Cassvan et al 1976) and between neglect and no-neglect patients (B, Gottlieb and Levine 1992).

Table 2
Correlation between the postural impairment in daily life on D30 after stroke onset (assessed using the PASS) and clinical deficits of 70 patients consecutively admitted in a neurorehab ward after a first hemisphere stroke [9]

Clinical measures	Pearson coefficients
Motricity – upper limb	$0.63; p = 10^{-6}$
Motricity – lower limb	$0.78; p < 10^{-6}$
Spatial neglect. omissions at the star cancellation test	$-0.53; p < 10^{-4}$
Sensitiveness – upper limb Semmes-Weinstein aesthesiometer	$-0.42; p = 0.002$
Sensitiveness – lower limb Semmes-Weinstein aesthesiometer	$-0.45; p < 10^{-3}$
Spasticity – upper limb Ashworth scale	$-0.14; p = 0.31$
Spasticity – lower limb Ashworth scale	$-0.14; p = 0.30$

of which to postural stability being notably enhanced by motion parallax [46]. To be optimised, this capture requires a voluntary anchoring of attention to the fixation point. Inattention to surroundings is the rule in neglect patients, with a coexistence of a spatial attentional bias and of a nonspatially lateralised loss of attentional capacity [96]. Regarding postural control, this nonspecific inattention to surroundings may translate into an impairment in the use of an additional allocentric referential to reduce the instability of the whole body. Measurements of eye movements during a balance task should help to test this speculation.

4.3. Posturographic features of neglect patients

Several papers report that patients with spatial neglect standing on posturographic force-platform(s) show a greater amount of sway and/or a greater weight bearing asymmetry than others [18,29,65,102]. The amount of sway reflects the postural instability, whereas the weight-bearing asymmetry is more complex [82], and less understood, although known for a while and a major focus in stroke rehabilitation [44]. The degree of weight-bearing asymmetry during quiet stance covaried with muscular weakness [101], the use of the nonparetic leg being perhaps partly favoured for safety and speed reasons thus resulting in 'disuse' of the paretic limb [39]. The influence of spatial neglect on the posturographic features of stroke patients may also be interpreted by referring to the existence of distortion in the co-ordinates used to distribute loading over the two legs while standing. According to Rode et al. [97], like the midsagittal plane representation, 'the postural reference' could be shifted toward the lesion in some stroke patients, explaining the weight bearing asymmetry. The fact that appropriate sensory manipulations such as vestibular stimulation or prism adaptation known to reduce neglect signs also reduce the asymmetric weight bearing asymmetry of standing stroke patients [98,115] strengthens the idea that it could be a postural signature of spatial neglect, especially of the body-neglect.

4.4. Spatial neglect and postural disorders in daily life

Both body orientation with respect to gravity and stabilisation of the centre of mass are perturbed in stroke patients. Taken together these two impairments explain why neglect patients show such a dramatic postural imbalance as compared to other stroke patients. In patients subjected to the rocking platform paradigm the *overall postural performance* takes into account the number of aborted trials as well as orientation and stabilisation indices in successful trials. In order to grade the influences of weakness, spasticity, sensory loss, spatial neglect, and hemianopia on the overall postural behaviour of 27 stroke patients submitted to the rocking platform paradigm, we performed a variable selection. The variable for explanation combined the *number of missed trials* due to balance loss together with *stability* and *orientation* of both the head and pelvis. Spatial neglect assessed by the behavioural CB scale [7] was the key factor, accounting for 59% of the postural behaviour with vision, and 74% without vision. These results confirm the strong association, not necessarily causal, between spatial neglect and postural disorders. Similar results are also found when postural disorders are assessed using a more ecological tool as the PASS (Table 2), motor weakness and spatial neglect representing the two best variables accounting for postural disorders in the lying, sitting and standing positions. A satisfactory postural control is required for walking, consequently walking recovery is slower in patients with a right stroke [23], or in those showing neglect [45] (Fig. 8).

5. Conclusion

Because they are both misoriented and unstable, patients with spatial neglect show a severe postural disability. These two postural impairments could be partly caused by a neglect phenomenon bearing on the somaesthetic and at a lower degree vestibular graviception, and also on the visual information serving body stabilisation through an exocentric frame of reference. This could correspond to a kind of postural neglect involving both the bodily and nonbodily domains of spatial neglect. The existence of distorsion(s) in the body scheme are also involved, especially to explain the weight-bearing asymmetry in standing, and more generally an impaired multisegmental postural coordination which leads to an impaired body stabilisation. Taken together these mechanisms explain why neglect patients show longer/worse recovery of postural-walking autonomy than other stroke patients.

References

[1] B. Amblard and A. Carblanc, Role of foveal and peripheral visual information in maintenance of postural equilibrium in man, *Percept Mot Skills* **51** (1980), 903–912.

[2] D. Anastasopoulos, A. Bronstein, T. Haslwanter, M. Fetter and J. Dichgans, The role of somatosensory input for the perception of verticality, *Ann N Y Acad Sci* **871** (1999), 379–383.

[3] D. Anastasopoulos and A.M. Bronstein, A case of thalamic syndrome: somatosensory influences on visual orientation, *J Neurol Neurosurg Psychiatry* **67** (1999), 390–394.

[4] D. Anastasopoulos, T. Haslwanter, A. Bronstein, M. Fetter and J. Dichgans, Dissociation between the perception of body verticality and the visual vertical in acute peripheral vestibular disorder in humans, *Neurosci Lett* **233** (1997), 151–153.

[5] M. Aoki, Y. Ito, P. Burchill, G.B. Brookes and M.A. Gresty, Tilted perception of the subjective upright in unilateral loss of vestibular function, *Am J Otol* **20** (1999), 741–747.

[6] C. Assaiante, A.R. Marchand and B. Amblard, Discrete visual samples may control locomotor equilibrium and foot positioning in man, *J Mot Behav* **21** (1989), 72–91.

[7] P. Azouvi, S. Olivier, G. de Montety, C. Samuel, A. Louis-Dreyfus and L. Tesio, Behavioral assessment of unilateral neglect: study of the psychometric properties of the Catherine Bergego Scale, *Arch Phys Med Rehabil* **84** (2003), 51–57.

[8] M. Bauermeister, H. Werner and S. Wapner, The effect of body tilt on tactual-kinesthetic perception of verticality, *Am J Psychol* **77** (1964), 451–456.

[9] C. Benaim, D.A. Pérennou, J. Villy, M. Rousseaux and J. Pélissier, Validation of a standardized assessment of postural control in stroke patient: the PASS, *Stroke* **30** (1999), 1862–1868.

[10] B. Bender and H.L. Teuber, Spatial organization of visual perception following injury to the brain, *Arch Neurol Psych* **58** (1948), 721–739 et 39–62.

[11] B. Bernspng and A.G. Fisher, Differences between persons with right or left cerebral vascular accident on the assessment of motor and process skills, *Arch Phys Med Rehabil* **76** (1995), 1144–1151.

[12] H. Birch, F. Proctor, M. Bortner and M. Lowenthal, Perception in hemiplegia: I. Judgment of vertical and horizontal

[13] A.R. Bisdorff, C.J. Wolsley, D. Anastasopoulos, A.M. Bronstein and M.A. Gresty, The perception of body verticality (subjective postural vertical) in peripheral and central vestibular disorders, *Brain* **119** (1996), 1523–1534.

by hemiplegic patients, *Arch Phys Med Rehabil* **41** (1960), 19–27.

[14] R. Bohannon, A. Cook, P. Larkin, W. Dubuc, M. Smith and M.E.A. Horton, The listing phenomenon of hemiplegic patients. *Neurology report* **10** (1986), 43–44.

[15] R. Bohannon, S. Walsh and M. Joseph, Ordinal and timed balance measurements: reliability and validity in patients with stroke, *Clin Rehabil* **7** (1993), 9–13.

[16] R.W. Bohannon, M.B. Smith and P.A. Larkin, Relationship between independent sitting balance and side of hemiparesis, *Phys Ther* **66** (1986), 944–945.

[17] A. Bohmer and J. Rickenmann, The subjective visual vertical as a clinical parameter of vestibular function in peripheral vestibular diseases, *J Vestib Res* **5** (1995), 35–45.

[18] I.V. Bonan, F.M. Colle, J.P. Guichard, E. Vicaut, M. Eisenfisz, P. Tran Ba Huy and A.P. Yelnik, Reliance on visual information after stroke. Part I: Balance on dynamic posturography, *Arch Phys Med Rehabil* **85** (2004), 268–273.

[19] T. Brandt, M. Dieterich and A. Danek, Vestibular cortex lesions affect the perception of verticality, *Ann Neurol* **35** (1994), 403–412.

[20] A.M. Bronstein, The interaction of otolith and proprioceptive information in the perception of verticality. The effects of labyrinthine and CNS disease, *Ann N Y Acad Sci* **871** (1999), 324–333.

[21] A.M. Bronstein, D.A. Perennou, M. Guerraz, D. Playford and P. Rudge, Dissociation of visual and haptic vertical in two patients with vestibular nuclear lesions, *Neurology* **61** (2003), 1260–1262.

[22] J.H. Bruell, M. Peszcznski and G.W. Albee, Disturbance of perception of verticality in patients with hemiplegia. A preliminary report, *Arch Phys Med Rehabil* **37** (1956), 677–679.

[23] A. Cassvan, P.L. Ross, P.R. Dyer and L. Zane, Lateralization in stroke syndromes as a factor in ambulation, *Arch Phys Med Rehabil* **57** (1976), 583–587.

[24] S. Chokron and M. Imbert, Variations of the egocentric reference among normal subjects and a patient with unilateral neglect, *Neuropsychologia* **33** (1995), 703–711.

[25] B. Clark and A. Graybiel, Perception of the postural vertical in normals and subjects with labyrinthine defects, *J Exp Psychol* **65** (1963), 490–494.

[26] F.M. Collen, The measurement of standing balance after stroke, *Physiotherapy Theory and Practice* **11** (1995), 109–118.

[27] C. Collin and D. Wade, Assessing motor impairment after stroke: a pilot reliability study, *J Neurol Neurosurg Psychiatry* **53** (1990), 576–579.

[28] C.J. Danells, S.E. Black, D.J. Gladstone and W.E. McIlroy, Poststroke pushing: natural history and relationship to motor and functional recovery, *Stroke* **35** (2004), 2873–2878.

[29] M. de Haart, A.C. Geurts, S.C. Huidekoper, L. Fasotti and J. Van Limbeek, Recovery of standing balance in postacute stroke patients: a rehabilitation cohort study, *Arch Phys Med Rehabil* **85** (2004), 886–895.

[30] G. Denes, C. Semenza, E. Stoppa and A. Lis, Unilateral spatial neglect and recovery from hemiplegia: a follow-up study, *Brain* **105** (1982), 543–552.

[31] E. Derenzi, P. Faglioni and G. Scotti, Judgement of spatial orientation in patients with focal brain damage, *J Neurol Neurosurg Psychiatry* **34** (1971), 489–495.

[32] R. Di Fabio and M. Badke, Relationship of sensory organization to balance function in patients with hemiplegia, *Phys Ther* **70** (1990), 542–548.

[33] R. Di Fabio and M. Badke, Stance duration under sensory conflict conditions in patients with hemiplegia, *Arch Phys Med Rehabil* **72** (1991), 292–295.

[34] J. Dichgans and M. Fetter, Compartmentalized cerebellar functions upon the stabilization of body posture, *Rev Neurol Paris* **149** (1993), 654–664.

[35] M. Dieterich and T. Brandt, Wallenberg's syndrome: lateropulsion, cyclorotation, and subjective visual vertical in thirty-six patients, *Ann Neurol* **31** (1992), 399–408.

[36] E. Duarte, E. Marco, J.M. Muniesa, R. Belmonte, P. Diaz, M. Tejero and F. Escalada, Trunk control test as a functional predictor in stroke patients, *J Rehabil Med* **34** (2002), 267–272.

[37] A. Edwards, Body sway and vision, *J Exp Psychol* **36** (1946), 526–535.

[38] A. El Fatimi, M. Masmoudi, M. Loigerot, M. Fares, J. Villy, C. Benaim, J. Pélissier and D.A. Pérennou, Prévalence et circonstances des chutes chez l'hémiplégique vasculaire: étude prospective sur quatre ans dans une unité de rééducation neurologique, *Ann Réadapt Méd Phys* **44** (2001), 462.

[39] M. Engardt, T. Ribbe and E. Olsson. Vertical ground reaction force feedback to enhance stroke patients' symmetrical bodyweight distribution while rising/sitting down, *Scand J Rehab Med* **25** (1993), 41–48.

[40] L. Feigin, B. Sharon, B. Czaczkes and A.J. Rosin, Sitting equilibrium 2 weeks after a stroke can predict the walking ability after 6 months, *Gerontology* **42** (1996), 348–353.

[41] A. Forster and J. Young, Incidence and consequences of falls due to stroke: a systematic inquiry,. *Bmj* **311** (1995), 83–86.

[42] F.P. Franchignoni, L. Tesio, C. Ricupero and M.T. Martino, Trunk control test as an early predictor of stroke rehabilitation outcome, *Stroke* **28** (1997), 1382–1385.

[43] E. Gentaz, M. Badan, M. Luyat and N. Touil, The manual haptic perception of orientations and the oblique effect in patients with left visuo-spatial neglect, *Neuroreport* **13** (2002), 327–331.

[44] A.C. Geurts, M. de Haart, I.J. Van Nes and J. Duysens, A review of standing balance recovery from stroke, *Gait Posture* **22** (2005), 267–281.

[45] D. Gottlieb and D. Levine, Unilateral neglect influences the postural adjustments after stroke, *J Neuro Rehab* **6** (1992), 35–41.

[46] M. Guerraz, V. Sakellari, P. Burchill and A.M. Bronstein, Influence of motion parallax in the control of spontaneous body sway, *Exp Brain Res* **131** (2000), 244–252.

[47] V. Gurfinkel and Y. Levik, Perceptual and automatic aspects of the postural body scheme, in: *Brain and Space*, J. Paillard, ed., Oxford Science Publications: Oxford, 1991, pp. 147–162.

[48] J. Held, E. Pierrot-Desselligny, B. Bussel, M. Perrigot and M. Mahler, Devenir des hémiplégies vasculaires par atteinte sylvienne en fonction du côté de la lésion, *Ann Réadaptation Méd Phys* **18** (1975), 592–604.

[49] S. Hesse, M. Schauer, M. Malezic, M. Jahnke and K.H. Mauritz, Quantitative analysis of rising from a chair in healthy and hemiparetic subjects, *Scand J Rehabil Med* **26** (1994), 161–166.

[50] F. Hlavacka, T. Mergner and M. Krizkova, Control of the body vertical by vestibular and proprioceptive inputs, *Brain Res Bull* **40** (1996), 431–434.

[51] F. Horak and J. MacPherson, Postural orientation and equilibrium, in: *Handbook of physiology*, L.B. Rowell and J.T. Sheperd, eds, Oxford University Press: New York, 1996, pp. 255–292.

[52] C.L. Hsieh, C.F. Sheu, I.P. Hsueh and C.H. Wang, Trunk control as an early predictor of comprehensive activities of daily living function in stroke patients, *Stroke* **33** (2002), 2626–2630.

[53] D. Hyndman, A. Ashburn and E. Stack, Fall events among people with stroke living in the community: circumstances of falls and characteristics of fallers, *Arch Phys Med Rehabil* **83** (2002), 165–170.

[54] M. Ioffe, On the functions of the motor cortex in reorganization of postural coordinations, *Journal of Higher Nervous Activity* **47** (1997), 86–92.

[55] L. Jorgensen, T. Engstad and B.K. Jacobsen, Higher incidence of falls in long-term stroke survivors than in population controls: depressive symptoms predict falls after stroke, *Stroke* **33** (2002), 542–547.

[56] H.O. Karnath, S. Ferber and J. Dichgans, The origin of contraversive pushing: evidence for a second graviceptive system in humans, *Neurology* **55** (2000), 1298–1304.

[57] H.O. Karnath, S. Ferber and J. Dichgans, The neural representation of postural control in humans, *Proc Natl Acad Sci USA* **97** (2000), 13931–13936.

[58] H.O. Karnath, L. Johannsen, D. Broetz and W. Kuker, Posterior thalamic hemorrhage induces pusher syndrome, *Neurology* **64** (2005), 1014–1019.

[59] H.O. Karnath, P. Schenkel and B. Fischer, Trunk orientation as the determining factor of the contralateral deficit in the neglect syndrome and as the physical anchor of the internal representation of body orientation in space, *Brain* **114** (1991), 1997–2014.

[60] G. Kerkhoff, Multimodal spatial orientation deficits in left-sided visual neglect, *Neuropsychologia* **37** (1999), 1387–1405.

[61] G. Kerkhoff and C. Zoelch, Disorders of visuospatial orientation in the frontal plane in patients with visual neglect following right or left parietal lesions, *Exp Brain Res* **122** (1998), 108–120.

[62] M. Lacour, J. Barthelemy, L. Borel, J. Magnan, C. Xerri, A. Chays and M. Ouaknine, Sensory strategies in human postural control before and after unilateral vestibular neurotomy, *Exp Brain Res* **115** (1997), 300–310.

[63] C. Lafosse, E. Kerckhofs, M. Troch, P. Santens and E. Vandenbussche, Graviceptive misperception of the postural vertical after right hemisphere damage, *Neuroreport* **15** (2004), 887–891.

[64] C. Lafosse, E. Kerckhofs, M. Troch, L. Vereeck, G. Van Hoydonck, M. Moeremans, J. Broeckx and E. Vandenbussche, Contraversive pushing and inattention of the contralesional hemispace, *J Clin Exp Neuropsychol* **27** (2005), 460–484.

[65] Y. Laufer, D. Sivan, R. Schwarzmann and E. Sprecher, Standing balance and functional recovery of patients with right and left hemiparesis in the early stages of rehabilitation, *Neurorehabil Neural Repair* **17** (2003), 207–213.

[66] D. Lee and J. Lishman, Visual proprioceptive control of stance, *Journal of Human Movement studies* **1** (1975), 87–95.

[67] C. Mann, N. Berthelot-Berry and H. Dauterive, The perception of the vertical: I. Visual and non-labyrinthine cues, *J Exp Psychol* **39** (1949), 538–547.

[68] H.F. Mao, I.P. Hsueh, P.F. Tang, C.F. Sheu and C.L. Hsieh, Analysis and comparison of the psychometric properties of three balance measures for stroke patients, *Stroke* **33** (2002), 1022–1027.

[69] J. Massion, Postural control system, *Curr Opin Neurobiol* **4** (1994), 877–887.

[70] J. Massion and M. Woollacott, Posture and equilibrium, in: *Clinical disorders of balance posture and gait*, A.M. Bronstein, T. Brandt and M. Woollacott, eds, Arnold: London, 1996, pp. 1–18.

[71] N.E. Mayo, N.A. Korner-Bitensky and R. Becker, Recovery time of independent function post-stroke, *Am J Phys Med Rehabil* **70** (1991), 5–12.

[72] M. Mennemeier, A. Chatterjee and K.M. Heilman, A comparison of the influences of body and environment centred reference frames on neglect, *Brain* **117** (1994), 1013–1021.

[73] I. Miyai, R.L.R. Mauricio and M.J. Reding, Parietal-insular strokes are associated with impaired standing balance as assessed by computerized dynamic posturography, *J Neurol Rehabil* **11** (1997), 35–40.

[74] L. Nashner, Adaptating reflexes controlling human posture, *Exp Brain Res* **26** (1976), 59–72.

[75] L. Nyberg and Y. Gustafson, Patient falls in stroke rehabilitation. A challenge to rehabilitation strategies, *Stroke* **26** (1995), 838–842.

[76] J. Paillard, Cognitive versus sensorimotor encoding of spatial information, in: *Cognitive Processing and Spatial Orientation in Animal and Man*, P. Ellen and C. Blanc-Tinus, eds, Martinus Nijhoff: Dordrecht, 1987, pp. 43–77.

[77] E. Palmer, L. Downes and P. Ashby, Associated postural adjustments are impaired by a lesion of the cortex, *Neurology* **46** (1996), 471–475.

[78] C. Partridge and S. Edwards, Recovery curves as a basis for evaluation, *Physiotherapy* **74** (1988), 141–143.

[79] W. Paulus, A. Straube and T. Brandt, Visual stabilization of posture. Physiological stimulus characteristics and clinical aspects, *Brain* **107** (1984), 1143–1163.

[80] P.M. Pedersen, A. Wandel, H.S. Jorgensen, H. Nakayama, H.O. Raaschou and T.S. Olsen, Ipsilateral pushing in stroke: Incidence, relation to neuropsychological symptoms, and impact on rehabilitation. The Copenhagen Stroke Study, *Arch Phys Med Rehabil* **77** (1996), 25–28.

[81] D. Pérennou, Towards a better understanding and quantitative assessment of pushing, a postural behaviour caused by some strokes, *Ann Readapt Med Phys* **48** (2005), 198–206.

[82] D. Pérennou, Weight-bearing asymmetry in standing hemiparetic patients, *J Neurol Neurosurg Psy* **76** (2005), 621.

[83] D. Pérennou, B. Amblard, M. Laassel el, C. Benaim, C. Herisson and J. Pelissier, Understanding the pusher behavior of some stroke patients with spatial deficits: a pilot study, *Arch Phys Med Rehabil* **83** (2002), 570–575.

[84] D. Pérennou, B. Amblard, C. Leblond and J. Pelissier, Biased postural vertical in humans with hemispheric cerebral lesions, *Neurosci Lett* **252** (1998), 75–78.

[85] D. Pérennou, C. Benaim, E. Rouget, M. Rousseaux, J. Blard and J. Pélissier, Postural balance following stroke: towards a disadvantage of the right brain-damaged hemisphere, *Rev Neurol* **155** (1999), 281–290.

[86] D. Pérennou, C. Leblond, B. Amblard, J. Micaleff and J. Pélissier – Understanding the pusher syndrome, in *Second World Forum of Neurorehabilitation* (1999), Toronto.

[87] D. Pérennou, C. Leblond, B. Amblard, J. Micalef, E. Rouget and J. Pélissier, The polymodal sensory cortex is crucial for

controlling lateral postural stability: evidence from stroke patients, *Brain Res Bul* **53** (2000), 359–365.

[88] D. Pérennou, C. Leblond, B. Amblard, J.P. Micallef, C. Herisson and J.Y. Pelissier, Transcutaneous electric nerve stimulation reduces neglect-related postural instability after stroke, *Arch Phys Med Rehabil* **82** (2001), 440–448.

[89] D. Pérennou, G. Mazibrada, D. Playford, J. Rothwell, M. Gresty, R. Greenwood and A.M. Bronstein, Verticality perception in pusher patients: ipsi or contralesional bias? in *Proceedings of the Third world forum of Neurorehabilitation* (2002), Venice.

[90] D. Pérennou, D. Playford, M. Guerraz, G. Mazibrada, M. Gresty and A. Bronstein, Dissociation in the verticality perception after a stroke, in: *Proceedings of the ISPG 2001*, H. Kingma and J Duysens, eds, 2001.

[91] M. Perrigot, C. Bergeco, C. Fakacs, J. Bastard and J. Held, Hémiplégie vasculaire. Bilan et éléments du pronostic de la rééducation, *Ann Réadaptation Méd Phys* **23** (1980), 229–241.

[92] L. Pizzamiglio, G. Vallar and F. Doricchi, Gravity and hemineglect, *Neuroreport* **7** (1995), 370–371.

[93] L. Pizzamiglio, G. Vallar and F. Doricchi, Gravitational inputs modulate visuospatial neglect, *Exp Brain Res* **117** (1997), 341–345.

[94] A. Pouget and J. Driver, Relating unilateral neglect to the neural coding of space, *Curr Opin Neurobiol* **10** (2000), 242–249.

[95] O. Pyoria, U. Talvitie and J. Villberg, The reliability, distribution, and responsiveness of the Postural Control and Balance for Stroke Test, *Arch Phys Med Rehabil* **86** (2005), 296–302.

[96] I.H. Robertson. Do we need the lateral in unilateral neglect? Spatially nonselective attention deficits in unilateral neglect and their implications for rehabilitation, *Neuroimage* **14** (2001), S85–90.

[97] G. Rode, C. Tiliket and D. Boisson, Predominance of postural imbalance in left hemiparetic patients, *Scand J Rehab Med* **29** (1997), 11–16.

[98] G. Rode, C. Tiliket, P. Charlopain and D. Boisson, Postural asymmetry reduction by vestibular caloric stimulation in left hemiparetic patients, *Scand J Rehabil Med* **30** (1998), 9–14.

[99] M. Romberg, *Lehrbuch der nervenkrankheiten des menschen*, 1846, Berlin: Duncker.

[100] P. Rondot, F. Odier and D. Valade, Postural disturbances due to homonymous hemianopic visual ataxia, *Brain* **115** (1992), 179–188.

[101] C. Sackley, The relationship between weight bearing asymmetry after stroke, motor function and activities of daily living, *Physiotherapy Theory and Practice* **6** (1990), 179–185.

[102] C.M. Sackley, Falls, sway, and symmetry of weight-bearing after stroke, *Int Disabil Stud* **13** (1991), 1–4.

[103] A. Saj, J. Honore, T. Bernati, Y. Coello and M. Rousseaux, Subjective visual vertical in pitch and roll in right hemispheric stroke, *Stroke* **36** (2005), 588–591.

[104] A. Saj, J. Honore, J. Davroux, Y. Coello and M. Rousseaux, Effect of posture on the perception of verticality in neglect patients, *Stroke* **36** (2005), 2203–2205.

[105] K.J. Sandin and B.S. Smith, The measure of balance in sitting in stroke rehabilitation prognosis, *Stroke* **21** (1990), 82–86.

[106] I. Schindler and G. Kerkhoff, Head and trunk orientation modulate visual neglect, *Neuroreport* **8** (1997), 2681–2685.

[107] A. Shumway-Cook and F.B. Horak, Assessing the influence of sensory interaction of balance, *Phys Ther* **66** (1986), 1548–1550.

[108] M.T. Smith and G.D. Baer, Achievement of simple mobility milestones after stroke, *Arch Phys Med Rehabil* **80** (1999), 442–447.

[109] C. Solley, Reduction of error with practice in perception of the postural vertical, *J Exp Psychol* **52** (1956), 329–333.

[110] A. Straube, S. Krafczyk, W. Paulus and T. Brandt, Dependence of visual stabilization of postural sway on the cortical magnification factor of restricted visual fields, *Exp Brain Res* **99** (1994), 501–506.

[111] K. Taguchi, O. Sasaki, K. Sato, K. Nezu and M. Sakaguchi, Subjective vertical and vestibular lesion, *Acta Otolaryngol Suppl* **519** (1995), 201–203.

[112] D. Taylor, A. Ashurn and C. Ward, Asymmetrical trunk posture, unilateral neglect and motor performance following stroke, *Clin Rehabil* **8** (1994), 48–53.

[113] H. Teuber and M. Mishkin, Judgement of visual and postural vertical after brain injury, *Journal Psychology* **38** (1954), 161–175.

[114] C. Tilikete, G. Rode, N. Nighoghossian, D. Boisson and A. Vighetto, Otolith manifestations in Wallenberg syndrome, *Rev Neurol (Paris)* **157** (2001), 198–208.

[115] C. Tilikete, G. Rode, Y. Rossetti, J. Pichon, L. Li and D. Boisson, Prism adaptation to rightward optical deviation improves postural imbalance in left-hemiparetic patients, *Curr Biol* **11** (2001), 524–528.

[116] J.A. Tutuarima, J.H. Van der Meulen, R.J. de Haan, A. Van Straten and M. Limburg, Risk factors for falls of hospitalized stroke patients, *Stroke* **28** (1997), 297–301.

[117] C. Ugur, D. Gucuyener, N. Uzuner, S. Ozkan and G. Ozdemir, Characteristics of falling in patients with stroke, *J Neurol Neurosurg Psychiatry* **69** (2000), 649–651.

[118] F. Viallet, J. Massion, R. Massarino and R. Khalil, Coordination between posture and movement in a bimanual load lifting task: putative role of a medial frontal region including the supplementary motor area, *Exp Brain Res* **88** (1992), 674–684.

[119] D. Wade, R. Langton Hewer and V. Wood, Stroke: influence of patients sex and side of weakness on outcome, *Arch Phys Med Rehabil* **65** (1984), 513–516.

[120] D. Wade, V. Wood and R. Langton Hewer, Recovery after stroke- The first 3 months, *J Neurol Neurosurg Psychiatry* **48** (1985), 7–13.

[121] C.H. Wang, I.P. Hsueh, C.F. Sheu, G. Yao and C.L. Hsieh, Psychometric properties of 2 simplified 3-level balance scales used for patients with stroke, *Phys Ther* **84** (2004), 430–438.

[122] H.A. Witkin and S.E. Asch, Studies in space orientation. III. Perception of the upright in the absence of a visual field, *J Exp Psychol* **38** (1948), 603–614.

[123] J.S. Yates, S.M. Lai, P.W. Duncan and S. Studenski, Falls in community-dwelling stroke survivors: an accumulated impairments model, *J Rehabil Res Dev* **39** (2002), 385–394.

[124] A.P. Yelnik, A. Kassouha, I.V. Bonan, M.C. Leman, C. Jacq, E. Vicaut and F.M. Colle, Postural visual dependence after recent stroke: Assessment by optokinetic stimulation, *Gait Posture*, in press.

[125] A.P. Yelnik, F.O. Lebreton, I.V. Bonan, F.M. Colle, F.A. Meurin, J.P. Guichard and E. Vicaut, Perception of verticality after recent cerebral hemispheric stroke, *Stroke* **33** (2002), 2247–2253.

[126] V.M. Zatsiorsky and D.L. King, An algorithm for determining gravity line location from posturographic recordings, *J Biomech* **31** (1998), 161–164.

Treatment techniques

Development of a rehabilitative program for unilateral neglect

Luigi Pizzamiglio*, Cecilia Guariglia, Gabriella Antonucci and Pierluigi Zoccolotti
Department of Psychology, University of Rome "La Sapienza", Neuropsychological Laboratory, IRCCS Fondazione Santa Lucia, Rome

Received 10 April 2006
Revised 16 June 2006
Accepted 22 June 2006

Abstract. *Purpose*: The aim of the present paper is to review several studies which assessed the validity of a visuo-spatial training for the rehabilitation of neglect patients. In addition two peripheral stimulations (TENS and Optokinetic Stimulation) have been studied to assess the improvements of neglect disorders when used in combination with the visuo-spatial training. Also we analyzed the potential effect of training for attention on neglect and, viceversa, the effect of visuo-spatial training on attentional impairments.
Methods: the goals have been investigated by both group studies and descriptions of single cases.
Results: The visuo-spatial training produced significant improvements on the performance of neglect patients which generalized to every day living situations: the results showed to be stable over time and had positive effects on a variety of other neurological impairments. It was also shown that the improvements are confined to tasks involving spatial exploration of extrapersonal space, but did not extend to other neglect disorders, such as representational and personal neglect.
The use of peripheral stimulations, at variance with other studies in the literature, did not add any advantage as compared to the improvements produced by the visuo-spatial training. No transfer between training for neglect and attention was observed.
Conclusions: the present review pointed out that neglect disorders can be improved in a clinically meaningful way: the studies described also showed some limitations and proposed the need of further researches in order to extend the improvements to several other aspects of the neglect syndrome.

Keywords: Neglect rehabilitation, attention rehabilitation, sensory stimulation, attention disorders, recovery of functions

1. Introduction

In the late 1980s we were intrigued by reports of significant improvement in the performance of patients with unilateral neglect deficits. Following early descriptions of individual cases [1,2] group studies also showed clinically significant effects [3,4]. These behavioural improvements contrasted with the clinical impression of resistance to verbal prompts typical of neglect patients. When explicitly requested to look toward the left side these patients either do not modify their performance or modify it minimally and inconsistently. Furthermore, the patients appear unaware of their inability and, if requested, may formulate incoherent or minimising explanations of their disorder.

A rehabilitative approach to the unilateral neglect disorder is particularly important because the disturbance is very frequent among patients with right hemisphere lesions (e.g. [5]). Further, while some improvements were reported in early phases of the disease [6], both cross-sectional (e.g. [7]) and longitudinal (e.g. [8, 9]) studies showed that the disturbance is relatively stable two months after stroke. Also, because of the deficit in exploration, the patient fails to perform a variety of

---

*Corresponding author: Prof. Luigi Pizzamiglio, MD, Department of Psychology, University "La Sapienza", Via dei Marsi, 78, 00100 Roma, Italy. E-mail: luigi.Pizzamiglio@uniroma1.it.

tasks calling on processes not directly impaired as an effect of the brain injury such as eating, dressing, reading, writing, etc. There are consistent reports that neglect has an overall negative effect on patients' recovery from stroke [10]. In a large sample of unselected patients, it was shown that the presence of cognitive deficits (i.e., unilateral neglect) is one of the strongest prognostic factors. Patients with hemineglect have a significantly higher risk of poor functional outcome [11].

In planning our research program we aimed to obtain selective and stable improvements in scanning ability and to foster generalisation of in-lab improvements to daily life activities. As to the former, we stimulated exploration of left space by using lateralised sensory signals to capture the patient's attention. Low-level stimulation had already been mentioned by Lawson [1] and used more systematically by Weinberg et al. [4]. In contrast, with few exceptions [12] the use of semantic cues was unsuccessful in modifying patients' behaviour. Based on reports in the literature of the effects of various types of somatosensory stimulation in temporarily reducing neglect [13–15], in subsequent studies we used some of these paradigms (e.g., optokinetic stimulation and TENS) in conjunction with the rehabilitative program to evaluate their influence. Since neglect patients characteristically have inconsistent performance gains, we used a training program that was sufficiently long to allow systematic evaluation of learning and to detect plateaux in performance gains. Finally, to foster generalisation of training to everyday life activities we used a large variety of stimulus materials and tasks.

Here, we present the basic rationale behind our training program for neglect, as well as some findings obtained over the past fifteen years and a few possible lines for future research.

2. Neglect rehabilitation: Basic observations

The first step was to demonstrate the efficacy of our rehabilitation training in reducing neglect patients' scanning deficit. Thirteen patients with chronic unilateral neglect due to right hemisphere lesions were submitted to a number of training procedures aimed at fostering scanning of the left side of space [16].

Four procedures were devised: 1. Visual-spatial scanning; 2. Reading and copying training; 3. Copying of line drawings on a dot matrix; and 4. Figure description. All procedures required that the patient actively and sequentially scan various parts of the visual field in order to produce the correct response (find a number, read or copy a sentence, draw a line drawing, describe a figure). The procedures are described in detail elsewhere [17,18]. Here, we only mention that, being computer driven, the Visual-spatial scanning procedure was particularly suited for documenting the patient's learning during therapy. This procedure permits presenting sequences of digits at given positions in space in a large visual field (96° horizontally and 18° vertically); sequences of varying difficulty are used. The patient's task was to name the digit presented and to press a button as quickly as possible afterwards; reaction times provided a sensitive measure of the patient's scanning ability.

To execute the training program, some general criteria were followed: a) slow and progressive variation of the task elements (e.g., in reading, changing from one-line to two-line sentences) only when performance on the preceding task had become stable; b) extensive use of stimulation in different sensory modalities (verbal, acoustic, tactile) in the initial phases, and their slow reduction as the patient progressively developed autonomous compensatory strategies. The training was continued for eight consecutive weeks (five times a week).

A within-subject control was used. Each patient was examined once at least two months after the CVA and a second time one month later. Only patients who did not show improvements in scanning ability in this period were included in the study. In 7 of the 13 patients an additional follow-up evaluation was carried out at least five months after the end of the training program to make sure the improvements were stable.

Training effectiveness was evaluated by comparing the patient's performance on a battery of diagnostic tests before and after treatment. The tests a) measured scanning ability in a variety of stimuli and task conditions, b) evaluated perceptual and visual-spatial abilities, allegedly independent of scanning, and c) measured scanning ability in a naturalistic context.

Some main results emerged from the comparison of pre-post therapy performances. Overall, the group of patients improved dramatically in their ability to scan the left part of space, regardless of whether this involved sequentially cancelling out segments or letters, reading or exploring the Wundt-Jastrow illusion, i.e., a display able to expose asymmetrical bias in perceptual judgements [19]. However, individual differences in recovery were also apparent. These were not clearly associated with disease duration or with the site/dimension of the lesion. In fact, even patients with very stable deficits and very large hemispheric lesions benefited from therapy.

Note that scanning improvements were very clear on tasks that were similar to daily life situations (such as serving a cup of tea). To this aim, we developed a semi-structured scale that focuses on the qualitative/quantitative asymmetries present in the exploration of space [20,21]. This scale also evaluates the presence of neglect for personal space through the use of simple tasks such as combing hair and wearing eyeglasses. This allowed us to evaluate changes in the exploration of personal space related to the rehabilitative training. After therapy, neglect patients showed small changes in the exploration of the left part of their body. Indeed, the effects due to the rehabilitation training were confined to exploration of extrapersonal space. This finding is consistent with the structure of the training exercises, which encourage exploration of extrapersonal space. The development of training to improve personal neglect is a goal of future research.

In the patients available at follow-up, the continued presence of scanning improvements many months after the end of therapy confirmed the stability of the effects of the therapeutic intervention. These observations confirm previous findings by Weinberg and colleagues [4].

Due to the specific nature of the therapy, improvements did not extend to other visual-spatial abilities. Performances in discriminating unfamiliar faces, identifying Street-like figures or solving the Raven tasks were minimally modified after the training.

Important observations were also obtained by carefully examining patients' performances during the therapeutic training. As expected, reaction times to visual targets across space improved most in the first weeks of training; but significant improvements were also seen across all eight weeks of training (after the presentation of over 10,000 stimuli). This indicates that almost the entire training was necessary to consolidate the exploratory acquisitions. Apparently, generalisation occurs only when the patient is brought to a high level of over-learning. Antonucci et al. [22] observed that most studies reporting negative results used short treatment periods (1–2 weeks).

During the therapy, most (but not all) patients changed their attitude toward the deficit. Initially they were indifferent and anosognosic of the scanning impairment. However, when their performances in responding or detecting targets in left space improved the patients slowly became more conscious of their scanning difficulties. Increased awareness produces important changes in the patient-therapist relationship. The patients begin to take an active part in the training and to construct personal compensatory strategies. At the same time, depressive crises occasionally occur when patients, who were initially indifferent, begin to understand the severity of their deficits.

Overall, this first study indicated the potential effectiveness of a rehabilitative intervention on neglect. Patients with otherwise stable symptoms showed clinically meaningful gains both on standard and on ecologically valid tests. However, a number of questions remained open or were generated from this first research. First, it seemed important to confirm these findings by controlling for potential confounding variables, including spontaneous recovery. A related question concerns the duration of training. After we carried out the original study, the Italian National Health system drastically reduced the length of in-patient recovery, thus making it necessary to shorten the training period. Consequently, a decrease in rehabilitation outcomes was demonstrated in a study that compared large samples of patients admitted before and after the new Italian regulations. The precocious discharge of patients affects stabilisation of rehabilitative results, with significant worsening of daily living activities [23]. Furthermore, since neglect has a widespread effect on the individual, an analysis should be made of the potential effect of therapy on other behaviours. Most neglect patients suffer from unilateral motor deficits. The generality of scanning improvements raised the question of whether neglect training can foster motor rehabilitation in these patients. The presence of individual variability in response to training raised the question about whether training effectiveness could be improved, e.g., by adding different types of sensory stimulation. Besides their deficit in responding to contralesional stimuli, neglect patients often respond slowly to stimuli that appear in the non-neglected field. This clinical association of spatially defined and basic (non-lateralised) deficits raised the issue of functional independence. From the rehabilitative standpoint one wonders whether training of neglect affects basic attentional processes or whether training of basic attentional processes affects neglect.

Following is a description of some of the studies we conducted to answer these and related questions.

2.1. Controlling for spontaneous recovery

The within-subject design used in the first study was useful for controlling the individual variability of patients but it did not allow definitively excluding the contribution of spontaneous recovery. In a second study [22] we adopted a more classical randomised design to confirm the original findings. The specific training for neglect was compared to a general cognitive intervention. Twenty patients with neglect were randomly assigned to an "immediate" or a "delayed" training group. All patients were included in the study two months after stroke. They were administered the test battery both at admission and two months later, i.e., at the end of the specific training for neglect for the immediate group and at the end of the general cognitive treatment for the delayed one. At that time the latter group was given the specific therapy and re-tested two months later.

In general, the results confirmed the effectiveness of neglect rehabilitation. The patients' improvement was strictly linked to the timing of the training. The immediately trained group showed consistent improvements in scanning, quite similar to those previously observed. In spite of general cognitive stimulation the performance of the delayed training group on explorative tests did not change after the first two months. However, this group showed significant changes when subsequently submitted to the specific training.

Overall, it appears that therapeutic effects cannot be interpreted in terms of spontaneous recovery. On the contrary, effectiveness was similar in patients who started therapy at different times, indicating that it is not crucial when treatment following stroke actually begins.

2.2. Training for neglect in interaction with physical rehabilitation

The previous study also gave us the opportunity to evaluate the relationship between neglect training and physical rehabilitation [24]. It has often been reported that, motor deficits being equal, patients with neglect are among those who benefit least from physiotherapy [10].

All participants were in-patients with various degrees of motor impairment. They received physical rehabilitation, based on Bobath therapeutic exercises (two sessions daily, six days a week), independent of the neglect/general cognitive stimulation training. After the first cycle of therapy the neglect patients submitted to immediate neglect training showed significant improvements in mobility (as assessed by the Rivermead Mobility Index) while the patients who received the general cognitive stimulation did not show significant gains. Parallel results were obtained for daily living status (as assessed by the Barthel Index). These different effects were not due to differences in motor performance at the beginning of the study. After the second therapy cycle, the other "delayed" group (that received the neglect therapy) also showed significant motor improvements.

Overall, these findings indicated that both functional and motor recovery are significantly improved by the simultaneous presence of a treatment specifically focused on neglect.

2.3. The use of peripheral stimulation in the recovery of neglect

Of the neuropsychological impairments that follow focal brain lesions, unilateral neglect has the rather unique characteristic of being transiently reduced by a variety of appropriate sensory or sensory-motor stimulations. Unilateral caloric vestibular stimulation [13,25], optokinetic stimulation [14,26,27], vibration and transcutaneous electrical nervous stimulation (TENS) of the neck muscles [15,28] may temporarily improve or worsen a number of manifestations of the neglect syndrome. These include disorders of space exploration, hemianesthesia, anosognosia, impairment of position sense, imaginal hemineglect and displacement of the subjective midline [29]. In the case of optokinetic and vibration stimuli, the duration of the effect seems to be confined to the period of stimulation. The effects of vestibular and TENS may be longer, lasting about 20 min.

All of these sensory inputs (vestibular, visual and somatosensory/ proprioceptive) contribute to the dynamic balance of egocentric representations of personal and extrapersonal space. Unilateral lesions of patients with neglect produce a distortion of these representations towards the side of the lesion. Lateralised stimulation of one of the sensory channels can counterbalance this distortion, thus reducing the bias whereby the patient fails to perceive contralesional stimuli and to organise motor responses to them [29,30].

This view implies the existence of a neural substrate that integrates this sensory information into non-primarily sensory representations of space. Neurons responding to vestibular inputs and also to optokinetic and different somatosensory stimulations have been found in the parieto-insular vestibular areas [31,32]. The responsiveness of these neurons to different sensory inputs suggests that they represent the neural basis for integrating polymodal spatial information.

Several researchers have stressed the potential relevance of these stimulation techniques for rehabilitating unilateral neglect. However, only a few attempts have been made to test whether systematic stimulation with any of the above techniques induces a long-lasting effect on these patients' performances or a generalisation of these changes to everyday living situations. An empirical response to these questions is necessary in order to transform interesting experimental effects into systematic procedures for rehabilitating neglect disorders.

Two studies were designed to test the efficacy of TENS and of optokinetic stimulation.

2.4. Use of TENS in the recovery of neglect

The first research [30] was divided into two stages. The first stage consisted of 40 consecutive treatment sessions of chronic neglect patients with TENS applied for each one-hour session while the patient was receiving a non- specific cognitive stimulation. The second stage consisted of 40 sessions of specific treatment for neglect given to the same patients immediately after the first stage of the study.

Four patients participated in the study. They began the general cognitive intervention, together with the TENS stimulation. A professional therapist entertained the patients with puzzles, chess, card games and crossword puzzles. The patients were encouraged to explore the stimuli, but no specific directional cues were provided.

The stimulation was applied to the left side of the neck, below the occiput and just lateral to the spine; frequency of stimulation was 100 Hz, with a pulse width of 100 msec. TENS was administered for the entire duration of the treatment session. While all four patients showed clear sensitivity to TENS stimulation (reading and line bisection tests), the systematic repetition of this procedure for as long as 8 weeks of treatment did not produce stable and generalised changes in all patients. Only one of the four patients showed consistent improvement; the second patient performed better on tests for neglect but showed no functional improvements; no variations were observed in the remaining two cases.

At the end of the 8 weeks, all patients received "specific" training for neglect for the same amount of time and with the same frequency. After this training all four patients showed significant functional improvement, similar to patients observed in previous studies.

The transient re-balancing of the egocentric frames of reference produced by TENS through the stimulation of the neck proprioceptive receptors did not extend to stable recovery after two months of treatment. The lack of improvement produced by TENS cannot be interpreted as the inability of the four patients to improve their disorders. In fact, consistent recovery was observed when they were submitted to more "specific" treatment for unilateral neglect.

2.5. Use of Optokinetic stimulation in the recovery of neglect

The aim of the next study was to strengthen and/or accelerate the rehabilitation of neglect by combining a standard training for spatial scanning with a different form of sensory stimulation, namely, optokinetic (OK) stimulation [33].

The paradigm was a simple randomised design comparing two groups of patients with right hemisphere lesions and unilateral neglect. One group was treated with a combination of the two techniques, while the other group received only the standard treatment.

To evaluate the effectiveness of the training with or without OK stimulation we used a quantitative assessment of neglect disorders before and after treatment and a semi-quantitative and functional evaluation of the patients' improvement in everyday activities and in functional independence. We expected to find either acceleration of improvement during the combined training or extension of improvement to behaviours that tend to be less susceptible to standard treatment (i.e., personal neglect).

Twenty-two right hemisphere brain damaged patients with unilateral neglect were consecutively recruited in the three participating hospitals (in Italy, Holland and Finland). Pre- and post-treatment comparisons showed significantly improved performances in both groups of patients. However, no difference between the two groups of patients and no group by type of treatment interaction were found.

Overall, the results showed that the treatment produced a significant change, but that this improvement was not influenced by the use of OK stimulation.

In spite of these negative results, clinical observations suggest that individual patients may benefit greatly from OK stimulation. Zoccolotti et al. [34] described a patient who, in spite of persistent anosognosia throughout treatment, showed good recovery of visual scanning. In addition to the standard treatment for neglect, this patient received combined OK stimulation. The patient's recovery was slow, without any change in anosognosia, but by the end of the treatment his level of recovery was similar to that of the other neglect patients.

Overall, in spite of the transient sensitivity of unilateral neglect to OK stimulation, no significant group effect was observed in the long-term recovery of spatial exploration. Other studies demonstrated transient effects at much lower speeds of background movement [26,27,35–37]. Therefore, the use of low speed OK might be more effective in rehabilitation. Empirical studies (such as those reported in this issue by Kerkhoff et al. [37] and Sturm et al. [27]) are required to verify this possibility.

Unlike some of the cognitive disorders that follow brain lesions (such as language or memory deficits), many perceptual, motor, and imaginative manifestations of unilateral neglect can be dramatically, but only temporarily reduced by a number of lateralised sensory manipulations. The latter include caloric vestibular, optokinetic, cutaneous electrical stimulation and lengthening of the neck muscle by rotating the head over the trunk. However, the systematic use of such stimuli for a long period of time in rehabilitation treatment does not produce relevant advantages in the recovery of spatial disorders. Therefore, based on systematic therapeutic interventions, it can be concluded that neglect undergoes positive recovery that extends to activities of daily living. However, these positive changes are most likely due to a complete and slow reorganisation of the spatial experience induced by the specific neglect training program [16,22,24]. In contrast, in most patients the contribution of different lateralised forms of stimulation, such as TENS and OK, is not easily integrated with the perceived and organised responses activated by the specific training. This latter procedure involves active reorganisation of spatial processing, while passive stimulation does not seem to help in consolidating the compensatory neural connections within the residual intact brain.

Results in contrast with these conclusions were obtained using the neck muscle vibration technique. In a first study [38], a combination of an exploration training and the neck vibration for 15 consecutive sessions resulted in superior improvements as compared to the exploration training alone. In a second study using a multiple baseline paradigm [39], a significant amelioration of neglect was reported applying the neck vibration alone for 10 sessions of 20 minutes each; a long lasting effect was maintained at a follow-up.

2.6. Training of basic attention and neglect

Some recent studies suggest there may be a functional link between recovery of neglect and recovery of attentional "non-spatialised" disorders, such as disorders of sustained attention (see for example [40]). Robertson and co-workers carried out a study in which unilateral neglect was tested as a function of training for sustained attention. The hypothesis was that an increase in arousal would facilitate contralesional exploration. Patients learned a rhythmic, paced sequence that had to be mentally repeated during a visuo-spatial task. The authors observed significant improvement in sustained attention as well as in visuo-spatial exploration even though no patient had received specific training for neglect [40]. However, the effects of training were limited, in some cases lasting just few weeks, and they did not generalise to everyday living activities [40]. More recently, Thimm et al. [41] used training for alertness to rehabilitate seven right-brain damaged patients with neglect. The training was based on two sub-routines of the "AIXTENT" [42] program. The patients had to "drive" a car or a motorcycle as quickly as possible and to avoid crashing into obstacles that appeared suddenly on the screen. After three weeks of training, both alertness and neglect deficits were significantly reduced. However, four weeks after the end of training, the neglect returned to the pre-training level.

We recently carried out two studies [43,44] to test the hypothesis that the reduction of a basic "non-spatialised" attentional deficit would significantly improve unilateral neglect.

In the first study we tested seven chronic neglect patients affected by severe hemispatial neglect and severe attentional deficits. Before treatment the patients were submitted to a neuropsychological examination to exclude the presence of mental deterioration, an extensive assessment of neglect and an evaluation of the phasic and tonic components of attention. Three sub-tests of the Italian version of TEA.02 [45] were used, i.e., Vigilance, Alertness and Go/No-Go. All seven patients showed very severe alertness and vigilance deficits as well as very severe unilateral neglect. Patients were submitted to visual spatial training [16] for two months and then re-tested. Data showed a significant improvement of unilateral neglect on both standard neuropsychological and functional measures. On the contrary, RTs and the number of omissions or errors on the three sub-tests of the TEA remained substantially unchanged.

In the second study [44], a new group of seven right-brain damaged patients with neglect and attentional deficits was studied to verify whether "non-spatialised" training of the attentional deficit would produce significant improvement in unilateral neglect. If attentional phasic and tonic disorders are critical for producing stable chronic neglect, attentional training in which no effort is made to direct attention toward the neglected side should result in an improvement of neglect.

All patients were submitted to the same neuropsychological examination used in the previous study to assess the presence and severity of neglect and phasic and tonic attentional deficits before and after the vigilance and selective attentional sub-routines of the AIXTENT training [42].

Results showed significant improvement in three attentional sub-tests of TEA (Vigilance, Alertness and Go/NoGo).

As for exploratory performance, changes were observed in the Letter cancellation and Bell tests but not in the other tests of neglect (Line bisection, Wundt-Jastrow Area Illusion and Reading). Due to reduction of the selective attention impairment, after the training the patients were more accurate in exploring the right hemispace, as well as the portion of the left hemispace spared by neglect, but did not show any enlargement of their explorative field. This improvement of selective attention resulted in more accurate performances on the two neglect tests in which the selective components of attention are more directly involved due to the presence of targets within distracters. No improvement was observed on the other tests in which the selective attention component is less important (e.g., Line bisection)

Taken together these two studies demonstrate that unilateral neglect is not functionally related to other attentional deficits. Indeed, the improvement of unilateral neglect observed in other studies after attentional rehabilitation can be ascribed to two different factors. First, as shown by our second study [44] some of the tests for neglect include great involvement of selective attention processes. Second, the exercises used during the attentional training may include spatial components that direct attention towards the neglected side. For example, in Thimm et al's study [41] attention was treated by using exercises that simulate driving a car or a motorcycle. The patients had to drive as quickly as possible and to avoid obstacles. In order to complete these tasks, attention has to be directed towards the entire visual field.

The frequent association of vigilance, alertness, sustained and selective attention deficits and neglect may be due to the anatomical contiguity of areas involved in different attentional processes and areas involved in directing attention in space. It is also clear that the two kinds of attentional deficits (phasic/tonic vs spatial) strongly interact to produce the alterations of explorative deficits. Not only do neglect patients fail to attend to the contralesional side of space, they are also less efficient in maintaining attention or in promptly attending to stimuli in the non neglected space.

These factors suggest that in rehabilitating neglect care must be taken to treat the "non-spatialised" disorders, in addition to the specific treatment of neglect training for vigilance, alertness, sustained and selective attention defects, whenever these are present.

2.7. General remarks

The structured procedure developed in our laboratory proved successful in improving unilateral neglect patients' ability to explore the contralesional hemifield. The improvements, repeatedly observed in the literature, apply to an unselected population of chronic patients, including those with severe impairments associated with very large lesions of the right hemisphere. The results are stable over time and extend to everyday activities that require sequential exploration of the neglected hemifield.

However, an important issue has to do with the specificity of these improvements. In the early studies reviewed in this paper very few changes were observed in spatial abilities that do not directly involve spatial scanning. Therefore, a goal for future research is to develop training for other manifestions of unilateral neglect, such as personal and representational neglect. Also, our data do not support the idea that a) the specific training developed produces significant changes in coexisting attentional deficits, such as phasic and tonic alertness disorders, vigilance and selective attention, and b) training for these attentional impairments extends to neglect. These considerations imply that additional training is needed to treat these disorders.

A second comment concerns the possibility of using different kinds of peripheral stimulations, such as vestibular, OK, etc., to speed up or to improve the results of neglect rehabilitation. Our data refer to TENS and OK stimuli used in isolation or in conjunction with specific training. The negative results obtained were certainly not due to the limited duration of the rehabilitation; both techniques were administered for 8 consecutive weeks. One possible explanation is that in order to achieve significant and stable results neglect patients must be engaged in a long and active attempt to reorganise their ability to explore the entire space. Passive exposure to different peripheral stimuli alone does not allow the central nervous system to reorganise or to develop compensatory strategies to overcome neglect. However, the few examples reported suggest that in some cases, in which the beginning of treatment or the severity of anosognosia creates unusual difficulties, one of the described peripheral stimulations may help modify the disorder, particularly in the early stages of treatment. Note that other kinds of peripheral manipulations, such as the use of prismatic lenses, are also promising (see the presentation of other papers in this issue).

A final consideration has to do with patient selection. We treated unselected samples of in-patients that often included patients with large lesions and very severe disorders. As we conducted the European study reported above (and read the works of other laboratories) we noted that in other countries primarily outpatients were studied. Some of the limitations of the presented results may be related to this important difference in the source of patients as well as to the time limits imposed on rehabilitation by some public and private health systems. Patient selection is certainly an important variable when comparing the observations collected in different clinical settings and using different approaches. Finally, the observation of significant improvements in very severe cases underscores the importance of not overlooking this type of patient in the rehabilitation practice.

References

[1] I.R. Lawson, Visual-spatial neglect in lesion of the right cerebral hemisphere. A study in recovery, *Neurology* **12** (1962), 23–33.

[2] X. Seron and P. Tissot, Essai de reduction d'une agnosie spatiale unilaterale gauche, *Acta Psychiat Belgica* **73** (1973), 448–457.

[3] L. Diller and W.A. Gordon, Interventions for cognitive deficits in brain-injured adults, *J Consult Clin Psychol* **49** (1981), 822–834.

[4] J. Weinberg, L. Diller, W.A. Gordon, L.J. Gerstman, A. Lieberman, P. Lakin, G. Hodges and O. Ezrachi, Visual scanning training effect on reading-related tasks in acquired right brain-damage, *Arch Phys Med Rehab* **58** (1977), 479–486.

[5] D.B. Hier, J. Mondlock and L.R. Caplan, Behavioral anormalities after right hemisphere stroke, *Neurology* **33** (1983), 337–344.

[6] G. Gainotti, Les manifestations de négligence et d'inattention pour l'hémispace, *Cortex* **4** (1968), 64–91.

[7] P. Zoccolotti, G. Antonucci, A. Judica, P. Montenero, L. Pizzamiglio and C. Razzano, Incidence and evolution of the hemineglect disorder in chronic patients with unilateral right brain damage, *Int J Neurosci* **47** (1989), 209–216.

[8] D.C. Campbell and J.M. Oxbury, Recovery from unilateral spatial neglect? *Cortex* **12** (1976), 303–312.

[9] A. Colombo, E. De Renzi and M. Gentilini, The time course of visual hemi-inattention, *Archiv fur Psychiatrie und Nervenkrankheiten* **29** (1982), 644–653.

[10] G. Denes, C. Semenza, E. Stoppa and A. Lis, Unilateral spatial neglect and recovery from hemiplegia – a follow-up study, *Brain* **105** (1982), 543–552.

[11] S. Paolucci, G. Antonucci, L. Emberti Gialloreti, M. Traballesi, S. Lubich, L. Pratesi and L. Palombi, Predicting stroke in patients' rehabilitation outcome: the prominent role of neuropsychological disorders, *Eur Neurol* **36** (1996), 385–390.

[12] K.M. Stanton, K.M. Yorkston, V.T. Kenyon and D.R. Benkelman, Language utilization in teaching reading to left neglect patients, in: *Clinical Aphasiology Conference Proceedings*, R.H. Brookshire, ed., Mineapolis, BRK Publishers, 1981.

[13] A.B. Rubens, Caloric stimulation and unilateral visual neglect, *Neurology* **35** (1985), 1019–1024.

[14] L. Pizzamiglio, R. Frasca, C. Guariglia, C. Incoccia and G. Antonucci, Effect of optokinetic stimulation in patients with visual neglect, *Cortex* **26** (1990), 535–540.

[15] G. Vallar, M. Rusconi, S. Barozzi, B. Bernardini, D. Ovadia, C. Papagno and A. Cesarani, Improvement of left visuo-spatial hemineglect by left-sided transcutaneous electrical stimulation, *Neuropsychologia* **33** (1995), 73–82.

[16] L. Pizzamiglio, G. Antonucci, C. Guariglia, A. Judica, P. Montenero, C. Razzano and P. Zoccolotti, Cognitive Rehabilitation of the hemineglect disorders in chronic patients with unilateral right brain damage, *J Clin Exp Neuropsyc* **14** (1992), 901–923.

[17] A. Judica, G. Galati and P. Zoccolotti, *Metodiche per la diagnosi ed il trattamento riabilitativo del paziente eminattento*, Roma: IRCCS Ospedale di Riabilitazione Santa Lucia, 1996.

[18] L. Pizzamiglio, G. Antonucci, C. Guariglia, A. Judica, P. Montenero, C. Razzano and P. Zoccolotti, *La rieducazione neurocognitiva della eminattenzione in pazienti con lesione cerebrale unilaterale*, Milano: Masson, 1990.

[19] M. Massironi, G. Antonucci, L. Pizzamiglio, M.V. Vitale and P. Zoccolotti, The Wundt-Jastrow illusion in the study of spatial hemi-inattention, *Neuropsychologia* **26** (1988), 161–166.

[20] P. Zoccolotti and A. Judica, Functional evaluation of hemineglect by means of a semi-structured scale: personal extrapersonal differentiation, *Neuropsychol Rehabil* **1** (1991), 33–44.

[21] P. Zoccolotti, G. Antonucci and A. Judica, Psychometric characteristics of two semi-structured scales for the functional evaluation of hemi-inattention in extra-personal and personal space, *Neuropsychol Rehabil* **2** (1992), 179–191.

[22] G. Antonucci, C. Guariglia, A. Judica, L. Magnotti, S. Paolucci, L. Pizzamiglio and P. Zoccolotti, Effectiveness of neglect rehabilitation in a randomized group study, *J Clin Exp Neuropsyc* **17** (1995), 383–389.

[23] S. Paolucci, M. Traballesi, L. Emberti Gialloreti, L. Pratesi, S. Lubich, G. Antonucci and C. Caltagirone. Changes in functional outcome in inpatient stroke rehabilitation resulting from new health policy regulations in Italy, *Eur J Neurol* **5** (1998), 17–22.

[24] S. Paolucci, G. Antonucci, C. Guariglia, L. Magnotti, L. Pizamiglio and P. Zoccolotti, Facilitatory effect of neglect rehabilitation on the recovery of left hemiplegic stroke patients: a cross-over study, *J Neurol* **243** (1996), 308–314.

[25] S. Cappa, R. Sterzi, G. Vallar, and E. Bisiach, Remission of hemineglect after vestibular stimulation, *Neuropsychologia* **25** (1987), 775–782.

[26] G. Kerkhoff, I. Schindler, I. Keller and C. Marquarot, Visual background motion reduces size distortion in spatial neglect, *Neuroreport* **10** (1999), 319–323.

[27] W: Sturm, M. Thimm and G.R. Fink Alertness-training in neglect -Behavioural and imaging results, *Restorative Neurology and Neuroscience*, present issue, in press.

[28] H.O. Karnath, Transcutaneous electrical stimulation and vibration of the neck muscles in neglect, *Exp Brain Res* **105** (1995), 321–324.

[29] G.Vallar, C. Guariglia and M.L. Rusconi, Modulation of the neglect syndrome by sensory stimulation, in: *Parietal lobe contributions to orientation in 3D space Heidelberg*, P. Thier and H.O. Karnath, eds, Spinger-Verlag, 1996.

[30] L. Pizzamiglio, G. Vallar and L. Magnotti, Transcutaneous Electrical stimulation of the neck muscles and Hemineglect rehabilitation, *Restor Neurol Neuros* **10** (1996), 197–203.

[31] O.J. Grusser, M. Pause and U. Schreiter, Localization and responses of neurones in the parieto-insular vestibular cortex of awake monkeys (macaca fascicularis), *J Physiol* **430** (1990), 537–557.

[32] O.J. Grusser, M. Pause and U. Schreiter, Vestibular neurones in the parieto-insular cortex of the monkey (macaca fascicularis): visual and neck receptor responses, *J Physiol* **430** (1990), 559–583.

[33] L. Pizzamiglio, L. Fasotti, M. Jehkonen, G. Antonucci, L. Magnotti, D. Boelen and S. Asa, The use of Optokinetic Stimulation in rehabilitation of the hemineglect disorder, *Cortex* **40** (2004), 441–450.

[34] P. Zoccolotti, C. Guariglia, L. Pizzamiglio, A. Judica and C. Razzano, Good recovery of visual scanning in a patient with persistent anosognosia, *Int J Neurosci* **62** (1992), 93–104.

[35] J.B. Mattlingley, J.L. Bradshow and J.A. Bradshow, Horizontal visual motion modulates focal attention in left unilateral spatial neglect, *J Neurol Neurosur Ps* **57** (1994), 1228–1235.

[36] G. Kerkhoff, Multiple perceptual distortion in leftsided visual neglect, *Neuropsychology* **38** (2000), 1073–1086.

[37] G. Kerkoff, I. Keller, V. Ritter and C. Marquardt. Repetetive optokinetic stimulation induces long lasting recovery fron visual neglect, *Restorative Neurology & Neuroscience*, in press, present issue.

[38] I. Schindler, G. Kerkhoff, H-O Karnath, I. Keller and G. Goldenberg, Neck muscle vibration induces lasting recovery in spatial neglect, *J Neurol Neurosurg Psychiatry* **73** (2002), 412–419.

[39] L. Johannsen, H. Ackermann and H.-O. Karnath, Lasting amelioration of spatial neglect by treatment with neck muscle vibration even without concurrent training, *J Rehab Med* **35** (2003), 249–253.

[40] I. Robertson, R. Tegnér, K. Tham, A. Lo and I. Nimmo-Smith, Sustained attention training for unilateral neglect: Theoretical and rehabilitation implications, *J Clin Exp Neuropsyc* **17** (1995), 416–430.

[41] M. Thimm, J.R. Fink, J. Küst, H. Karbe and W. Sturm, Impact of alertness training on spatial neglect: A behavioural and fMRI study, *Neuropsychologia* **44** (2006), 1230–1246.

[42] W. Sturm, W. Hartje, B. Orgass and K. Willmes, Computer-assisted rehabilitation of attention disorders, in: *Development in the assessment and rehabilitation of brain damaged patients*, F. Stachowiak, ed., 1993, Narr, Tübingen.

[43] L. Piccardi, D. Nico, I. Bureca, A. Matano and C. Guariglia, Efficacy of visuo-spatial training in right-brain damaged patients with spatial hemineglect and attention disorders, *Cortex* (2006), in press.

[44] D. Nico, L. Piccardi, I. Bureca, A. Matano and C. Guariglia, *Efficacy of attentional training on visuo-spatial neglect*, in preparation.

[45] P. Zimmermann and B. Fimm, *Test for Attentional Performance (TAP)*, English version 1.02. Herzogenrath: Psytest, 1995.

Neglect and prism adaptation: A new therapeutic tool for spatial cognition disorders

Gilles Rode[a,b,c,*], Thomas Klos[d], Sophie Courtois-Jacquin[a,b,c], Yves Rossetti[b,c,e] and Laure Pisella[b,c]
[a]*Service de rééducation neurologique, Hospices Civils de Lyon, Hôpital Henry Gabrielle, 20 route de Vourles, 69230 St Genis Laval, France*
[b]*INSERM U534, Espace et Action, UMR-S 534, Institut National de la Santé Et de la Recherche Médicale, 16 avenue Lépine, Case 13, F-69676 Bron, France*
[c]*Université Claude Bernard LYON 1, IFNL, Institut Fédératif des Neurosciences de Lyon, Hôpital Neurologique, Bât B13, 59 Bd Pinel, 69394 LYON cedex, France*
[d]*Zentrum für Neurologie und neurologische Rehabilitation (ZNR), Klinikum am Europakanal, Am Europakanal 71, 91056 Erlangen, Germany*
[e]*Mouvement et Handicap, Rééducation Neurologique, Hôpital Henry Gabrielle, Hospices Civils de Lyon – IFNL, Route de Vourles, St Genis Laval, France*

Received 17 March 2006
Revised 6 May 2006
Accepted 22 June 2006

Abstract. *Purpose:* A large proportion of right-hemisphere stroke patients show unilateral neglect, a neurological deficit of perception, attention, representation, and/or performing actions within their left-sided space, inducing many functional debilitating effects on everyday life, and responsible for poor functional recovery and ability to benefit from treatment. This spatial cognition disorder affects the orientation of behaviour with a shift of proprioceptive representations toward the lesion side.
Methods: This shift can be reduced after a prism adaptation period to a right lateral displacement of visual field (induced by a simple target-pointing task with base-left wedge prisms). The modification of visuo-motor or sensory-motor correspondences induced by prism adaptation involves improvement of different symptoms of neglect.
Results: Classical visuo-motor tests could be improved for at least 2h after adaptation, but also non-motor and non-visual tasks. In addition, cross-modal effects have been described (tactile extinction and dichotic listening), mental imagery tasks (geographic map, number bisection) and even visuo-constructive disorders. These cognitive effects are shown to result from indirect bottom-up effects of the deeper, adaptive realignment component of the reaction to prisms. Lesion studies and functional imaging data evoke a cerebello-cortical network in which each structure plays a specific role and not all structures are crucial for adaptation ability.
Conclusions: These cognitive effects of prism adaptation suggest that prism adaptation does not act specifically on the ipsilesional bias characteristic of unilateral neglect but rehabilitates more generally the visuo-spatial functions attributed to the right cortical hemisphere. These results reinforce the idea that the process of prism adaptation may activate brain functions related to multisensory integration and higher spatial representations and show a generalization at a functional level. Prism adaptation therefore appears as a new powerful therapeutic tool for spatial cognition disorders.

Keywords: Neglect, prism adaptation, rehabilitation, after-effect, right hemisphere

---

*Corresponding author: Pr. Gilles Rode, Hôpital Henry Gabrielle, Hospices Civils de Lyon, 20 route de Vourles, 69230 Saint-Genis-Laval, France. Tel.: +33 04 78 86 50 24; Fax: +33 04 78 86 50 30; E-mail: gilles.rode@chu-lyon.fr.

1. Neglect, a behavioural ipsilesional bias

Hemispatial neglect is classically defined as the patient's failure to report, respond to, or orient toward novel and/or meaning-ful stimuli presented to the side opposite the brain lesion [1]. This condition is frequently found in right-brain damaged patients, often in association with contralesional hemiplegia or hemiparesis. Neglect thus constitutes a space-oriented behaviour disorder with an ipsilesional bias toward the right side. This disorder may be illustrated by the clinical observation of the patient suffering from neglect. Spontaneously the patient displays an ocular and cephalic deviation toward the side right. When asking to orient his gaze toward the contralesional space, the pursuit movements are reduced and sometimes are unable to cross the central region. Moreover an asymmetry of ocular saccades may be also observed. This behavioural bias will be evidenced in a bisection task or in asking to the patient to point in a straight-ahead position in darkness. In this situation, a shift of pointing movements is demonstrated reflecting a shift of the proprioceptive egocentric reference towards the lesion side.

The strong core of neglect is that this behavioural ipsilesional bias is associated to a unawareness of the contralesional space with reduction of perception, action and attentional and/or representational processes performed within it [2,3]. The unilateral neglect patient is thus unable to compensate his illness by a voluntary orientation of attention unlike the patient with a hemianopia who could orient his gaze toward the blind hemi-field. These both factors explained that neglect induces many functional debilitating effects on everyday life and has been shown to be responsible for poor functional recovery and reduced ability to benefit from treatment of impaired motor functions [4,6].

2. Reduction of behavioural bias after rehabilitation

Numerous attempts to improve neglect have been made over the last forty years. The main question which remains debated is how one could reduce the behavioural bias of neglect and corollary improve the consciousness of the left peripersonal and personal space (see review [7]). Two theoretical tracks may be thus distinguished in rehabilitation of neglect: a 'top-down' and a 'bottom-up' approach. The first is a pragmatic clinical approach which is aimed at improving the perceptual and behavioural biases by acting on the patient's awareness of the deficit, i.e. at the highest cognitive levels, including visual scanning training, cueing or sustained attention training [8,9]. The second physiological approach is aimed at modifying the sensorimotor level by passive sensory manipulations, or visuomotor adaptation which allow to bypass the central awareness deficit and directly influence the highest cognitive levels of space and action representation (see reviews [10,11]).

These two levels of representation, sensori-motor and cognitive are supported by the posterior parietal cortex particularly the inferior parietal lobule (BA thirty nine and forty). The inferior parietal lobule is a sensorimotor interface between space representation and action. The damage of these areas involves a severe and persistent contralesional neglect [12,13]. Damage of other areas, as BA areas 6, 8 and forty-four and superior temporal sulcus could also produce neglect [14, 16]. Such an interaction between space representation and action may be experimentally provoked by prismatic adaptation procedure. The aim of this paper is thus to review the different studies showing that a prismatic adaptation (PA) may reduce the behavioural bias of neglect and awareness deficit according a bottom-up track.

3. Experimental behavioural bias after prism exposure in normals

In normal subjects a transient behavioural bias may be experimentally induced by a prism adaptation procedure [17,18]. This optical manipulation may produce a shift of proprioceptive representations, evidenced by the displacement of manual straight-ahead pointing in the dark in the direction opposite to the visual shift produced by the prisms. The exposure to an optical alteration of the visual field involved initially a disorganization of visuo-motor behaviour which could be corrected through visuo-motor adaptation. The shift of proprioceptive representations constitutes one major compensatory effect of short-term wedge-prism exposure. Negative after-affects also include a measure of the total after-effect by open loop pointing and of the visual after-effect by requiring subjects to set a visual target to their straight-ahead. After-effects reflect the plasticity of coordinate transformations involved in multisensory and sensorimotor integration. They are used to assess and quantify the presence of true adaptation [18, 19]. In addition, subjects exhibit error reduction curves

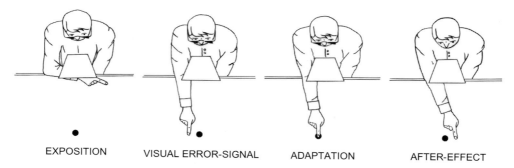

Fig. 1. Viusomotor adaptation procedure. **Exposition:** The patient wore a pair of goggles fitted with wide-field point-to-point prismatic lenses creating a rightward optical shift of 10°. Prism exposure consisted of 50 fast pointing movements made to visual targets presented either 10° to the left or 10° to the right of the body midline, given in pseudorandom order. A shelf was placed under the patient's chin to prevent viewing of the hand at its starting position, but allowing an unobstructed view of the targets and terminal pointing errors. This adaptation procedure took between 6–10 min. **Perception of visual error-signal:** At the start of the process, the subject will misreach to the right of the target, an error referred to as the direct effect. **Adaptation:** The error will swiftly diminish and disappear entirely as the participant adapts to the visual shift. **After-effect:** After removal of the prism, the subject will misreach in the opposite direction to the visual shift, an error referred to as the after-effect.

during the prism exposure period, which also reflects the ability to strategically compensate for the optical shift [18,19]. These adaptive realignment and strategic contribution to the compensation of the optical shift have been ascribed to distinct neuroanatomical substrates [18,20]: the strategic component mainly relies on the parietal cortex [21,23] whereas the adaptive realignment component relies on the cerebellum [19,24]. The relevant point for unilateral neglect rehabilitation is that after an optical deviation of the visual field to the right, subjects show a systematic leftward deviation of visuo-motor responses with the adapted limb. The hypothesis proposed by Rossetti et al. [25,26] was to use this after-effect as method to help the neglect patient to orient his behaviour toward the neglected side. An interesting and additional question was to specify whether a lower-order visuo-motor action may influence higher-level spatial representation.

4. After-effect and improvement of neglect after PA

In the first study, Rossetti et al. [25] have clearly demonstrated that a short period of pointing toward targets viewed through prisms that displaced the visual field 10 degrees in the rightward direction (50 pointing movements for an exposure period of two to five minutes) involved a shift in manual straight-ahead pointing toward the left side in the dark (see Fig. 1).

Prior to prism exposure six patients pointed, on average, about 9 degrees to the right (ipsilesional side), but after exposure the same test showed an average pointing of 2 deg rightward: an after-effect of about 8 deg or 70 percent compensation for the 10 deg optical displacement. This after-effect is much larger than the 30 percent shown by normal control participants, showing that neglect patients, in spite of brain damage were more affected by the adaptation than the controls were. Surprisingly neglect symptoms were ameliorated for six patients exposed to prism adaptation. Improvement was evidenced in visuo-manual tasks as line bisection [27], copy drawing [28], line cancellation [29], daisy drawing and text reading. Aspects of object-based neglect and space-based neglect were equally improved by the adaptation procedure.

From this previous paper, 18 different studies were published about the effects of prism adaptation on symptoms of neglect and possible underlying mechanisms. Eighty-three right brain damaged patients entirely benefit from this treatment with different results on after-effects, clinical effects and duration of improvement (See Table 1).

The table clearly shows that the amount of the after-effect varies from 2.7° [30] to 14° [31,32] with a mean value of 7.1°. It appears that the quantitative relationship between the amplitude of after-effect and neglect amelioration is not obvious. As shown by numerous studies, the main interest of PA is that the effects produced by a single 5-min session of adaptation last for much longer than any other rehabilitation method. Two group studies showed fully sustained effects after at least 2 h [25] and 1 day [33], respectively. Case studies reported even more prolonged improvements, lasting for about 4 days [34,35]. It is possible that some patients are improved for a longer period than others [36].

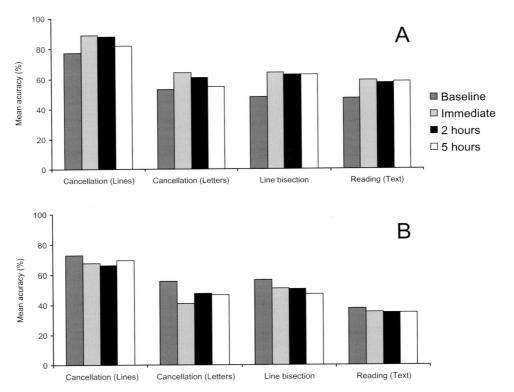

Fig. 2. Effect of prism adaptation on neglect assessed by cancellation tests [29,56], line bisection [27] and text reading (3 columns, 140 words) in a sample of 10 right brain-damaged patients. Baseline before adaptation, immediately upon 10′ prism removal, 2 hours later and 5 hours later (Fig. 2A). The study was controlled by a sample of 10 right brain-damaged patients treated by goggles made of window glass (Fig. 2B). Patients were randomly assigned and matched on age (61.4 vs. 60.2) and gender (5/5 vs. 6/4). The mean duration of disease was 2.7 vs. 2.6 months. All differences between experimental and control group reached significant levels. Line cancellation $p < 0.05$ immediate, $p < 0.01$ (2 hours) and $p < 0.05$ (5 hours). Letter cancellation $p < 0.001$ immediate, and $p < 0.05$ (2 hours and 5 hours). Line bisection $p < 0.005$, all conditions. Text reading $p < 0.005$ immediate, $p < 0.001$ (2 hours) and $p < 0.01$ (5 hours).

But the best prospect for rehabilitation purposes is to repeat adaptation sessions. Recently a treatment with prismatic lenses in twice-daily sessions over a period of 2 weeks was applied in a group of seven neglect patients compared with a control group. The results showed an improvement in the experimental patient's performance after PA, which was maintained during a 5-week period after treatment. This long-term improvement of neglect symptoms was found in standard as well as in behavioural tests and in all spatial domains [30].

Recently ineffectiveness of PA was reported in ten right brain damaged patients with neglect assessed by visuomotor and visuo verbal tasks [37]. In this study the partial improvement which was observed with repetition of tests could be related to a learning effect or an increase of vigilance or sustained attention. This factor was taken into account in the only randomised controlled clinical trial in a sample of 10 right-brain damaged patients with neglect [38,39]. The authors extended the study of Rossetti et al. [25] using identical procedures: Post tests were measured at 2 and 5 hours post adaptation and further testing was employed. Patients were sampled from different stages of rehabilitation, showing neglect for more than 3 months. The experimental group was compared to a control group of patients treated by goggles made of window glasses. The results showed a clear difference between experimental and control groups, in favour of a selective effect of PA on unilateral neglect (see Fig. 2).

5. What are the neural mechanisms involved by PA?

This point was recently assessed by Serino et al. [40] in a group of 16 neglect patients submitted to a PA treatment for 10 daily sessions compared to a control group. Effects of PA were assessed by the recovery of neglect (measured by the B.I.T. Conventional and Behavioural scales, a reading task but also an eye movement analy-

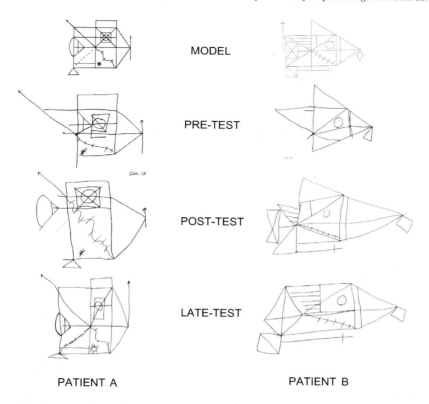

Fig. 3. Effect of prism adaptation on neglect and constructional apraxia in two right brain-damaged patients assessed by the Taylor's figure (patient A) and the Rey's figure (patient B) before adaptation (pre-test), immediately upon the 10° prism removal (post-test) and 2–4 hours later (late-test). Before adaptation, the figures displayed a neglect of the left part and graphic errors in the entire of drawing consistent with an associated constructional apraxia. After PA, improvement of the drawing was observed both for left neglect and visuo-constructive disorders.

sis). Moreover PA visuo-motor effects (the error reduction and the after-effect) were also measured. Serino et al. [40] showed that no correlation between recovery of neglect and after-effect. The after-effect has to be considered as the demonstration that the patient was able to adapt to a prismatic deviation of his visual environment but this should not be considered as a predictive factor of neglect recovery after PA. In this study on the other hand, a significant correlation between leftward oculo-motor deviations produced by PA and recovery of neglect was evidenced and even patients with greater leftward deviation of the first saccade displayed the greater improvement of visuo-spatial tasks. For these authors it is therefore possible to speculate that the increase in the amplitude of the first leftward saccade obtained after PA produces also a shifting of visual attention towards the left side of the visual field. However Ferber et al. [31] reported in a neglect patient exposed to a prismatic deviation, a shift of the exploratory eye movement toward the left but a persistent deficit in awareness of the left side assessed by the ability of the patient to judge the happiness of vertically arranged pairs of chimeric faces composed of half-smiling and half-neutral faces.

The effects of PA from a low-order visuo-motor to a high-order level rely also probably on other mechanisms.

6. Prism adaptation, a bottom-up track

The first findings which can not be explained by a modification of exploratory eye movements concern the effects of PA on sensory neglect, particularly in the tactile and auditory domains where no visuo-manual response could be involved. Mac Intosh et al. [36] in a single case study of a chronic patient showed that PA involves improvement not only of visual components of neglect, but also non-visual haptic neglect assessed by tactile exploration of a circle. Maravita et al. [41] reported in four neglect patients an improvement of contralesional visual and tactile extinction. Same results are reported in the auditory domain. Indeed following a right-brain-damage, unilateral omissions of auditory

Table 1
Review of relevant papers studying the effects of prism adaptation in right brain damaged patients with neglect

Studies	Cases	After-effect (degrees)	Clinical effects	Duration of effect
Rossetti et al., 1998 (25)	6	8°	visuo-motor tasks (bisection, cancellation, drawing, reading)	> or = 2 h
Rode et al., 2001 (44)	2	9°	visuo-motor tasks (drawing) mental imagery task	immediate
Tilikete et al., 2001 (51)	5	no assessed	postural imbalance	immediate
Pisella et al., 2002 (35)	2	9°	visuo-motor tasks (bisection, cancellation, straight-ahead pointing)	96 h
Farnè et al., 2002 (33)	6	3°	visuo-motor tasks (bisection, cancellation) visuo-verbal tasks (object description; objects, words and no-words naming)	24 h
Frassinetti et al., 2002 (30)	6	2.7°	visuo-motor tasks (bisection, cancellation, drawing) behavioral measures	5 weeks
MacIntosh et al., 2002 (36)	1	no given	visuo-motor tasks (bisection, cancellation, drawing) neglect dyslexia tactile spatial task	three repeated sessions
Ferber et al., 2003 (31)	1	14.3°	eye movement pattern	immediate
Maravita et al., 2003 (41)	4	8°	visuo-motor tasks (bisection, cancellation) tactile extinction	immediate
Dijkerman et al., 2003 (57)	3	no given	visuo-motor tasks (bisection, cancellation) perceptual size judgement ocular asymmetry	immediate
Klos et al., 2004 (39)	10	no assessed	visuo-motor tasks (bisection, cancellation, drawing, reading)	5 h
Berberovic et al., 2004 (58)	4	4.33°	attentional task judgement of temporal order	immediate
Angeli et al., 2004 (59)	8	4.12°	neglect dyslexia eye movement pattern	immediate
Rossetti et al., 2004 (46)	2	4.8° and 9.4°	mental number bisection task	immediate
Dijkerman et al., 2004 (60)	1	no given	visuo-motor tasks (bisection, cancellation) somatosensory deficit	immediate
Morris et al., 2004 (61)	4	7°	visuo-motor tasks (bisection)	immediate
Serino et al., 2005 (40)	16	3.6°	visuo-motor tasks (B.I.T.) reading task eye movement pattern	3 months
Rousseaux et al., 2006 (37)	10	4.8°	visuo-motor tasks (bisection, cancellation, drawing) reading	no effect
Jacquin-Courtois et al., 2006 (34)	1	6.72°	visuo-motor tasks (bisection, cancellation) wheelchair driving	96 h
Rode et al., 2006 (32)	1	14.8°	visuo-motor tasks (bisection, cancellation) spatial dygraphia	72 h
	93	**Mean: 7.1°**		

targets occur frequently in the situation where two auditory stimuli are presented simultaneously from the right and from the left, while no omission is observed when presenting one single stimuli, Jacquin-Courtois et al. [42] have thus studied effects of PA on left auditory extinction in two groups of right-brain damaged patients with neglect: the first receiving a classical prism treatment, the second performing the same pointing procedure, but wearing neutral glasses creating no optical shift. Effects of PA were assessed on conventional visuomotor tasks and a dichotic listening test immediately upon prism removal and 2 hours later. Results displayed a long-lasting improvement of both visuospatial deficit and auditory extinction, only in patients exposed to PA.

These results show that the beneficial effects of PA are not restricted merely to visuomotor tasks but can also affect perception in non visual modalities. These results suggest that the calibration of sensory-motor transformations induced by PA, which directly affects visual space representation and action, may also alter the orientation of attention in other sensory modalities. In all these experiments, the patients were blindfolded and it s difficult to explain that this orientation is consecutive to a leftward exploratory eye movements.

The second findings concern the effect of PA on manifestations of imaginal neglect. Rode et al. [43,44] explored the effect of prism adaptation on visual imagery in two neglect patients asked to evoke mentally the map of France. Before adaptation, both patients are unable to evoke town names on the left part of map; named towns were located to the right half of the map consistent with a left representational neglect. After adaptation, a clear-cut improvement is demonstrated, reflecting an ability of both patients to generate or explore a symmetrical inner representation of the map. This imagery task is explicitly spatial in nature. More recently, similar effects were obtained in a non explic-

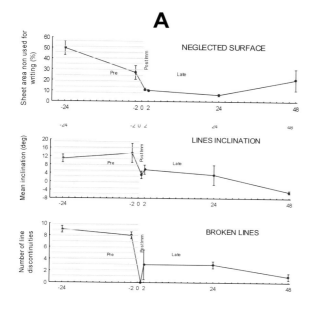

Fig. 4. Effect of prism adaptation on spatial dysgraphia. Temporal evolution of mean values of three distinct parameters of spatial dysgraphia (neglected surface, lines inclination and broken lines), measured in three writing tasks (writing-from-dictation on a A4 paper sheet, on a name-card and writing by copy on a A4 paper sheet) in a right-brain-damaged patient with neglect. The shadowed area represents the Pre-testing period gathering the two sessions realised by the patient before the single prism adaptation procedure.

itly mental task, a mental number-bisection task in two neglect patients. This task was recently described by Zorzi et al. [45] who reported that the mental bisection between two numbers was systematically shifted to the right (i.e. toward bigger numbers) in neglect patients, paralleling their bias when asked to mark the center of a physical line. The two neglect patients displayed a stable number-bisection bias during the first two sessions; after PA, the two patient's reliable bias was greatly improved, suggesting an effect of PA on highly cognitive task [46].

Both findings suggest that PA may influence the high level multimodal representations associated with spatial attention. The effects of PA may be considered as stimulating processes involved in brain plasticity related to multisensory integration and space representation. A supplementary question is to know whether PA favors the spontaneous recovery of neglect or facilitates the occurrence of selective compensation mechanisms. This question refers either to the cerebral plasticity naturally involved after the cerebral damage or to the cerebral plasticity specifically activated by the visuo-motor adaptation task. In normal subjects, neural structures considered to be involved in PA have long been restricted to the cerebellum [26,46], as shown by the inability of adaptation of patients with focal olivocerebellar lesion [19,47]. The posterior parietal cortex contralateral to the acting hand might be activated during adaptation to a prism-induced shift of the visual field [21]. The reciprocal connections between the deep cerebellar structures and the posterior parietal cortex provide an anatomical substrate that may support the cerebellar participation also in high-order processing [48,49].

In order to answer this question, Luauté et al. [23] performed a functional imaging PET study in five neglect patients after a prism exposure period. This study confirms a strong implication of the cerebellum which may be implied in the realignment of visuo-motor coordinates but also significant activations in different cortical and sub-cortical structures as the left thalamus, the left temporo-occipital cortex, the left medial temporal cortex and the right posterior parietal cortex. These activation patterns suggest that the low level sensori-motor adaptation may activate a distributed network between cerebellum, thalamus and cortical areas. This network may underline the cognitive effects of PA independently from modification of exploratory eye movements. Supplementary studies will be useful to precise the respective cerebral structures involved in the two components of PA (strategic and adaptative).

7. From neglect to spatial cognition

Two main lines of arguments can be used to argue that PA may produce effects that may be more specific to spatial cognition than to unilateral neglect per se. First, effects of PA have been demonstrated in normal subjects [50] Second, the effects found in the right brain damaged patients appear to be found on non-neglect symptoms and on on-neglect patients. The best example comes from a study where patients with right hemisphere lesion and no unilateral neglect were tested [51]. As patients with right hemisphere lesion, whether or not they present with neglect, tend to exhibit a postural balance biased to the right [51,52] attempted to improve postural balance in a group of patients with no or resolved neglect and found significant therapeutical effects of PA. This result has been interpreted as an indirect effect of PA on the central level of space representation. At a more directly high-level, the common characteristic of PA cognitive effects (especially the cross-modal and mental imagery effects) is the enlargement or the shift of space represented parallel to the reduction of the attentional bias. This disturbance refers to the general visuo-spatial functions attributed to the right cortical hemisphere. We could thus postulate that PA may improve more generally spatial cognition. The better symmetry (object-based neglect) and spatial organisation of drawing following prism adaptation in individuals e.g. in the Gainotti test (Rode et al. [11] Fig. 6 [25, p. 284]) suggest for example a possible effect of PA on visuo-constructive disorders (see Fig. 3).

This point was recently assessed in a neglect patient also showing a spatial dysgraphia following right brain damage. Spatial dysgraphia has been defined as "a disturbance of graphic expression due to an impairment of visuospatial perception resulting from a lesion in the nonlanguage-dominant hemisphere" [53,54]. According to these authors, four main features define spatial dysgraphia: (i) "right-page' preference: writing is crowded onto the right side of the page leaving an excessively wide "margin" on the left side; (ii) sloping lines (inclination): patients fail to write horizontally and produce oblique or wavy lines; (iii) broken lines: patients leave abnormally large space between words, thus leading to the fragmentation of the line into small segments and (iv) graphic errors: production of an uncorrect number of strokes for a given letter or of letters for a given word. The first feature reflects the left-sided neglect although the second and third reflect visuoconstructive disorders. After a PA procedure, an improvement of neglect was evidenced (with a reduction of the right page preference) as well as a long lasting reduction of sloping and broken lines (see Fig. 4).

The ability to place and orient correctly the words in the page and relatively to each others was durably improved; The positive effect of PA on visuo-constructive disorders suggests that PA does not act specifically on the ipsilesional bias characteristic of unilateral neglect but rehabilitates more generally the visuo-spatial functions attributed to the right cortical hemisphere [32]. Prism adaptation may thus enlarge or shift the part of space represented in the spared cortical hemisphere [55]. This different distribution of the representation of space between hemispheres could explain the improvement of both the right-oriented behavioural disorders and the visuo-constructive disorders.

8. Conclusions

These different cognitive effects (mental imagery, sensory cross-modal effect, visuo-constructive disorders) of PA suggest that PA does not act specifically on the ipsilesional bias characteristic of unilateral neglect but rehabilitates more generally the visuo-spatial functions attributed to the right cortical hemisphere. These reinforce the idea that the process of PA may activate brain functions related to multisensory integration and higher spatial representations and show a generalization at a functional level. Prism adaptation therefore appears as a therapeutic tool for spatial cognition disorders and a useful tool in the theoretical attempt to identify the underlying 'core' mechanisms of the neglect syndrome.

References

[1] K.M. Heilman, R.T. Watson and E. Valenstein, Neglect and related disorders, in: *Clinical Neuropsychology*, K.M. Heilman and E. Valenstein, eds, Oxford University Press, New York, NY, 1985, pp. 243–293.

[2] E. Bisiach, Unilateral neglect and related disorders, in: *Handbook of Clinical and Experimental Neuropsychology*, F. Denes and L. Pizzamiglio, eds, Hove: Psychology Press, 1999.

[3] G. Kerkhoff, Spatial hemineglect in humans, *Prog Neurobiol* **63** (2001), 1–27.

[4] G. Denes, C. Semenza, E. Stoppa and A. Lis, Unilateral spatial neglect and recovery from hemiplegia: a follow-up study, *Brain* **105** (1982), 543–552.

[5] K.J. Fullerton, D. McSherry and R.W. Stout, Albert's test: a neglected test of perceptual neglect, *Lancet* (1986) **327**, 430–432.

[6] M. Jehkonen, J.P. Ahonen, P. Dastidar, A.M. Koivisto, P. Laippala, J. Vilkki and G. Molnar, Visual neglect as a predictor of functional outcome one year after stroke, *Acta Neurol Scand* **101** (2000), 195–201.

[7] J. Luaute, P. Halligan, Y. Rossetti, G. Rode and D. Boisson, Visuo-spatial Neglect; a systematic review of current interventions and their effectiveness, *Neurosciences and biobehavioral reviews* (2006), in press.

[8] L. Diller and J. Weinberg, Hemi-inattention in rehabilitation: the evolution of a rational remediation program, *Adv Neurol* **18** (1997), 63–82.

[9] I.H. Robertson, J.B. Mattingley, C. Rorden and J. Driver, Phasic alerting of neglect patients overcomes their spatial deficit in visual awareness, *Nature* **395** (1998), 169–170.

[10] Y. Rossetti and G. Rode, Reducing spatial neglect by visual and other sensory manipulations: non-cognitive (physiological) routes to the rehabilitation of a cognitive disorder, in: *The Cognitive and Beural Bases of Spatial Neglect*, H.O. Karnath, A.D. Milner and G. Vallar, eds, 2000, pp. 375–396, Oxford University Press, New York.

[11] G. Rode, L. Pisella, Y. Rossetti, A. Farne and D. Boisson, Bottom-up transfer of sensory-motor plasticity to recovery of spatial cognition: visuomotor adaptation and spatial neglect, *Prog Brain Res* **142** (2003), 273–287.

[12] G. Vallar, Extrapersonal visual unilateral spatial neglect and its neuroanatomy, *Neuroimage* **14**(1 Pt 2) (2001), S52–S58.

[13] P.W. Halligan, G.R. Fink, J.C. Marshall and G. Vallar, Spatial cognition : evidence from visual neglect, *Trends in Cognitive Sciences* **7** (2003), 125–133.

[14] H.O. Karnath, S. Ferber and M. Himmelbach, Spatial awareness is a function of the temporal not the posterior parietal lobe, *Nature* **411** (2001), 950–953.

[15] H.O. Karnath, B.M. Fruhmann, W. Kuker and C. Rorden, The Anatomy of Spatial Neglect based on Voxelwise Statistical Analysis: A Study of 140 Patients, *Cereb Cortex* (2004).

[16] D.J. Mort, P. Malhotra and S.K. Mannan l, The anatomy of visual neglect, *Brain* **126**(Pt 9) (2003), 1986–1997.

[17] Y. Rossetti, K. Koga and T. Mano, Prismatic displacement of vision induces transient changes in the timing of eye-hand coordination, *Percept Psychophys* **54** (1993), 355–364.

[18] G.M. Redding, Y. Rossetti and B. Wallace, Applications of Prism Adaptation: A Tutorial in Theory and Method, *Neuroscience and Biobehavioral Reviews* **29** (2005), 431–444.

[19] M.J. Weiner, M. Hallett and H.H. Funkenstein, Adaptation to lateral displacement of vision in patients with lesions of the central nervous system, *Neurology* **33**(6) (1983), 766–772.

[20] G. M. Redding and B. Wallace, Adaptive spatial alignment and strategic perceptual-motor control, *J Exp Psychol Hum Percept Perform* **22** (1996), 379–394.

[21] D.M. Clower, J.M. Hoffman, J.R. Votaw, T.L. Fabert, R. Woods and G.E. Alexander, Role of posterior parietal cortex in the recalibration of visually guide reaching, *Nature* **383** (1996), 618–621.

[22] L. Pisella, C. Michel, H. Grea, C. Tilikete, A. Vighetto and Y. Rossetti, Preserved prism adaptation in bilateral optic ataxia: strategic versus adaptive reaction to prisms, *Exp Brain Res* **156** (2004), 399–408.

[23] J. Luaute, C. Michel, G. Rode, L. Pisella, S. Jacquin-Courtois, N. Costes, F. Cotton, D. LeBars, D. Boisson, P. Halligan and Y. Rossetti, Functional anatomy of the therapeutic effects of prism adaptation on left neglect, *Neurology* **66** (2006), 1859–1867.

[24] L. Pisella, Y. Rossetti, C. Michel, G. Rode, D. Boisson, D. Pelisson and C. Tilikete, Ipsidirectional impairment of prism adaptation after unilateral lesion of anterior cerebellum, *Neurology* **65** (12 Jul. 2005), 1:150–152.

[25] Y. Rossetti, G. Rode, L. Pisella, A. Farne, L. Li, D. Boisson and M.T. Perenin, Prism adaptation to a rightward optical deviation rehabilitates left hemispatial neglect, *Nature* **395** (1998), 166–169.

[26] M. Jeannerod and Y. Rossetti, in: *Visual Perceptual Defects*, C. Kennard, ed., Tindall, London, 1993, pp. 439–460.

[27] T. Schenkenberg, D.C. Bradford and E.T. Ajax, Line bisection with neurologic impairment, *Neurology* **30** (1980), 509–517.

[28] G. Gainotti, P. Messerli and R. Tissot, Qualitative analysis of unilateral spatial neglect in relation to laterality of cerebral lesions, *J Neurol Neurosurg Psychiat* **35** (1972), 545–550.

[29] M.L. Albert, A simple test of neglect, *Neurology* **23** (1973), 658–664.

[30] F. Frassinetti, V. Angeli, F. Meneghello, S. Avanzi and E. Ladavas, Long-lasting amelioration of visuospatial neglect by prism adaptation, *Brain* **125** (2002), 608–623.

[31] S. Ferber, J. Danckert, M. Joanisse, H.C. Goltz and M.A. Goodale, Eye movements tell only half the story, *Neurology* **60** (2003), 1826–1829.

[32] G. Rode, L. Pisella, L. Marsal, S. Mercier, Y. Rossetti and D. Boisson, Prism Adaptation Improves Spatial Dysgraphia Following Right Brain Damage, *Neuropsychologia* **44** (2006), 2487–2493.

[33] A. Farne, Y. Rossetti, S. Toniolo and E. Ladavas, Ameliorating neglect with prism adaptation: visuo-manual and visuo-verbal measures, *Neuropsychologia* **40** (2002), 718–729.

[34] S. Jacquin-Courtois, G. Rode, D. Boisson and Y. Rossetti, Wheel-chair driving improvement following visuo-manual prism adaptation, *Cortex*, in press, (2006).

[35] L. Pisella, G. Rode, A. Farne, D. Boisson and Y. Rossetti, Dissociated long lasting improvements of straight-ahead pointing and line bisection tasks in two unilateral neglect patients, *Neuropsychologia* **40** (2002), 3:327–334.

[36] R.M. McIntosh, Y. Rossetti and A.D. Milner, Prism adaptation improves chronic visual and haptic neglect, *Cortex* **38** (2002), 309–320.

[37] M. Rousseaux, T. Bernati, A. Saj and O. Kozlowski, ineffectiveness of prism adaptation on spatial neglect signs, *Stroke* **37** (2006), 542–543.

[38] S. Geggus, Effektivität von Prismenadaptation bei der Therapie von hemispatialem Neglect. Unpublished Diploma-Theses, University of Würzburg.

[39] T. Klos, S. Geggus and P. Pauli, Improvement of visuospatial neglect by prism adaptation. Paper presented at the annual meeting of the German society of neuropsychology (GNP), Munich, Sept. 2nd to 5th, 2004.

[40] A. Serino, V. Angeli, F. Frassinetti and E. Ladavas, Mechanisms underlying neglect recovery after prism adaptation, *Neuropsychologia*, in press, (2005).

[41] A. Maravita, J. McNeil, P. Malhotra, R. Greenwood, M. Husain and J. Driver, Prism adaptation can improve contralesional tactile perception in neglect, *Neurology* **60**(11) (2003), 1829–1831.

[42] S. Courtois-Jacquin, Y.Rossetti, G. Rode, C. Fischer, C. Michel, C. Allard and D. Boisson, Effect of prism adaptation on auditory extinction: an attentional effect? International Symposium on neural control of space coding and action production, *INSERM Lyon Mars* (2001), poster.

[43] G. Rode, Y. Rossetti, L. Li and D. Boisson, The effect of prism adaptation on neglect for visual imagery, *Behavioural Neurology* **11** (1998), 251–258.

[44] G. Rode, Y. Rossetti and D. Boisson, Prism adaptation improves representational neglect, *Neuropsychologia* **39**(11) (2001), 1250–1254.

[45] M. Zorzi, K. Priftis and C. Umilta, Brain damage: negelct disrupts the mental number line, *Nature* **417** (2002), 198–139.

[46] Y. Rossetti, S. Jacquin-Courtois, G. Rode, H. Ota, C. Michel and D. Boisson, Does action make the link between number and space representation? Visuo-manual adaptation improves number bisection in unilateral neglect, *Psychol Sci* **15**(6) (2004), 426–430.

[47] T.A. Martin, J.G. Keating, H.P. Goodkin, A.J. Bastian and W.T. Thatch, Throwing while looking through prisms, I Focal olivocerebellar lesions impair adaptation, *Brain* **119** (1996), 1183–1198.

[48] J.D. Schmaahmann, Dysmetria of thought: clinical consequences of cerebellar dysfunction on cognition and affect, *Trends Cogn Sci* **2** (1998), 362–371.

[49] Y. Rossetti, L. Pisella, C. Colent, G. Rode, C. Tilikete, A. Vighetto, D. Boisson and D. Pelisson, A cerebellar therapy for a parietal deficit? (abstract), in: *Action and visuo-spatial attention. Neurobiological Bases and Disorders*, PH.H. Weiss, ed., Life Sciences, Reihe Lebenswissenschaften, Forschungszentrum Jülich GmbH, Germany, 2000, p. 21.

[50] C. Michel, Simulating unilateral neglect in normals: myth or reality? in: *Plasticity in Spatial Neglect: Recovery and Rehabilitation*, G. Kerkhoff and Y. Rossetti, eds, Restorative Neurology and Neuroscience, in press, 2006.

[51] C. Tilikete, G. Rode, Y. Rossetti, L. Li, J. Pichon and D. Boisson, Prism adaptation to rightward optical deviation improves postural imbalance in left hemiparetic patients, *Current Biology* **11** (2001), 524–528.

[52] G. Rode, C. Tilikete and D. Boisson, Predominance of postural imbalance in left hemiparetic patients, *Scand J Rehabil Med* **29**(1) (Mar. 1997), 11–16.

[53] H. Hécaen, R. Angelergues and J.A. Douzenis, Les agraphies, *Neuropsychologia* **1** (1963), 179–208.

[54] H. Hecaen and P. Marcie, Disorders of written language following right hemisphere lesions: spatial dysgraphia, in: *Hemisphere function in the human brain*, S.S.J. Diamond and J.G. Beaumont, eds, London: Elek, 1974, pp. 345–366.

[55] G.M. Redding and B. Wallace, Prism adaptation and unilateral neglect: Review and analysis, *Neuropsychologia* **44**(1) (2006), 1–20.

[56] M. Mesulam, A cortical network for directed attention and unilateral neglect, *Annals of Neurology* **10** (1981), 309–325.

[57] H.C. Dijkerman, R.D. McIntosh, Y. Rossetti, C. Tilikete, R. C. Roberts and A.D. Milner, Ocular Scanning and Perceptual Size Distortion in Hemispatial Neglect: Effects of Prism Adaptation and Sequential Stimulus Presentation, *Experimental Brain Research* **153**(2) (2003), 220–230.

[58] N. Berberovic, L. Pisella, A.P. Morris and J.B. Mattingley, Prismatic adaptation reduces biased temporal order judgements in spatial neglect, *NeuroReport* **15** (2004), 1199–1204.

[59] V. Angeli, M.G. Benassi and E. Ladavas, Recovery of oculomotor bias in neglect patients after prism adaptation, *Neuropsychologia* **42** (2004), 1223–1234.

[60] H.C. Dijkerman, M. Webeling, J.M. ter Wal, E. Groet and M.J. Van Zandvoort, A long-lasting improvment of somatosensory functon after prism adaptation, a case study, *Neuropsychologia* **42** (2004), 1697–1702.

[61] A.P. Morris, A. Kritikos, N. Berberovic, L. Pisella, C.D. Chambers and J. Mattingley, Prism adaptation and spatial attention: a study of visual search in normals and patients with unilateral neglect, *Cortex* **40** (2004), 703–721.

Repetitive optokinetic stimulation induces lasting recovery from visual neglect

G. Kerkhoff[a,*], I. Keller[b], V. Ritter[c] and C. Marquardt[d]
[a] *Clinical Neuropsychology Unit, Saarland University, Saarbrücken, Germany*
[b] *Neurologische Klinik, Bad Aibling, Germany*
[c] *Neurological rehabilitation clinic, Ulm University, Germany*
[d] *EKN-Neuropsychology Research Group, Hospital Bogenhausen, München, Germany*

Received 6 December 2005
Revised 16 February 2006
Accepted 22 June 2006

Abstract. *Purpose*: To evaluate whether repetitive optokinetic stimulation with active pursuit eye movements leads to substantial and greater recovery from visual neglect as compared to conventional visual scanning training.
Methods: Two groups of five patients with leftsided hemineglect were consecutively collected and matched for clinical and demographic variables as well as neglect severity. One group received five treatment sessions of repetitive optokinetic stimulation (R-OKS) within one week, while the other group received the same amount of conventional visual scanning training (VST) using identical visual stimuli and setup. All patients were treated in a single-subject baseline design with treatment-free intervals before (14 days) and after specific neglect therapy (14 days). Dependent variables were the improvements in digit cancellation, visuoperceptual and visuomotor line bisection and visual size distortion during treatment. The transfer of treatment effects was assessed by a paragraph reading test.
Results: The results showed superior effects of OKS treatment in all five patients which generalized across all tasks administered and remained stable at follow-up. In contrast, no significant improvements were obtained after VST training in any of these tasks, except in line bisection.
Conclusion: We conclude that the presentation of *moving* visual stimulus displays with active smooth pursuit eye movements can be more efficient than conventional visual scanning training using *static* visual displays.

Keywords: Brain damage, neglect, visual motion, rehabilitation, therapy, recovery

Abbreviations: OKS: optokinetic stimulation, VST: visual scanning training

1. Introduction

Hemineglect denotes the impaired or lost ability to react to or process sensory stimuli (visual, auditory, tactile, olfactory) presented in the hemispace contralateral to the lesioned cerebral hemisphere. Despite recovery of the most obvious signs of hemineglect in the first 2–3 months after stroke a considerable portion of neglect patients – especially those with *large* right-hemispheric lesions – remains severely impaired in visual scanning, reading and functional activities of daily living (ADL) [10,14]. Furthermore, neglect patients have a delayed recovery from hemiplegia [3], often display postural problems [31] and suffer from a poor long-term outcome as compared to patients without neglect. Few neglect patients recover in a way that allows them to live independently or even return to work. Since its

*Corresponding author: Prof. Dr. G. Kerkhoff, Clinical Neuropsychology Unit, Saarland University, Faculty of Social Sciences, Postbox 15 11 50; D-66041 Saarbrücken, Germany. E-mail: kerkhoff@mx.uni-saarland.de.

introduction by Diller and colleagues [4] visual scanning training (further abbreviated VST) has been used successfully as a treatment for neglect [1]. However, VST is often laborious, requires numerous treatment sessions (i.e. about 40 [16]) shows little transfer to activities of daily living [29] and has no effect on non-visual neglect [35]. Another drawback of VST is that it is based on *top-down mechanisms* requiring a conscious compensatory strategy – which is often difficult for the acute patient due to unawareness of the symptoms. Consequently, treatments based on *bottom-up mechanisms* which do not require explicit awareness of the deficits may be more successful in these patients.

In the last decade a variety of sensory stimulation techniques (for review, see [18]) have shown that virtually every aspect of neglect behaviour can be significantly, though transiently improved by such techniques. The basic idea underlying all sensory stimulation approaches in neglect patients is that neglect results from a disrupted representation and/or transformation of spatial coordinates into a common frame of reference necessary for accurate orientation of the subject in space. Since multiple sensory and proprioceptive informations are fed into such a hypothetical reference frame, many of these input channels have been used to manipulate the neglect symptomatology by varying this input.

One of these techniques, optokinetic stimulation (OKS [27]) or repetitive optokinetic stimulation [17]), is based on visual displays of numerous stimuli all moving coherently to the patient's neglected side. This technique positively affects several aspects of the neglect syndrome. Leftward OKS temporarily reduces the ipsilesional line-bisection error [22,27], alleviates the ipsilesional deviation of the subjective visual straight ahead [13] and it transiently decreases visual size-distortion in neglect patients [19]. Moreover, OKS effects are not limited to *visual* neglect. Vallar and colleagues described significant positive effects of leftward large-field OKS on position-sense in the contra- and ipsilesional arm of patients with leftsided neglect [37,38]. Furthermore, grip-strength could be temporarily improved in two patients with leftsided hemiparesis and leftsided neglect by viewing large-field OKS moving to the neglected side [39]. Finally, leftward OKS temporarily reduces tactile extinction of the contralesional hand [24]. Interestingly, OKS induced by high velocities is not necessary to obtain modulatory effects on neglect, or is inefficient [26]. Beneficial effects occur also with low velocities ($<10°$/sec [22]), and relatively small stimulus displays ($30° \times 20°$ [34]). Although this might induce optokinetic nystagmus, it may be questioned whether the crucial effect is based on the nystagmus or other factors (see Discussion).

Despite the modulatory but mostly *transient* effects of OKS on all aspects of the neglect syndrome few studies have been conducted to use it for the treatment of neglect. Here, we report the results of a pilot study with ten neglect patients to evaluate the therapeutic potential of *repetitive* optokinetic stimulation (OKS) in comparison with Visual Scanning Training (VST) in neglect therapy. In addition to asking whether OKS has measurable and permanent therapeutic effects we were also interested to learn whether such effects generalize across different domains of the neglect syndrome, i.e. cancellation, reading, visuomotor and visuoperceptual line bisection as well as size distortions.

2. Patients and methods

2.1. Patients

Ten patients with leftsided chronic neglect (time post lesion >2 months) were tested with a battery of neglect screening tests (Table 1). The first five patients were allocated to the group receiving optokinetic stimulation (OKS), the next five patients (termed VST-group) were collected to match the patients in the OKS-group with regards to clinical and demographic variables as well as neglect severity in the baseline tests.

2.2. Tests

Cancellation tests: Patients were instructed to cancel with a pen in their right hand, two types of digits (i.e. all tokens of "1" and "9") distributed randomly among 200 single digits ranging from "0" – "9" presented on a 29×21 cm white piece of paper in front of the patient. Three tests were performed at each measurement point. The number of omissions in the left and right hemifield was counted (max. 20 per hemifield).

Reading tests: To examine the transfer to a non-trained but important activity of daily living, 25 parallel paragraph reading tasks were developed for the assessment of neglect dyslexia. Each text had on average 55 words (range: 52–58) arranged in 6 lines with irregularly indented margins on both sides (arial font, point size 12, double line spacing, size of the text: 25 cm horizontal and 9 cm vertical). Reading texts were presented centrally on a 17" PC monitor at a distance of 0.4 m from the patient. Five texts were presented suc-

Table 1
Demographic and clinical data of 10 neglect patients in the two treatment groups. In cancellation, the number of omissions on the left/right side of the page are listed (Cutoff: max 10% per hemifield); Line bisection: horizontal deviation from true midline in mm (Cutoff: +/− 5 mm); neglect dyslexia: omissions in a 180 word reading test. MCI: middle cerebral artery infarction; ICB: intracerebral bleeding; T: temporal, P: parietal, O: occipital, BG: basal ganglia

Patient code	Treatment	Age, Gender	Etiology, Months since Lesion	Lesion location	Motor/ sensory loss left side	Visual field, Field Sparing (°)	Cancell. Omissions L/R (%)	Line bisection deviation L/R (mm)	Neglect-dyslexia
OKS-1	OKS	50, m	MCI-R, 5	T,P	+/+	left quadran-tanopia, 6°	60/20	+8	moderate
OKS-2	OKS	74, f	MCI-R, 3	P	+/+	left hemianopia, 3°	100/70	+80	severe
OKS-3	OKS	54, m	MCI-R, 3	T, P	+/+	left hemianopia, 4°	30/00	+41	severe
OKS-4	OKS	55, m	MCI-R, 3	T, BG	+/+	left quadran-tanopia, 10°	30/00	−2	moderate
OKS-5	OKS	37, f	MCI-R, 3	T, P	+/+	left hemi-amblyopia 5°	30/00	0	no
Median/ mean	–	54 yrs	3 months	–	–	–	50/18	+27.4 mm	–
VST-1	VST	69, m	MCI-R, 2	T, P	+/+	left hemianopia 3°	50/10	+25	severe
VST-2	VST	50, m	MCI-R, 3	T, BG	+/+	left hemianopia, 5°	90/40	−11	moderate
VST-3	VST	60, m	MCI-R, 2	T, O	+/+	left hemianopia, 8°	50/20	+13	severe
VST-4	VST	57, f	ICB-R, 5	T,P	+/+	left hemianopia 3°	80/10	+39	moderate
VST-5	VST	53, f	MCI-R, 3	T,P	+/+	left hemianopia 4°	30/00	+70	moderate
Median/ mean	–	57 yrs	3 months	–	–	–	60/16	+31.6 mm	–

cessively on each measurement. Two types of errors were analysed: omissions of words (space-based errors) and substitutions of words or word-parts (word- or object-centered errors). In addition reading time was recorded with a stopwatch.

Line bisection: Visuoperceptual horizontal line-bisection was tested with VS, a computerized test system for the analysis of spatial perception [17]. A 25 × 1 cm yellow horizontal bar was presented centrally on a screen at a distance of 40 cm from the patient. On the right side of the bar a small vertical slit was visible (0.2 cm wide) which had to be positioned towards the patient's subjective midline position. No manual performance was allowed by the patient, who indicated verbally to the examiner how to position the slit into the midline position. Ten trials were performed on each measurement. Visuomotor line bisection was tested with a paper and pencil test. A 20 cm long and 5 mm wide black horizontal line was presented centrally on a 29 × 21 cm large white piece of paper. The patient was instructed to bisect the line with a pencil using his/her right hand. Three trials were performed at each measurement point on separate test sheets.

All tests were untimed; only in the paragraph reading test reading times were taken with a stopwatch.

2.3. Repetitive optokinetic stimulation (OKS)

Visual stimuli were presented on a 17" PC monitor (eccentricity: 22.4° horizontal, 17.4° vertical). The patients were instructed to look at computer-generated random displays of 30–70 dots (2–4 cm in diameter) on a dark background, using specifically designed software (EyeMove, www.Medical-Computing.de). All dots moved coherently towards the left, contralesional hemispace with a speed of 7.5–50°/s. Movement speed was varied from trial to trial to keep patients alert. Subjects were encouraged to make smooth pursuit movements towards the direction of the motion and return with their eyes repeatedly to the ipsilesional side of the screen. No head movements were allowed. Every 10 minutes a break was given for a few minutes without OKS-stimulation. Thus, in every therapy session 4 runs of OKS à 10 minutes duration were practiced (see Fig. 1A)

2.4. Visual scanning treatment (VST)

The five control patients received the same amount of neglect treatment as the OKS group, using the same device and stimuli (see above), yet with the important difference that all visual stimuli displayed on the screen remained *stationary*. Patients were instructed to scan the stimuli in a systematic way starting on the left top to the right bottom of the screen (see Fig. 1B). Scanning strategies were repeatedly explained to the patients and the timing of treatment and breaks was identical to the OKS group. Patients were encouraged to make (saccadic) eye movements and scan to the left side as far as possible. Head movements were not allowed. Thus, in every therapy session 4 runs of VST à 10 minutes duration were practiced. Hence, the crucial difference between the two treatments lay in the moving vs. stationary character of the visual stimuli, and subsequently,

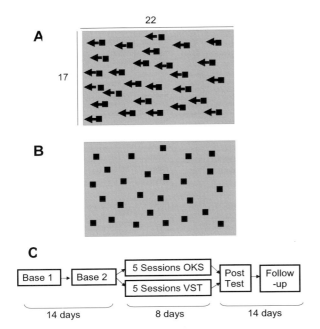

Fig. 1. Schematic illustration of the setup for the optokinetic stimulation training (A) and the visual scanning treatment (B), and the design of the study (C). For details see text. Note, that the arrows in Fig. A only show the direction of motion, they were not visible for the patient.

in the type of eye movements exacted by the patient (saccades in the VST vs. pursuit eye movements and saccades in the OKS group).

2.5. Design

Every patient was studied in a single subject baseline design with a treatment-free interval of 14 days *before* the specific neglect therapy (OKS or VST) and an identical follow-up period of 14 days after this period. During the 14-day baseline period all subjects were tested three times (twice in the bisection and size distortion tasks, respectively) in all neglect tests to exclude effects of spontaneous recovery and/or test repetition or the influence of other therapies. The follow-up period served to test the stability of improvements. The day after the last baseline assessment specific neglect treatment was started (either OKS or VST) and performed for five sessions (à 45 minutes, delivered in a period of seven to ten days). All neglect tests were repeated on the day after the fifth treatment session and 14 days after this post-test a follow-up investigation was performed (see Fig. 1C). Apart from the specific neglect treatment, all patients received standard occupational therapy and physiotherapy – but no neglect nor attentional nor reading training – throughout the *complete* course of the study (hence during baseline, treatment and follow-up periods in both treatment groups).

3. Results

Due to the small samples all statistical analyses were run separately for both patient groups with nonparametric tests over all single trials in the five patients of each group. Friedman nonparametric analyses of variance were used to test for overall effects over time and paired comparisons were performed with Wilcoxon-tests (two-tailed, $p < 0.05$, Bonferroni-correction).

3.1. Comparison of the two treatment groups before neglect therapy

Both treatment groups were comparable with respect to clinical and demographic variables (see Table 1). In addition, we compared the two treatment groups via Mann-whitney tests with respect to the outcome variables on the last baseline measurement before specific neglect treatment was started. No significant differences were obtained for any of the seven outcome variables detailed in the results section (largest U-value: 182.0, smallest p-value: 0.075). Taken together, these results show that both groups were comparable regarding demographic and clinical variables as well as neglect severity before treatment.

3.2. Cancellation

In the OKS group the Friedman-test revealed a significant main effect over time for the number of left-sided (contralesional) omissions ($\chi^2 = 34.4$, $df = 4$, $p < 0.0001$). Post-hoc Wilcoxon-tests revealed no significant change between the first and third baseline $z = -1.9$, $p > 0.05$). After OKS treatment the percentage of leftsided omissions in cancellation had significantly decreased relative to the third baseline ($z = -3.7$, $p < 0.0001$; see Fig. 2A). These improvements were maintained from the post-test to the follow-up test ($z = -1.1$, $p > 0.05$). In contrast, no significant effect was found for the number of rightsided (ipsilesional) omissions ($\chi^2 = 6.5$, $df = 4$, $p > 0.05$). This result was mainly due to the small percentage of rightsided omissions in three neglect patients with moderate visual neglect (ceiling effect). The mean percentage of rightsided omissions ranged between 8.3%

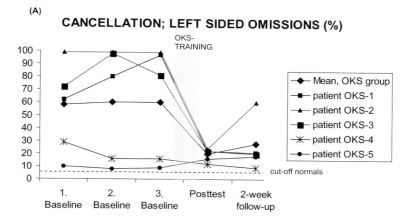

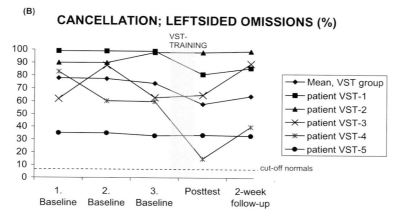

Fig. 2. Effects of repetitive optokinetic stimulation (OKS, **A**) and visual scanning training (VST, **B**) on the percentage of contralesional (leftsided) omissions in digit cancellation. Single graphs of five patients are displayed (individual mean values and group mean; see legend). Note the stability of deficits over the baseline period, and the significant reduction of omissions after treatment which remained stable at follow-up. The shaded area indicates the treatment period, the dotted line shows the normal cutoff in this task. For patient codes see Table 1.

and 28% in the five patients over the five measurement points.

In the VST group the Friedman-test revealed no significant effect over time for the number of left-sided (contralesional) omissions ($\chi^2 = 6.541$, $df = 4$, $p > 0.05$; see Fig. 2B). Furthermore, no significant effect for the number of rightsided (ipsilesional) omissions was found over time ($\chi^2 = 8.473$, $df = 4$, $p > 0.05$) although there was a nonsignificant trend towards a reduction of rightsided omissions after VST-training (exact $p = 0.076$). The mean percentage of rightsided omissions ranged from 19% to 39 % in the 5 patients over all measurement points.

3.3. Line bisection

For *perceptual* line bisection (on the PC screen) there was a significant effect over time in the OKS group ($\chi^2 = 46.5$, $df = 3$, $p < 0.001$). Subsequent Wilcoxon-tests revealed a significant deterioration in performance from the first to the second baseline ($z = -4.5$, $p < 0.001$). After OKS the rightsided deviation in line bisection was significantly reduced as compared to the second baseline ($z = -5.3$, $p < 0.001$; see Fig. 3A). These improvements were maintained from the post-test up to the follow-up ($z = -0.7$, $p > 0.05$).

In the VST group there was also a significant effect over time in perceptual line bisection ($\chi^2 = 29.6$, $df = 3$, $p < 0.0001$). Subsequent Wilcoxon-tests revealed a significant deterioration in performance from the first to the second baseline ($z = -2.9$, $p < 0.005$). After VST the rightsided deviation in line bisection was significantly reduced as compared to the second baseline ($z = -5.5$, $p < 0.0001$; see Fig. 3B). These improvements remained stable from the post-test up to the follow-up test ($z = -1.2$, $p > 0.05$).

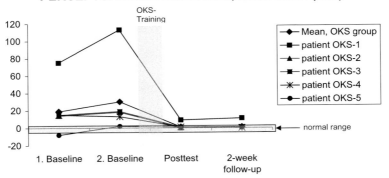

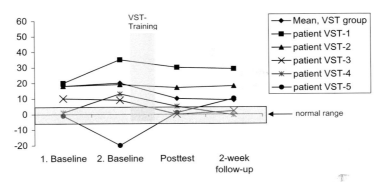

Fig. 3. Effects of repetitive optokinetic stimulation (OKS, **A**) and visual scanning training (VST, **B**) on visuoperceptual, horizontal line bisection. The deviation from the true midline is displayed (in mm; $-/+$ denote left-/rightward deviations from the true midline). Note the deterioration of deficits over the baseline period, and the significant reduction of the deviation after treatment which remained stable at follow-up. The shaded area indicates the treatment period, the striped area indicates the normal range. Patient codes as in Fig. 2.

For manual (visuomotor) line bisection there was a significant effect over time in the OKS group ($\chi^2 = 19.8$, $df = 3$, $p < 0.0001$). Post-hoc Wilcoxon-tests revealed no significant difference in performance between the first and the second baseline ($z = -0.1$, $p > 0.05$). After OKS therapy visuomotor line bisection had significantly improved as compared to the second baseline ($z = -2.6$, $p < 0.005$; see Fig. 4A). These improvements were maintained between the post- and follow-up test ($z = -0.2, p > 0.05$).

In the VST group no significant effect over time was observed for *visuomotor* line bisection ($\chi^2 = 0.3$, $df = 3$, $p > 0.05$; see Fig. 4B).

3.4. Size distortion

A significant main effect over time was found in the OKS group for the extent of the visual size distortion in the length judgment task ($\chi^2 = 19.0$, $df = 3$, $p < 0.0001$). No significant change was observed between the first and second baseline ($z = -1.6$, $p > 0.05$). After OKS-therapy the size distortion was significantly reduced as compared to the second baseline ($z = -4.1$, $p < 0.0001$; see Fig. 5A). These improvements were maintained from the post-test up to the follow-up test ($z = -2.0$, $p > 0.05$). Three of the five patients showed the typical size distortion during baseline (overreproduction of the horizontal length of the bar in the contralesional, left hemispace). This deficit improved in all three cases after treatment. The other two cases showed no stable size distortion before treatment and did not show any consistent change over time.

No significant effect over time was found for the extent of the visual size distortion in the VST group ($\chi^2 = 3.2$, $df = 3$, $p > 0.05$; see Fig. 5B). Four of the five patients showed the typical size distortion over nearly all measurement dates, with the exception of patient VST-2 who scored in the normal range in the first baseline test. In none of these four patients a

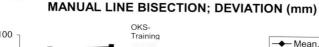
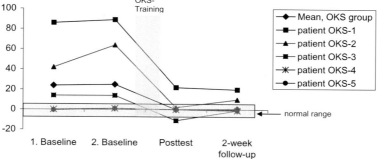
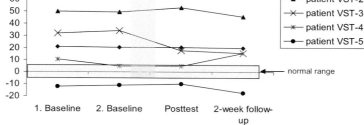

Fig. 4. Effects of repetitive optokinetic stimulation (OKS, **A**) and visual scanning training (VST, **B**) on visuomotor (manual), horizontal line bisection. Note the stability of deficits over the baseline period, and the significant reduction of the deviation after treatment which remained stable at follow-up. The shaded area indicates the treatment period, the striped area indicates the normal range. Patient codes as in Fig. 2.

significant change was observed after VST. The fifth patient in the VST group did not show a consistent size distortion over the four measurement points.

3.5. Reading

The Friedman-test revealed a significant main effect over time for the number of omissions ($\chi^2 = 34.4$, $df = 4$, $p < 0.0001$). No significant change was observed between the first and third baseline ($z = -1.9$, $p > 0.05$) although there was a trend for a nonsignificant deterioration from the first to the third baseline test (see Fig. 6A). After OKS reading had improved significantly in the posttest as compared to the third baseline ($z = -3.7$, $p < 0.0001$). These improvements were maintained from the post-test up to the follow-up ($z = -1.1$, $p > 0.05$).

In contrast, no improvement was observed regarding object-based reading errors (substitutions; $\chi^2 = 4.3$, $df = 4$, $p > 0.05$). The mean error rates for substitutions were: Base 1: 2.7%, Base 2: 2.0%, Base 3: 2.7%, Posttest: 2.3%, Follow-up: 2.1%).

Finally, mean reading times (per condition) were compared over the five measurements. There was no significant effect over time ($\chi^2 = 6.5$, $df = 4$, $p > 0.05$) showing that the reduction of omissions after treatment reported above did not occur as a result of increased time spent during the reading tasks. However, there was a numerical but statistical nonsignificant trend for longer reading times at the post- und follow-up test. The mean reading times (per text) for the five measurements were: Base(line) 1: 58.9 s (seconds), Base 2: 54.8 s, Base 3: 61.1 s, Posttest: 70.5 s, Follow-up-test: 76.4 s.

In the VST group no significant effect over time was observed for the number of omissions in the paragraph reading test ($\chi^2 = 6.8$, $df = 4$, $p > 0.05$). Likewise, no significant change over time was observed with respect to object-based reading errors (substitutions; $\chi^2 = 2.1$, $df = 4$, $p > 0.05$). The mean er-

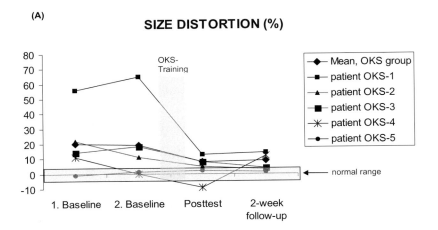

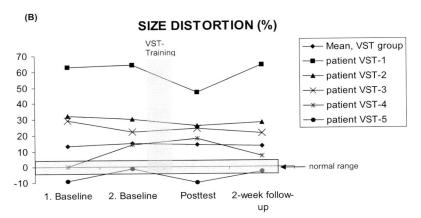

Fig. 5. Effects of repetitive optokinetic stimulation (OKS, **A**) and visual scanning training (VST, **B**) on the horizontal visual size distortion (+/− denotes over- or underestimation of the left line segment in % compared to the reference bar). Single graphs of five patients are displayed (individual mean values and group mean). Note the stability of the size distortion over the two baselines in three neglect patients, and their improvement after OKS. Two subjects did not show size distortions. Patient codes as in Fig. 2.

ror rates for substitutions were: Base 1: 2.9%, Base 2: 2.3%, Base 3: 1.7%, Posttest: 2.8%, Follow-up: 2.9%). Finally, mean reading times (per condition) were compared over the five measurement dates. There was a significant effect over time ($\chi^2 = 10.0$, $df = 4$, $p < 0.05$). Wilcoxon tests showed that the reading time increased significantly from the second to the third baseline ($z = -2.5$, $p < 0.05$). Furthermore, the reading time at the follow-up was significantly longer as that during the first ($z = -2.2$, $p > 0.05$) and the second baseline ($z < 0.05$). All other paired comparisons were not significantly different (largest $z = -1.559$, smallest $p = 0.119$). The mean reading times (per text) for the five measurements were: Base(line) 1: 57.6 seconds (s), Base 2: 53.3 s, Base 3: 62.9 s, Posttest: 58.6 s, Follow-up-test: 64.9 s.

3.6. Mean improvements and their stability

In order to make the improvements and stability of the obtained improvements during therapy more comparable we computed the average change (in %) after training as compared to averaged pre-treatment baseline values for each test and treatment group separately (Table 2). Similarly, we computed a measure of stability by comparing the mean change (in %) from averaged pre-treatment baseline values to the follow-up-test. When both measures yield similar values this indicates relative stability of the treatment effects. As is obvious from Table 2 the values for improvement and stability are nearly identical for most test variables in both groups, but in toto are about five times higher in the OKS group than in the VST group.

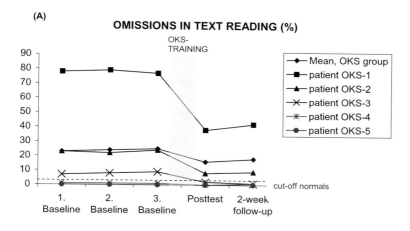

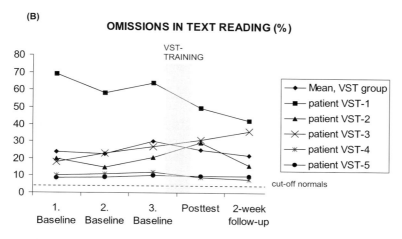

Fig. 6. Effects of repetitive optokinetic stimulation (OKS, **A**) and visual scanning training (VST, **B**) on the percentage of omissions in paragraph reading. Single graphs of five patients in the group receiving repetitive optokinetic stimulation (OKS) are displayed (individual mean values and group mean). Note the stability of neglect in reading during the baseline period in all patients. Patient codes as in Fig. 2.

4. Discussion

Two main findings are apparent from this pilot study: 1) repetitive OKS has therapeutic effects in a wide variety of visual neglect tasks, showing that the obtained improvements generalize across several domains of neglect, different tasks as well as different input/output modes (i.e. in line bisection). Furthermore, OKS is more effective than conventional visual scanning training. 2) OKS has similar therapeutic effects as other novel therapeutic techniques, i.e. attentional and limb activation training [28,30], neck muscle vibration [35] or prism adaptation [8]. The subsequent discussion will deal with these two main aspects.

4.1. General therapeutic effects of OKS

To our knowledge this is the first successful study showing significant therapeutic effects after a small number of OKS treatment sessions in patients with moderate to severe visual neglect. Previous authors using slow visual motion have indeed suggested that *repetitive* motion stimuli might constitute a promising treatment technique [22], although a recent study did not obtain additional positive effects of OKS training in neglect therapy [26]. The improvements obtained in the present study clearly demonstrate that this may be achieved. The improvements covered different domains of neglect (cancellation, reading and visuospatial tasks) as well as different input/output modes as in *visuoperceptual* vs. *visuomotor* line bisection. Moreover, improvements were also obtained in a highly relevant task for daily living, i.e. paragraph reading. The fact that omissions (space based errors) could be reduced significantly whereas the less frequent substitutions were not affected by OKS treatment shows that the therapeutic effects are quite specific and cannot be explained by unspecific effects (i.e. arousal, test repetition).

Furthermore, leftsided omissions in cancellation were considerably reduced. The reason for the non-significant change of rightsided (ipsilesional omissions) in the OKS group lies in the simple fact that three of the five neglect patients showed only very rarely omissions on the right side of the test sheet and therefore could not improve further on this side after treatment (due to a ceiling effect).

With respect to line bisection, improvements were obtained for visuomotor *and* visuoperceptual line bisection tests indicating that the therapeutic effect transferred from perceptual tasks to those that require overt motor responses. Interestingly, OKS positively affected the visual size distortion in all three patients who showed such perceptual distortions before therapy. This result fits neatly to the positive but *transient* modulatory effect of leftsided OKS on visual size distortions in neglect reported recently by us [34]. It contrasts with the finding, that neck muscle vibration has neither a transient ("on-line") [34], nor a permanent effect on line bisection [35].

Despite the clearcut results reported here with OKS therapy some methodological caveats have to be kept in mind. First, our samples were relatively small and matched. Instead of a randomized allocation of subjects to one of the two treatments – which is feasible in studies with larger samples ($n > 25$) – the small sample size necessitated an individual matching of patients in the two treatment groups according to clinical and demographic variables. This was done to achieve relatively homogenous subgroups with respect to clinical variables and neglect severity. Clearly, this induces a risk of a selection bias [21], although we tried to parallel both samples as far as possible. Subsequent studies using OKS as neglect therapy should adopt a randomized control group design based on larger samples (see Lincoln and Bowen, this volume, for a detailed discussion of these aspects [21].

4.2. Comparison of OKS with other neglect treatments

When comparing the effects of the present study with other neglect treatments there are accordances as well as divergencies. OKS has similar therapeutic effects on visual neglect as attentional training [28], prism adaptation [7,8,32] and neck muscle vibration [11]. Nevertheless, few studies have so far *directly* compared the efficiency of these novel techniques with another *specific* neglect treatment, i.e. conventional VST. Most often, a novel treatment has been compared with an unspecific therapy or with a "no-treatment-group" receiving what is called "standard occupational and physiotherapy". Such a strategy clearly favours the more specific neglect treatment. The present study indicates that neglect therapy based on repetitive sensory stimulation is more effective than VST, although the latter is at least partially effective, too [1]. However, the effects of these "bottom-up" therapeutic techniques seem to be superior to those obtained with "top-down" compensatory strategies such as VST, or reach similar improvements in a considerably shorter time period. However, there are also limitations of these new "bottom-up"-techniques. Neither neck-vibration [35], nor OKS (present study), nor prism adaptation [6] seem to affect object-centered neglect phenomena, i.e. substitution errors in paragraph reading. Although these errors constituted only 3% of all reading errors in our patients other treatment approaches have to be developed for neglect patients with pronounced object-centered neglect of this type. Furthermore, the lack of OKS-treatment impact on object-centered neglect nicely illustrates the dissociability of space- and object-related attentional mechanisms.

4.3. What is the crucial effect of OKS therapy?

With respect to the putative mechanism of OKS in neglect therapy two hypotheses may be advocated, which are also compatible with each other. First, OKS or coherent background motion with slower velocities (even with small stimulus displays) may facilitate the directing of attention towards neglected regions of space [22]. This improved attention allocation leads to subsequent improvements in all visual neglect tasks requiring systematic leftward exploration, as in cancellation, reading, size comparisons or line bisection. This view is corroborated by the observation that forcing the patients' attention to the contralesional side produces a change in the degree of size distortion in patients with visual neglect [5]. A recent optokinetic treatment study [36] clearly corroborates this hypothesis. In this study, Sturm, Thimm and Fink found significant improvements in behavioural neglect tasks, including a visual attention test, after 3 weeks of optokinetic stimulation in seven patients with visual neglect, using the same device and test stimuli as we used in the present study (EYEMOVE). Moreover, they obtained evidence of a significant re-activation in posterior cortical regions (including angular gyrus, temporo-occipital areas, precuneus and posterior cingulate gyrus [36], induced by

Table 2

The mean improvement in performance (in %) after treatment (OKS = optokinetic stimulation versus visual scanning training = VST) as compared to averaged pre-treatment baseline values is indicated. Furthermore, we computed the mean change in performance at the follow-up investigation as compared to the averaged pre-treatment-baseline values as a measure of the stability of treatment effects (stability). Note, that the averaged improvements are higher for all test variables after optokinetic treatment, and that there similar values for stability and improvement in this group indicating stability of the improvements achieved during treatment. In contrast, the improvements in the visual scanning group were considerably smaller. −indicates deterioration, +indicates improvement

Test Variable	Improvement OKS	Improvement VST	Stability OKS	Stability VST
Cancellation, omissions left side	+65.0	+23.0	+65.0	+13.7
Line Bisection Perceptual	+95.8	+27.7	+100	+33.3
Line Bisection Manual	+100	00	+100	00
Size Distortion	+50.0	+3.7	+45.0	+3.7
Reading, omissions	+21.7	+5.3	+17.4	+13.6
Mean (all tests)	+66.5	+11.9	+65.5	+12.9

OKS. In contrast to our study, the improvements remained only partially stable at the follow-up investigation 4 weeks after cessation of the neglect treatment in their patients. While the question of long-term stability of optokinetic neglect therapy clearly requires further in-depth-studies with longer follow-up-periods (i.e. 2–6 months) the fMRI-results of Sturm et al. [36] corroborate our earlier hypothesis [18] according to which repetitive optokinetic stimulation re-activates many of those cortical regions activated by the same stimulation in healthy subjects. These regions include those posterior cortical regions identified by Sturm et al. [36], as well as subcortical regions like the basal ganglia and the thalamus. More precisely, leftward optokinetic stimulation might *initially* activate the undamaged left hemisphere – as suggested recently [5] and *consecutively* via callosal fibers the damaged right hemisphere in patients with left neglect.

Another hypothesis which is well compatible with the scenario outlined above is that OKS facilitates the generation of a more accurate egocentric space representation by providing directional, visual motion input to this disturbed spatial representation in neglect patients. Since the visual motion system remains largely intact even after large cortical lesions [33], most of this system remains functional in neglect. In accordance with this hypothesis multiple activation sites in the lesioned and intact hemisphere were found with full-field OKS in an imaging study of hemianopic subjects without neglect [2]. Thus, global directional motion – even in a blind hemifield – might constitute a strong modulatory input to the visual motion system in the dorsal visual stream, thereby influencing spatial attention and perception in patients. Another interesting variable which has been completely neglected so far is the potential role of smooth pursuit eye movements which are elicited when following moving visual stimuli during OKS. Interestingly, Gur and Ron [9] were able to show a significant improvement in functional visual tasks after a feedback-based training of smooth pursuit eye movements in patients with closed head trauma, but without neglect. A recent functional imaging study with healthy subjects showed that smooth pursuit eye-movements as well as optokinetic nystagmus activate a largely overlapping neural network including the visual cortex, human area MT, the frontal and supplementary eye fields, parietal cortex and cerebellar regions of both hemispheres [20]. We hypothesized recently [18] that the partial *re*-activation of some of these regions can be induced by repetitive optokinetic stimulation in neglect patients and might constitute the physiological-anatomic correlate of the improvements seen in behavioural neglect tests in these patients. Indeed, this hypothesis was largely confirmed recently [36], as argued above. Furthermore, Sturm et al. [36] results strongly suggest that the strict dichotomy between neglect treatments based on attention training and neglect treatments based on sensory stimulation manoeuvers may be unnecessary and contraproductive since both types of treatment may lead to behaviourally equivalent improvements, although the physiological-anatomic mechanisms leading to these improvements may be quite different. We therefore believe that it is more fruitful for future research to combine different treatment approaches and evaluate whether this combination evokes greater improvements on the behavioural level.

Our positive results of OKS treatment in neglect are at variance with a recent study [26] using an individually adapted form of optokinetic stimulation in neglect patients who did not benefit significantly from this add-on-treatment which was given in addition to conventional scanning training. The reasons for these discrepant results are not clear at the moment. Future studies, using eye movement recording devices, will have to pinpoint precisely the crucial therapeutic mechanism(s), and evaluate whether OKS therapy has also beneficial therapeutic effects on functional measures, activities of daily living, on the unawareness and finally on *nonvisual* neglect. As many patients with visual neglect also show auditory [25] and tactile neglect [12] the aspect of crossmodal therapeutic efficiency deserves more attention in future studies. Both neck vibration [35] and prism adaptation [23] have crossmodal effects on tactile neglect which are not obtained with VST training [35]. In summary, the display of contralesionally moving visual stimuli via conventional PC technology provides an easy-to-use and effective therapeutic technique for patients with visuospatial neglect. In the future, randomized treatment studies will have to elucidate the precise mechanisms of action and evaluate possible crossmodal (haptic, auditory, representational) therapeutic effects of this method on multimodal neglect.

Acknowledgements

We are grateful to two reviewers for helpful comments on a previous version of the manuscript.

References

[1] G. Antonucci, C. Guariglia, A. Judica, L. Magnotti, S. Paolucci, L. Pizzamiglio and P. Zoccolotti, Effectiveness of Neglect Rehabilitation in a Randomized Group Study, *Journal of Clinical and Experimental Neuropsychology* **17** (1995), 383–389.

[2] Th. Brandt, S.F. Bucher, K.C. Seelos and M. Dieterich, Bilateral functional MRI activations of the basal ganglia and middle temporal/medial superior temporal motion-sensitive areas – Optokinetic stimulation in homonymous hemianopia, *Archives of Neurology* **55** (1998), 1126–1131.

[3] G. Denes, C. Semenza, E. Stoppa and A. Lis, Unilateral spatial neglect and recovery from hemiplegia. A follow-up study, *Brain* **105** (1982), 543–552.

[4] L. Diller and J. Weinberg, Hemi-inattention in rehabilitation: The evolution of a rational remediation program, *Advances in Neurology* **18** (1977), 63–82.

[5] F. Doricchi, I. Siegler, G. Iaria and A. Berthoz, Vestibo-ocular and optokinetic impairments in left unilateral neglect, *Neuropsychologia* **40** (2002), 2084–2099.

[6] A. Farné, Y. Rosetti, S. Toniolo and E. Ladavas, Ameliorating neglect with prism adaption: visuo-manual and visuo-verbal measures, *Neuropsychologia* **40** (2002), 718–729.

[7] A. Farnè, Y. Rossetti, S. Toniolo and E. Ladavas, Ameliorating neglect with prism adaptation: visuo-manual and visuo-verbal measures, *Neuropsychologia* **40** (2002), 718–729.

[8] F. Frassinetti, V. Angeli, F. Meneghello and E. Làdavas, Long-lasting amelioration of visuospatial neglect by prism adaptation, *Brain* **125** (2002), 608–623.

[9] S. Gur and S. Ron, Training in oculomotor tracking: occupational health aspects, *Israel Journal of Medical Science* **28** (1992), 622–628.

[10] M. Jehkonen, J.-P. Ahonen, P. Dastidar, A.-M. Koivisto, P. Laippala, J. Vikki and G. Molnár, Visual neglect as a predictor of functional outcome one year after stroke, *Acta Neurologica Scandinavia* **101** (2000), 195–201.

[11] L. Johannsen, H. Ackermann and H.-O. Karnath, Lasting amelioration of spatial neglect by treatment with neck muscle vibration even without concurrent training, *Journal of Rehabilitation Medicine* **35** (2003), 249–253.

[12] H.O. Karnath and M.-T. Perenin, Tactile exploration of peripersonal space in patients with neglect, *NeuroReport* **9** (1998), 2273–2277.

[13] H.-O. Karnath, Optokinetic stimulation influences the disturbed perception of body orientation in spatial neglect, *Journal of Neurology, Neurosurgery, and Psychiatry* **60** (1996), 217–220.

[14] N. Katz, A. Hartman-Maeir, H. Ring and N. Soroker, Functional disability and rehabilitation outcome in right hemisphere damaged patients with and without unilateral spatial neglect, *Archives of Physical Medicine & Rehabilitation* **80** (1999), 379–384.

[15] I. Keller, J. Ditterich, T. Eggert and A. Straube, Size distortion in spatial neglect, *NeuroReport* **11** (2000), 1655–1660.

[16] G. Kerkhoff, Rehabilitation of Visuospatial Cognition and Visual Exploration in Neglect: a Cross-over Study, *Restorative Neurology and Neuroscience* **12** (1998), 27–40.

[17] G. Kerkhoff, Multiple perceptual distortions and their modulation in patients with left visual neglect, *Neuropsychologia* **38** (2000), 1073–1086.

[18] G. Kerkhoff, Transient modulation and rehabilitation of spatial neglect by sensory stimulation, *Progress in Brain Research* **142** (2003), 257–281.

[19] G. Kerkhoff, I. Schindler, I. Keller and C. Marquardt, Visual background motion reduces size distortion in spatial neglect, *NeuroReport* **10** (1999), 319–323.

[20] C.S. Konen, R. Kleiser, R.J. Seitz and F. Bremmer, An fMRI study of optokinetic nystagmus and smooth-pursuit eye movements in humans, *Experimental Brain Research* **165** (2005), 203–216.

[21] N.B. Lincoln and A. Bowen,The need for randomised treatment studies in neglect research, *Restor Neurol Neurosci* (2006).

[22] J.B. Mattingley, J.L. Bradshaw and J.A. Bradshaw, Horizontal visual motion modulates focal attention in left unilateral spatial neglect, *Journal of Neurology, Neurosurgery, and Psychiatry* **57** (1994), 1228–1235.

[23] R.D. McIntosh, Y. Rossetti and A.D. Milner, Prism adaptation improves chronic visual and haptic neglect: a single case study, *Cortex* **38** (2002), 309–320.

[24] D. Nico, Effectiveness of sensory stimulation on tactile extinction, *Experimental Brain Research* **127** (1999), 75–82.

[25] F. Pavani, M. Husain, E. Ladavas and J. Driver, Auditory deficits in visuospatial neglect patients, *Cortex* **40** (2004), 347–365.

[26] L. Pizzamiglio, L. Fasotti, M. Jehkonen, G. Antonucci, L. Magnotti, D. Boelen and S. Asa, The use of optokinetic stimu-

lation in rehabilitation of the hemineglect disorder, *Cortex* **40** (2004), 441–450.

[27] L. Pizzamiglio, R. Frasca, C. Guariglia, C. Incoccia and G. Antonucci, Effect of optokinetic stimulation in patients with visual neglect, *Cortex* **26** (1990), 535–540.

[28] I. Robertson and T. Manly, Cognitive routes to the rehabilitation of unilateral neglect, in: *The Cognitive and Neural Bases of Spatial Neglect*, H.-O. Karnath, A.D. Milner and G. Vallar, eds, Oxford University Press, Oxford, 2002, pp. 365–374.

[29] I.H. Robertson, Cognitive rehabilitation: attention and neglect, *Trends in Cognitive Sciences* **3** (1999), 385–393.

[30] G. Rode, L. Pisella, Y. Rossetti, A. Farnè and D. Boisson, Bottom-up transfer of sensory-motor plasticity to recovery of spatial cognition: visuomotor adaptation and spatial neglect, in: *Progress in Brain Research*, C. Prablanc, D. élisson and Y. Rossetti, eds, Elsevier Science B.V., 2003, pp. 273–287.

[31] G. Rode, C. Tiliket and D. Boisson, Predominance of postural imbalance in left hemiparetic patients, *Scandinavian Journal of Rehabilitation Medicine* **29** (1997), 11–16.

[32] Y. Rossetti, G. Rode, L. Pisella, A. Farné, D. Boisson and M.-T. Perenin, Prism adaptation to a rightward optical deviation rehabilitates left hemispatial neglect, *Nature* **395** (1998), 166–169.

[33] Th. Schenk and J. Zihl, Visual motion perception after brain damage: I. Deficits in global motion perception, *Neuropsychologia* **35** (1997), 1289–1297.

[34] I. Schindler and G. Kerkhoff, Convergent and divergent effects of neck proprioceptive and visual motion stimulation on visual space processing in neglect, *Neuropsychologia* **42** (2004), 1149–1155.

[35] I. Schindler, G. Kerkhoff, H.-O. Karnath, I. Keller and G. Goldenberg, Neck muscle vibration induces lasting recovery in spatial neglect, *Journal of Neurology, Neurosurgery, and Psychiatry* **73** (2002), 412–419.

[36] W. Sturm, M. Thimm and G.R. Fink, Alertness-Training in Neglect – Behavioural and Imaging Results, *Restorative Neurology and Neuroscience* (2006).

[37] G. Vallar, G. Antonucci, C. Guariglia and L. Pizzamiglio, Deficits of position sense, unilateral neglect, and optokinetic stimulation, *Neuropsychologia* **31** (1993), 1191–1200.

[38] G. Vallar, C. Guariglia, L. Magnotti and L. Pizzamiglio, Optokinetic Stimulation Affects Both Vertical and Horizontal Deficits of Position Sense in Unilateral Neglect, *Cortex* **31** (1995), 669–683.

[39] G. Vallar, C. Guariglia, D. Nico and L. Pizzamiglio, Motor deficits and optokinetic stimulation in patients with left hemineglect, *Neurology* **49** (1997), 1364–1370.

Alertness-training in neglect: Behavioral and imaging results

W. Sturm[a,*], M. Thimm[a], J. Küst[d], H. Karbe[d] and G.R. Fink[b,c]
[a]*Department of Neurology, Section Clinical Neuropsychology, University Hospital RWTH Aachen, Germany*
[b]*Institute of Medicine, Research Centre Jülich, Germany*
[c]*Department of Neurology, Cognitive Neurology, University Hospital RWTH Aachen, Germany*
[d]*Neurological Rehabilitation Centre Godeshöhe, Bonn, Germany*

Received 9 November 2005
Revised 7 February 2006
Accepted 22 June 2006

Abstract. *Purpose*: It has been proposed that the right hemisphere alerting network co-activates, either directly or via the brainstem, the spatial attention system in the parietal cortex. The observation that measures of impaired alertness and sustained attention can be used to predict the outcome of neglect might suggest such a relationship, too. The aim of the present study was to investigate the effects of alertness training on hemispatial neglect.
Method: A three-week computerised alertness training was applied to patients with chronic (>3 months) stable visuospatial hemineglect. Training effects were investigated both in a single case and in a group of 7 patients by means of neuropsychological tests and functional magnetic resonance imaging (fMRI).
Results: After the training, the patients showed a significant improvement in a neglect test battery above any natural fluctuation during a three-week baseline phase. Improvements in the neglect tasks were accompanied by an increase of both right and left hemisphere frontal, anterior cingulate and superior parietal activation, areas known to be associated with both alertness and spatial attention. Four weeks after the end of the training, the patients' neglect test performance had mostly returned to baseline. Despite decreases of activation in some of the initially reactivated areas, increases in neural activity bilaterally in frontal areas, in the right anterior cingulate cortex, the right angular gyrus and in the left temporoparietal cortex remained. An Optokinetic Stimulation Training (OKS) in a control group of another 7 neglect patients led to comparable behavioral results. After the training, however, there was a reactivation mainly in posterior parts of both hemispheres suggesting training specific functional reorganization.
Conclusion: The limited stability of the behavioral and reactivation results over time demonstrates that a three-week alertness or OKS training alone does not result in long lasting behavioral improvements and stable reactivation patterns in every patient. We rather suggest that combining alertness and spatial attention oriented training procedures might lead to a more stable amelioration of neglect symptoms.

Keywords: Neglect, spatial attention, functional reactivation, recovery of function, stroke, plasticity

1. Introduction

Attention is not a unitary function but can be divided into several subsystems, among them alertness and spatial attention. Alertness is concerned with the internal control of wakefulness and arousal. Spatial attention operates to enhance perception at particular spatial locations and seems to depend on a predominantly

*Corresponding author: Prof. Dr. Walter Sturm, Department of Neurology, Section Clinical Neuropsychology, University Hospital RWTH Aachen, Pauwelsstraße 30, D 52074 Aachen, Germany. Tel.: +49 241 8089826; Fax: +49 241 8082598; E-mail: sturm@neuropsych.rwth-aachen.de.

right-lateralized cortical network. Findings from lesion studies and functional imaging data suggest that the cognitive control of alertness (intrinsic or endogenous alertness) also relies on a right-lateralized network, involving the frontal and the parietal lobe as well as subcortical structures. Intrinsic alertness is defined as the internal control of arousal in the absence of an external cue [55] whereas phasic alertness represents the ability to increase response readiness for a short time period after a warning stimulus [39]. A typical task to assess intrinsic alertness is a simple reaction time (RT) measurement [38] without a preceding warning stimulus. Some authors have defined even short periods of endogenously maintaining vigilant responding as sustained attention.

Lesion studies in stroke patients revealed an important role of the right hemisphere for intrinsic alertness; several studies [19,25,40] have reported a dramatic increase in simple visual and auditory reaction time (RT) after RH-lesions. In a PET-study concerned with this basic attention function, Sturm and co-workers found an extended right hemisphere network including frontal (anterior cingulate gyrus, dorsolateral prefrontal cortex), inferior parietal, thalamic (pulvinar and possibly the reticular nucleus), and brainstem (pontomesencephalic tegmentum) structures, when participants waited for and rapidly responded to a centrally presented white dot [55] or to a 1000 Hz tone signal [57]. The similarity of activation patterns under visual, auditory and somatosensory stimulation [23] lends support to a supramodal right-hemisphere network for the control of intrinsic alerting. The notion of a fronto-parietal alertness network was also supported by an auditory vigilance task [33]). In contrast, short term phasic (exogenous) alerting elicited by warning cues either activates a left [9] or at least less lateralized fronto-parietal network [59]. Thiel and co-workers [61] found bilateral extrastriate but no lateral parietal and no frontal activations for phasic alerting.

In contrast to attention intensity, aspects of spatial attention have been investigated by functional imaging studies using e.g. covert orienting tasks. Corbetta et al. [4] showed that the detection of lateralised stimuli was associated with bilateral activation of the superior parietal and frontal cortex with the parietal activation being more pronounced in the right hemisphere regardless of the side of stimulus presentation. Similar results were found by other groups [30,13,5] and led to the assumption of a right hemisphere accentuated frontoparietal network for spatial attention. Other studies required the subjects to discriminate changes of bilaterally and simultanously presented objects [17, 68]. These tasks induce activation of the contralateral occipital cortex and suggest a close interaction between the spatial attention network and extrastriatal regions most likely reflecting a top-down modulation of early visual processing [3,12–14,51,52].

In addition to the mentioned studies which showed the localisation of alerting and spatial attention functions, some studies investigated the functional reactivation of impaired attentional networks. Longoni et al. [26] and Sturm et al. [57] examined the effects of the AIXTENT alertness training in right hemisphere stroke patients *without* neglect. Those patients who responded behaviorally to the training showed reactivation of the right hemisphere alertness network, especially the right dorsolateral or medial prefrontal cortex while performing an intrinsic alertness task. In contrast, a computerised memory training neither led to a behavioral improvement in alertness tasks nor to a functional reactivation in alertness related regions.

Other studies of the functional reactivation of impaired attention networks found that the remission of neglect depends on functional metabolic recovery of the intact areas of the right hemisphere and the left parietal lobe [31,34,63]. Pizzamiglio et al. [36], using a visuospatial task in a PET-study, showed that recovery from spatial neglect was associated with a recruitment of right superior parietal, parieto-occipital and bilateral inferior frontal cortex.

Spatial neglect subsequent to right hemisphere lesions is closely associated with non spatial deficits of attention like intrinsic alertness and sustained attention [7,42,43,45]. Several studies have shown that the degree to which sustained attention is impaired is a strong predictor for the persistence of neglect [18,46, 50].

According to Posner and Petersen [41], three interrelated mechanisms underlie human attention: orienting, selection, and alerting/sustained attention. Orienting is thought to be mediated by a "posterior attention system" comprising, among other areas, structures in the posterior parietal lobe. Selection involves an "anterior attention system" possibly based anatomically on the anterior cingulate gyrus and supplementary motor areas, and is closely related both functionally and anatomically, to the posterior attention system. The alerting or sustained attention system is responsible for providing an adequate level of arousal. The authors also propose a specialisation of the right hemisphere – particularly the right prefrontal cortex and the right anterior cingulate gyrus – for this alerting function. They furthermore suppose that noradrenaline (NA) may be the most important transmitter to subserve alerting since lesion studies in rats [48,49] provide evidence for a right hemisphere bias in the NA system, originating in the locus coeruleus and projecting most strongly to frontal areas, but also spreading to the parietal cortex. Based on the latter data it has been suggested that the NA-based, alerting/sustained attention system may exert a modulatory effect on the posterior attention system of the right hemisphere [41]. This alerting effect could, for example, result from a co-activation of the posterior attention system either directly or via the brainstem [11]. This notion was corroborated in a PET study by Coull et al. [8] where clonidine, an $\alpha 2$-adrenoceptor agonist and noradrenaline antagonist increased the modulatory effects of frontal, particularly cingulate cortex on projections from the locus coeruleus to parietal cortex during attentional tasks. Sturm and co-workers [58,59] in an fMRI study found highly overlapping networks for alerting and orienting. In ten normal subjects a covert visual orienting task (responding to the onset of visual targets presented randomly at unpredictable locations in both visual fields while fixating a central square, adopted from the subtest "neglect" from the Testbattery of Attention Performance TAP, see below) and an alertness task (responding to the same targets, but now presented centrally inside the fixation square) were performed. Contrasting the two tasks with a rest condition – putting aside motor and primary visual activations – demonstrated activation clusters in dorsolateral prefrontal regions, in the anterior cingulate gyrus, in the superior and inferior parietal cortex as well as in the superior temporal gyrus, and in the thalamus (top left and right of Fig. 1).

For both tasks, these activation foci were stronger in the right hemisphere.

Compared to the alertness condition, the task of covert orienting of attention induced stronger bilateral activations in regions of the superior parietal cortex (Fig. 1, bottom left). A conjunction analysis for the spatial attention and the alertness task confirmed the involvement of highly overlapping, mostly right hemisphere networks in the control of the two attentional functions (Fig. 1, bottom right).

The postulated interaction between the anterior alerting and the posterior spatial attention network leads to the hypothesis that an alertness training may improve spatial neglect in right hemisphere stroke patients. First evidence supporting this hypothesis comes from a study by Robertson et al. [44]. In that study, an attention training based on a self-instruction technique and on

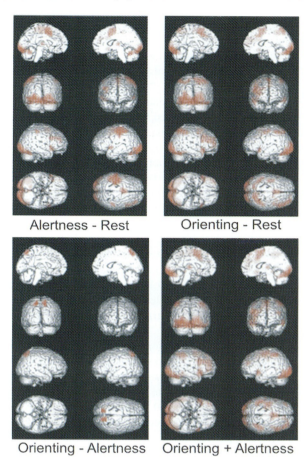

Fig. 1. Overlapping networks for orienting and alerting. Top left: alertness minus rest; top right: orienting (neglect task) minus rest; bottom left: orienting (neglect task) minus alertness, bottom right: orienting + alertness (conjunction analysis).

an enhancement of "phasic" alertness resulted in an improvement of neglect symptoms in all patients. In another study, Robertson et al. [47] temporarily ameliorated the spatial bias of neglect patients by means of phasic alerting.

In the following we will present the results of behavioral and imaging studies based on the above mentioned theoretical framework, which we have carried out during the last years. All aimed at the amelioration of neglect symptoms by enhancing the patients' cognitive control of alertness. In a control group study, an optokinetic stimulation training was carried out.

2. Treating neglect by alertness training

In contrast to the above mentioned attempts to ameliorate neglect, the computerised alertness training method used in our studies "AIXTENT" [53] addresses "intrinsic" alertness. Intrinsic alertness refers to the top-down aspect of alertness, i.e. the cognitive control of wakefulness and arousal which does not rely on external "warning" stimuli. "AIXTENT" has been successfully applied in the treatment of impaired attention functions in stroke patients [54], traumatically brain injured patients [56] and patients suffering from multiple sclerosis [37]. On a computer screen, the patient is shown either a car or a motorcycle driving on a road. The patient has to handle two response keys: one for speed and the other one for braking. The objective is both to drive the vehicle as fast as possible and to stop it just in time to avoid crashing into obstacles. The goal of the training is the improvement of the alertness level indicated by an impaired response time level in a standardized alertness test. In our studies we hypothezised that right hemisphere stroke patients suffering from both spatial neglect and alertness deficits might benefit from the "AIXTENT" training with respect to their neglect symptoms.

In addition to testing for behavioral effects of the alertness training, we also investigated the associated neural (re)activation pattern ("plasticity") using serial fMRI. In right hemisphere stroke patients presenting with chronic stable spatial neglect and deficits of intrinsic alertness we expected reduced activation of right frontal and parietal areas while performing a task of alerting and spatial attention. After treating patients with a three-week alertness training we expected increased frontal and parietal activations either ipsilesionally (right) or contralesionally (left) reflecting a training induced functional (re)activation ("plasticity") associated with a training induced amelioration of neglect symptoms ("recovery of function").

2.1. Pilot single case study

In a pilot study, a 69-year old female patient after a right hemisphere stroke with lesions in the right caudate nucleus, the right internal capsule, the right nucleus lentiformis and in the right parietal and temporal operculum, who after more than two years still presented with a severe left sided neglect, was treated by the AIXTENT alertness training [59]. For some tasks (letter cancellation, fast responses to stimuli presented in the right and left visual field under extinction conditions) even some of the stimuli in the right half of the display were neglected (see Fig. 2). We treated the patient for 14 days with one hour sessions each. Besides her neglect symptoms, the patient also showed a severe alertness deficit with very slow response times (45 2ms median response time; intraindividual variability: percentile rank 4) before the training. No spatial orienting or other neglect oriented training procedures were administered during the study phase.

Twice before (baseline testing) and once after the training an alertness test (visual response time) and four neglect tests were carried out (line bisection, line cancellation, letter cancellation, fast responses to stimuli presented in the right and left visual field under extinction conditions – subtest Neglect of the TAP by Zimmermann and Fimm [69]; for a detailed description of the tasks see section "group study" below). During the four week baseline phase there was no change of performance for any of the tasks, all indicating severe alertness deficits (see above) and neglect symptoms. After the training there was a slight improvement in the response time of the alertness task (432 ms) and a significant improvement in the intraindividual response time variability (percentile rank 10). There was a considerable improvement for every single neglect task (line bisection: pre 17.1% mean shift to the right, post 6.7%; line cancellation: pre 5 left ommissions, post no left ommissions, pre-post change $p = 0.023$ one-tailed, Fisher's exact test), with the strongest effects for the letter cancellation and the Neglect test of the TAP (see Fig. 2; letter cancellation: pre 20 left, 11 right ommissions, post 14 resp. 0. Pre-post-change left $p = 0.010$, right $p = 0.0006$ one-tailed, Fisher's exact test; Neglect test: pre 22 left, 14 right ommissions, post 17 resp. 5. Pre-post change left $p = 0.024$, right $p = 0.007$ one-tailed, Fisher's exact test; Fig. 2).

Before and after the training, fMRI activation studies were carried out using a neglect task similar to the hemifield response test (Neglect test of the TAP) mentioned above. Before the training, the patient did not respond to any left sided stimuli and even neglected many stimuli in the right hemifield during the activation phase. The SPM analysis (Neglect test minus rest) revealed virtually no activation of the right hemisphere (except for some "tiny" right frontal and inferior parietal "spots") but also a very reduced left sided activation pattern (superior parietal cortex, inferior temporal gyrus; Figure 3, top left) compared to the pattern normal subjects show while performing the same task (see Fig. 1, top right). After the training, there was a large right and a much smaller left prefrontal activation, as well as a much more pronounced left hemisphere parietal focus. Also both right and left occipital areas showed much more activity than before the training (Fig. 3, top

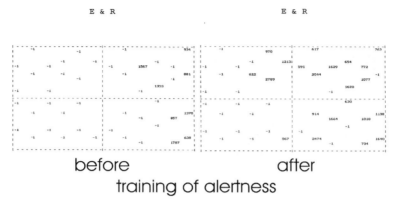

Fig. 2. Top: letter cancellation, bottom: neglect task of the TAP (− = no response to stimuli presented at that position). Left before (pre2) and right after (post1) alertness training of the single patient in the pilot study.

right). Furthermore, there was an extended activation of right thalamic structures, showing no activity before the training at all. The bottom part of Fig. 3 depicts the changes in activation from before to after the training. It seems that the alertness training improved the function of at least part of the right frontal alerting network which probably coactivated parietal and even occipital areas as hypothesized by Fernandez-Duque and Posner [11], thus leading to a substantial improvement of neglect symptoms behaviorally.

2.2. Group study

In a prospective study, seven (two female, five male) right-handed patients with cortical and subcortical right hemisphere vascular lesions were included [62]. The patient characteristics are detailed in Table 1.

Median age was 65 years (range 44 to 77 years). All patients presented with stable neglect symptoms and an intrinsic alertness deficit for at least 3 months post stroke (median time 5 months, range 3 to 31 months). For inclusion, patients had to show neglect symptoms in at least two tasks taken from the "Neglect Test" (NET) [10] or the "Test Battery of Attentional Performance" (TAP) [69] described later in detail and a percentile rank <20 for the median RT in the subtest "Alertness" (simple visual reaction time task without warning signal, i.e. "intrinsic alertness") of the TAP. Exclusion criteria were left hemisphere infarction, epilepsy and any severe internal medical disease.

If at the end of a three week baseline period the inclusion criteria still held, a first fMRI measurement was carried out, using the same neglect paradigm as in the single case study reported above. During the following three weeks, patients underwent 14 daily sessions of the AIXTENT alertness training each session lasting 45 minutes. One day ("post 1") and four weeks ("post 2") after this training period, again a neuropsychological assessment and fMRI were carried out to assess both short and long term effects of the training on spatial neglect.

2.3. Neuropsychological assessment

Intrinsic alertness (alerting without exogenous warning cues) was investigated by means of the subtest "Alertness" of the computerised attention test battery TAP. Patients were instructed to respond as fast as possible to a simple centrally presented visual stimulus ("X") by pressing a response key with the right index finger.

Neglect symptoms were assessed by subtests of the TAP ("neglect", "visual field" and "visual scanning") and by subtests of the NET, a German version of the Behavioral Inattention Test "BIT" [66], including letter, star and line cancellation, line bisection, clock drawing, text reading, copying of simple line drawings.

In the TAP subtest "neglect", patients were instructed to fixate a central square (size 3.8°) on a black screen. Around the square in each visual hemifield the dis-

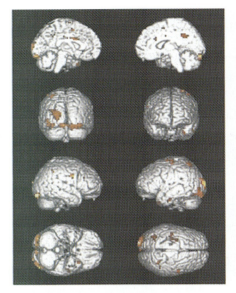
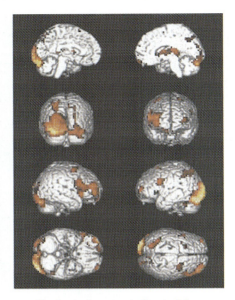

Neglect minus rest before training   Neglect minus rest after training

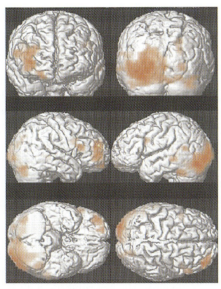

After minus before training

Fig. 3. Top left: Neglect minus rest before alertness training in the single case study, right top: neglect minus rest after the alertness training. Bottom: change of activation after minus before training.

play showed 24 randomly distributed white distractors (small, hardly legible two and three-digit numbers). These stimuli were introduced to enhance possible neglect symptoms by distraction. In the gaps between these distractors a peripheral three digit flickering target appeared at random locations in either the left or the right visual field within 13 degrees from the central square. Patients were instructed to press a key with the right index finger as soon as they detected the target. In each visual half field 22 targets were presented at different positions. Dependent variable was the number of detected stimuli in the left visual half field.

To generate a baseline before the training, this test was performed outside the scanner (at pre1 and pre 2) while training effects were investigated inside the scanner (at pre 2, post 1 and post 2) in order to allow

Table 1
Patient characteristics

Pat	Sex	Age	Lesion (all right hemisphere)
D.N.	M	77	Infarction of the anterior part of the MCA: predominantly subcortical
L.F.	M	72	Incomplete MCA infarction: parietal, temporal; cerebellar infarct
H.G.	M	51	Incomplete MCA infarction: central region, putamen, insula
I.S.	W	68	Incomplete MCA infarction: inf. parietal, temporal, premotor frontal, putamen, caudatum
I.J.	W	65	Incomplete MCA infarction: sup. parietal, parts of inf. parietal and temporal, prefrontal, putamen, capsula, caudatum
C.R.	M	49	Infarction of the temporooccipital and temporoparietal junction, prefrontal, basal ganglia
K.A.	M	44	Complete MCA infarction

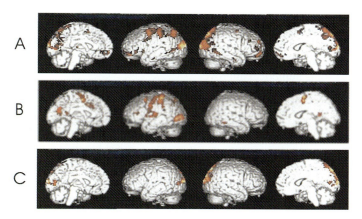

Fig. 4. Activation patterns before the alertness training at the end of the baseline (pre2) a) neglect task minus rest, b) alertness task minus rest, c) neglect task minus alertness task.

for a direct correlation with the imaging data.

2.4. fMRI activation tasks

Neglect task: A slightly modified version of the subtest "neglect" of the TAP (see above) was used as an activation paradigm in a box-car fMRI design. This task has previously been shown to activate in normal subjects bilateral fronto-parietal networks with a right hemispheric preponderance [58,59].

Alertness task: This task was set up to control for primary sensory and motor activation and for the alertness aspects of the neglect task. Patients had to respond to the same stimuli as in the neglect task. The only difference in the alertness task was the *location* of the stimuli, which were presented centrally, i.e. inside the fixation square, so that no spatial distribution of attention was necessary. In fact, this task is a typical visual simple reaction time task, thus tapping the cognitive control of intrinsic (unwarned) alertness. It is known to activate a network comparable to the neglect task described above but with a more inferior parietal cortex activation [59].

For details of the fMRI data acquisition and statistical evaluation of both behavioral and imaging data see Thimm et al. [62].

3. Results

3.1. Behavioral data

Our design enabled us to use the patients as their own control group. Therefore we compared the overall improvements resulting from the training period (post 1 vs. pre 2) with any spontaneous changes during the baseline period (pre 2 vs. pre 1). While there were significant ameliorations in a total of 10 neglect subtests across the seven patients after the training (10 of 31 originally impaired subtests = 32), only 3 neglect subtests (3 of 32 impaired subtests = 9%) revealed an improvement of neglect symptoms during the baseline period before the training.

The number of improved test results after the training was significantly larger than that after the baseline phase (Fisher's exact test: $p = 0.026$).

In the fMRI neglect task immediately after the training (post1), two patients (H.G., I.J.) detected significantly more left sided visual stimuli than before the training. The other patients showed at least some numerical improvement at post1 (D.N., I.S., C.R., K.A.) or remained stable (L.F.). A group analysis revealed a significantly increased number of detected left sided stimuli ($p = 0.04$) but not for the detection of right sided stimuli ($p = 0.16$). Four weeks later (post2), another group analysis revealed that these effects did not persist (compared to pre2), although two patients showed some further numerical improvement compared to post 1 (D.N., L.F., see Table 2a).

Outside the scanner, five patients (D.N., L.F., H.G., I.S., K.A.) showed a significant improvement in at least one neglect task at post1 and long term effects (at post2) were found in three patients (D.N., L.F., I.S.).

In the fMRI alertness task immediately after the training (post1), one patient (D.N.) showed significantly faster reaction times than before the training. Four patients showed at least some numerical improvements (H.G., I.J., I.S., C.R.). There was no significant stable long term improvement in reaction times 4 weeks later at post 2.

3.2. Imaging data

The activation provoked by the neglect task (minus rest) performed during fMRI immediately before the start of the alertness training revealed the areas involved in alerting, spatial distribution of attention, visual processing and responding to the presented stimuli. This analysis showed activation of a bilateral network comprising the parieto-occipital cortex and frontal areas, similar to, albeit less extended and less lateralised, the network described in normals for the same task [58, 59]. Subcortical activations were found in the left basal ganglia (Fig. 4a). The group contrast "alertness task minus rest" at the same session revealed the areas involved in alerting, visual processing and responding to the presented stimuli in the fMRI alertness task. It showed activation of bilateral (posterior) cingulate cortex, the right middle temporal gyrus, and wide spread left hemisphere areas (Fig. 4b).

Subtracting the alerting, visual and motor components of the neglect task by contrasting "neglect task minus alertness task" isolated the areas specifically related to spatial attention. Before the training, activations were found bilaterally in the precuneus and cuneus and the left middle occipital gyrus (Fig. 4c) corresponding to the spatial attention network found in normals [58] but less extended.

3.3. Increase of neural activity immediately after the training (post1 > pre2)

Improvements in the performance of the neglect task were associated with an increase of neural activity bilaterally in the superior and middle frontal gyrus, the medial frontal and anterior cingulate cortex, precuneus, cuneus and middle occipital gyrus, in the right angular gyrus and in the left precentral gyrus, insula and basal ganglia (Fig. 5a).

Training effects related specifically to spatial attention without structures involved in alertness were investigated contrasting "(neglect post 1 minus alertness post 1) minus (neglect pre 2 minus alertness pre 2)". Increased neural activity was found in the left middle frontal gyrus only (Fig. 5b).

3.4. Stability four weeks after the end of the training (post1 > post2)

Corresponding to the decrease of performance on the behavioral level, four weeks after the end of the training there were decreases of neural activity in the following areas:

The contrast "neglect post 1 minus neglect post 2" showed decreases of neural activity in bilateral frontal, occipital, temporal and parietal areas (Fig. 6a).

Contrasting "(neglect post 1 minus alertness post 1) minus (neglect post 2 minus alertness post 2)" revealed decreases of activation specifically related to *spatial attention (without alertness)*. Decreases of neural activity were found in the right superior frontal gyrus, the left inferior frontal gyrus, inferior temporal gyrus, middle occipital gyrus and posterior cingulate cortex (Fig. 6b).

3.5. Remaining long term effects on neural activity four weeks after the training (post2 > pre2)

Persistent effects associated with alerting and spatial attention (contrast "neglect post 2 minus neglect pre 2") were found bilaterally in the superior and middle frontal gyrus, the right anterior cingulate cortex and the right angular gyrus and in the left middle temporal gyrus, supramarginal gyrus and lingual gyrus (Fig. 7a).

In a single subject analysis 4 weeks after the training the patient with the best long term improvement in the scanner task (D.N.) also showed the strongest long term increase of neural activity.

Persistent effects specifically associated with spatial attention without alertness (contrast "(neglect post 1 minus alertness post 1) minus (neglect pre 2 minus alertness pre 2)") were found for the left superior temporal gyrus and left inferior occipital gyrus (Fig. 7b).

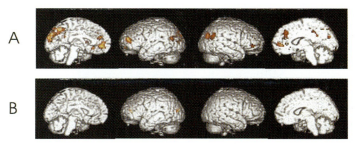

Fig. 5. Increase of activation immediately after the alertness training compared to the state at the end of the baseline (post1 > pre2) a) neglect task minus rest, b) neglect task minus alertness task.

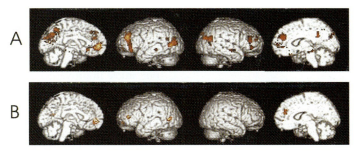

Fig. 6. Decrease of activation four weeks after the end of the alertness training compared to the state immediately after the training (post2 < post1) a) neglect task minus rest, b) neglect task minus alertness task.

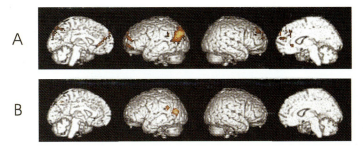

Fig. 7. Remaining increase of activation four weeks after the end of the alertness training compared to the state immediately before the training (post2 > pre2) a) neglect task minus rest, b) neglect task minus alertness task.

4. Treating neglect by Optokinetic Stimulation (OKS) training

In a second approach parallel to our alertness training, again 7 patients suffering from chronic left sided hemineglect (>3 months) were treated by an optokinetic stimulation training which has successfully been introduced by Kerkhoff [21,22]. For inclusion, the same criteria held and the same test procedures were carried out as for the alertness study. Patients were instructed to conduct eye pursuit movements towards stimulus patterns of 30–70 dots moving coherently from the right to the left side. No head movements were allowed. The optokinetic stimulation treatment is part of the treatment program EYEMOVE, http://www.medicalcomputing.de. The same study design with a three week baseline and a subsequent three week training period as for the alertness training was chosen.

Following treatment, all 7 patients showed significant ameliorations of their neglect in some of the tests. The rate of improved test performances after the training was significantly larger than after the baseline period (Fisher's exact test $p < 0.05$).

A longitudinal fMRI study with the same neglect paradigm as used in the alertness study was carried out. Improvements on the behavioral level were associated with bilaterally increased activation in the posterior cingulate gyrus and the precuneus as well as left hemisphere activation in the angular gyrus and temporo-occipital areas (BA 22). The changes of activation from the fMRI session immediately before to the session immediately after the training are depicted in Fig. 8.

5. Long term stability of OKS training effects

At the time being, only part of the OKS training group underwent a fourth neuropsychological and third fMRI session four weeks after the end of the training. Thus, the results for that period are not yet available. As, however, can be seen from single cases, there also seems to be a decrease of performance and activation despite some remaining reactivation as reported for the alertness training.

6. Discussion

The aim of the pilot and the group study presented here was to investigate the impact of a computerized, gamelike alertness training ("AIXTENT") in patients suffering from chronic, stable spatial neglect both on the behavioral and neural level. In a parallel approach, a comparable number of patients was treated by Optokinetic Stimulation (OKS) Training.

For the alertness training, immediately after the training task performance in the single case study was improved in all neglect measurements as well as in six of the seven patients of the group study in at least one of the neglect subtests. Altogether, the patient group showed an improvement in 32% of the impaired subtests, which was a significantly higher percentage than the gain of 9% during the pre-training baseline phase. Four weeks later, however, most of the improvement had disappeared again.

The improvement observed immediately after the alertness training phase is unlikely to result purely from effects of repeated testing or spontaneous recovery since improved test results were significantly more numerous after the training period than after the pre-training baseline period of equal duration. Furthermore, the positive training effects in many cases disappeared again during the post-training period. Finally, all patients had presented with stable chronic neglect symptoms over at least three months, so it is unlikely that spontaneous recovery of function could explain the positive behavioral effects observed immediately after the training.

The behavioral results corroborate the hypothesis that improved neglect is mediated by improved alertness: One patient showed significantly faster reaction times immediately after the training and four patients improved at least numerically. In parallel to the results of the neglect tasks positive training effects on the alertness task tended to disappear again during the post training period.

Robertson et al. [44] also found that a sustained attention training based on a self-instruction technique resulted in an improvement of neglect symptoms in all patients. Their and our results thus support the hypothesis that the persistance of spatial neglect after right hemisphere lesions is at least in part based on sustained attention or alertness deficits and can be improved by attention training. However, neither in their nor in our study improvement in neglect could consistently be demonstrated in all neglect tests. It is well known that patients differ from each other in their pattern of impairments in neglect tests [15,16] and this also seems to hold for the recovery from neglect and especially for the training procedure used here: the alerting system seems to interact with the posterior attention system rather than with specific visuospatial processes.

The rate of improved test performance, compared to the session immediately after the end of the training, four weeks later decreased to 10%. This lack of stability is a problem often reported in different kinds of neglect rehabilitation training such as visual scanning, limb activation, prism adaptation, caloric and optokinetic stimulation or neck vibration treatment [35]. Some of these studies did not investigate the stability of training effects at all and those who did often reported poor long term effects. Regarding the alertness approach, Robertson et al. [44] reported a stable improvement in several neglect tests for an interval of 2 weeks which is shorter than the interval in our study (4 weeks).

In a longitudinal fMRI study parallel to the repeated behavioral measurements we investigated the impact of the alertness training on the increase of brain activity. Before starting the training, we investigated the functional networks of alertness and spatial attention in all of our patients. Performing the neglect task which comprises both alertness and spatial attention, patients amongst other areas activated the right superior and middle frontal gyrus. These are parts of the right hemisphere alertness network previously shown to be involved in the performance of alertness and sustained attention tasks [2,32,33,55,59]. There were, however, only very small frontal activations in our neglect pa-

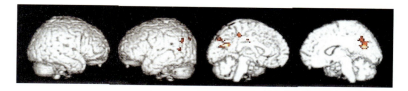

Fig. 8. Increase of activation during the performance of the neglect task (minus rest) immediately after the OKS training compared to the state at the end of the baseline (post1 > pre2).

tients and we did not find any activation of the right anterior cingulate cortex, right thalamic or inferior parietal areas as in healthy subjects performing an alertness task [55]. For our fMRI alertness task there was less right hemisphere activation yet than in the neglect task. Only the (posterior) cingulate and the middle temporal gyrus but no frontal areas at all were activated, reflecting a dysfunction of the alertness network in our patients presenting with extended, mostly parietal lesions.

Our patients, however, bilaterally activated the precuneus and cuneus, which may reflect the close interaction between the spatial attention network and extrastriatal regions of the visual system [3,12–14,51,58,61] in a situation where the normal networks have become dysfunctional.

After the alertness training we found an increase of neural activity for the right superior and middle frontal gyrus, medial frontal and anterior cingulate cortex, angular gyrus, and precuneus. This "re-activation" of structures known to be crucial both for alerting and orienting are likely to indicate neural plasticity within the right-hemisphere attentional network. Right frontal areas were already activated before the training and the additional increase in neural activity after the training emphasises the role the right frontal cortex plays in the cognitive control of alerting. The anterior cingulate cortex is often regarded as an essential regulating component of the alertness network [28] and has been associated with anticipation and preparation of attentional activity [24,29,55]. In an event-related fMRI study Thiel et al. [61] investigated the subsystems of a visuospatial Posner-type attention task and found the anterior cingulate cortex to be also involved in spatial orienting. The right angular gyrus is one of the most important areas in the development of spatial neglect [27] and has consistently been shown to be involved in maintaining attention to spatial locations [20, 64]. Finally, the right precuneus has previously been implicated in the neurorehabilitation of neglect [36].

We also observed left hemisphere increases of neural activity after the alertness training. These training effects were similar to the activation pattern of the right hemisphere. Training-related effects were found in frontal and anterior cingulate areas, the middle occipital gyrus, precuneus and cuneus. Furthermore, there were activations in the insula and basal ganglia. Since there was no behavioral increase in the detection of right sided stimuli we suggest that these increases in neural activity may either be associated with the improvement of the detection of left sided stimuli after the alertness training or reflect a generally increased impact of the alerting system on bilateral attention systems involved in the bilateral detection task we used for the fMRI study.

For the alertness task, too, after the training there was an increase of activity in bilateral frontal, parietal and occipital areas again reflecting the close relationship between the alerting and spatial attention network.

After subtracting the neural activity provoked by the alertness task from the neglect task, there only remained an increase of neural activity exclusively in the left middle frontal gyrus. This demonstrates that the right hemisphere activation pattern after the training is best interpreted as reflecting a training induced re-activation of the network for top-down control of alertness.

The results suggest that functional recovery from spatial attention deficits after an alertness treatment is based on a (re)activation of ipsilesional and contralesional areas which are part of the attentional networks. Other studies also found evidence for both kinds of (re)activation either of areas remote but connected to the damaged area [31,34,63] or of the damaged area itself [36]. In a SPECT study with right hemisphere stroke patients, Pantano et al. [31] found increased activation of left anterior and right posterior regions induced by a two month neglect rehabilitation treatment. These regions included the areas we found in our study. In a PET study of patients with predominantly subcortical lesions, Pizzamiglio et al. [36] found that after a training patients showed recovery of those regions activated in healthy controls performing the same task. Sturm and coworkers [57] did the same alertness training used in our study in right hemisphere stroke patients. In patients who behaviorily responded to the training, they found increased perilesional right frontal activation which can be interpreted as a reactivation of the network usually involved in alerting and sustained attention. In contrast to short term "phasic alerting", which has been shown to be beneficial in neglect [47], our alertness training aims at an improvement of the more cognitively controlled "intrinsic" aspect of alertness, probably improving the patients' awareness for their deficits and encouraging them to maintain an alert state in order to improve their monitoring of the task given (like in the Robertson et al. [44] study using a self instruction technique to improve sustained attention).

Four weeks after the training, and in parallel to the return of the behavioral performance to pre-training levels, we found a decrease of neural activity. The pattern of long term decreases was similar to the pattern of increases observed immediately after the training. This corroborates the association between behavioral recovery from visuospatial neglect and the function of the areas discussed. Four weeks after the training there, however, still were remaining increases of neural activity compared to the pre-training session. In the neglect task, these increases were bilateral in frontal areas, in the right anterior cingulate cortex and the right angular gyrus. Furthermore there was an increase in the left temporoparietal cortex and lingual gyrus. This might reflect a stable or even increasing behavioral improvement which behaviorally could be observed in at least one of our patients (D.N.) who also showed the strongest long term increase of activity on the single subject level.

One could argue that increases in neural activity after the training not necessarily can be attributed to the training itself but could also be an effect of repeated measurements or any unspecific computer activity. Therefore we investigated the retest reliability of the neglect paradigm used in our patients in a pilot study with 12 healthy subjects [62]. In the repeated fMRI sessions 3 and 7 weeks after the first fMRI session, there were no increases of neural activity in any region of the brain compared with the first session. Thus we can assume that any increase of neural activity observed post-training in the patients is associated with the improvement in task performance induced by the training.

The group treated by an Optokinetic Stimulation Training (OKS) showed a comparable amount of behavioral improvement as our alertness training patients. Interestingly, the changes in activation after the training showed a completely different pattern than that of the alertness training group. While in the latter group the most prominent changes took place in frontal regions, the OKS training led to changes confined to posterior regions including the angular gyrus, temporo-occipital areas (BA 22), precuneus and posterior cingulate gyrus. Thus, despite comparable behavioral results, the two training methods seem to have impact on two different parts of the spatial attention system, one addressing predominantly the frontal, the other one the posterior part of the system.

The neurophysiological results reported above imply that the functional reactivation of an alertness (or of an OKS) training is not sufficient for a significant long term improvement in visuospatial neglect. The crucial areas might be those bilateral frontal and/or parietal areas which showed an increased activation at the first post-training session when patients also showed improved task performance but less extended or no activation at the follow-up when patients' performance had returned to pre-training levels. Especially, superior parietal and frontal regions reflect top-down control of spatial attention [6]. The data thus suggest that both alertness and OKS training are sufficient to induce short lasting activation of areas crucial for the spatial distribution of attention but that either training alone might not be powerful enough to lead to a stable improvement of the cognitive attentional control and to a permanent functional reactivation of the areas involved. One then might speculate that a combination of both training procedures or of training procedures addressing similar aspects of spatial attention and alertness could be more efficient, if, for example, the alertness training could be used as a pre-activator on neglect related areas that might be stabilised by an additional neglect specific training. In principle, a beneficial effect of combining different neglect treatment methods on long term outcome has been suggested by Brunila and co-workers [1] and Wilson and colleagues [67].

At the time being we are investigating the behavioral and neurobiological impact of a combination of a recent version of the AIXTENT alertness training and a newly developed computerized visuospatial training procedure on visuospatial neglect.

Acknowledgements

These studies were supported by a grant from the Deutsche Forschungsgemeinschaft to G.R.F. and W.S. (DFG-KFO 112) and by the Interdisciplinary Center for Clinical Research (IZKF), University Hospital RWTH Aachen (TV 13).

References

[1] T. Brunila, N.B. Lincoln, A. Lindell, O. Tenovuo and H. Hämäläinen, Experiences of combined visual training and arm activation in the rehabilitation of unilateral visual neglect, A clinical study, *Neuropsychological Rehabilitation* **12** (2002), 27–40.

[2] R.M. Cohen, W.E. Semple, M. Gross, H.J. Holcomb, S. Dowling and T.E. Nordahl, Functional localization of sustained attention, *Neuropsychiatry, Neuropsychology, and Behavioral Neurology* **1** (1988), 3–20.

[3] M. Corbetta, F.M. Miezin, S. Dobmeyer, G.L. Shulman and S.E. Petersen, Selective and divided attention during visual discriminations of shape, color, and speed, functional anatomy by positron emission tomography, *Journal of Neuroscience* **11** (1991), 2383–2402.

[4] M. Corbetta, F.M. Miezin, G. Shulman and S.E. Petersen, A PET study of visuospatial attention, *Journal of Neuroscience* **13** (1993), 1202–1226.

[5] M. Corbetta and G.L. Shulman, Human cortical mechanisms of visual attention during orienting and search, Philosophical Transactions of the Royal Society of London, Series B, *Biological Sciences* **353** (1998), 1353–1362.

[6] M. Corbetta and G.L. Shulman, Control of goal-directed and stimulus-driven attention in the brain, *Nature Reviews Neuroscience* **3** (2002), 201–215.

[7] H.B. Coslett, D. Bowers and K. Heilman, Reduction in cerebral activation after right hemisphere stroke, *Neurology* **37** (1987), 957–962.

[8] J.T. Coull, C.D. Frith, R.J. Dolan, R.S. Frackowiak and P.M. Grasby, The neural correlates of the noradrenergic modulation of human attention, arousal and learning, *The European Journal of Neuroscience* **9** (1997), 589–598.

[9] J.T. Coull, A.C. Nobre and C.D. Frith, The noradrenergic alpha2 agonist clonidine modulates behavioral and neuroanatomical correlates of human attentional orienting and alerting, *Cerebral Cortex* **11** (2001), 73–84.

[10] M. Fels and E. Geissner, *Neglect-Test (NET)*, Hogrefe, Göttingen, 1996.

[11] D. Fernandez-Duque and M.I. Poster, Relating the mechanisms of orienting and alerting, *Neuropsychologia* **35** (1997), 477–486.

[12] G.R. Fink, P.W. Halligan, J.C. Marshall, C.D. Frith, R.S.J. Frackowiak and R.J. Dolan, Where in the brain does visual attention select the forest and the trees? *Nature* **382** (1996), 626–628.

[13] G.R. Fink, R.J. Dolan, P.W. Halligan, J.C. Marshall and C.D. Frith, Space-based and object-based visual attention, shared and specific neural domains, *Brain* **120** (1997), 2013–2028.

[14] G.R. Fink, P.W. Halligan, J.C. Marshall, C.D. Frith, R.S.J. Frackowiak and R.J. Dolan, Neural mechanisms involved in the processing of global and local aspects of hierarchically organized visual stimuli, *Brain* **120** (1997), 1779–1791.

[15] P.W. Halligan and J.C. Marshall, Graphic neglect – more than the sum of the parts? *NeuroImage* **14** (2001), 91–97.

[16] P.W. Halligan, G.R. Fink, J.C. Marshall and G. Vallar, Spatial cognition, Evidence from visual neglect, *Trends in Cognitive Sciences* **7**(3) (2003), 125–133.

[17] H.J. Heinze, G.R. Mangun, W. Burchert, H. Hinrichs, M. Scholz, T.F. Münte, A. Gös, M. Scherg, S. Johannes, H. Hundeshagen, M.S. Gazzaniga and S.A. Hillyard, Combined spatial and temporal imaging of brain activity during visual selective attention in humans, *Nature* **372** (1994), 543–546.

[18] H. Hjaltason, R. Tegner, K. Tham, M. Levander and K. Ericson, Sustained attention and awareness of disability in chronic Neglekt, *Neuropsychologia* **34** (1996), 1229–1223.

[19] D. Howes and F. Boller, Simple reaction time, evidence for focal impairments from lesions of the right hemisphere, *Brain* **98** (1975), 317–332.

[20] M. Husain and C. Rorden, Non-spatially lateralized mechanisms in hemispatial neglect, *Nature Reviews Neuroscience* **4** (2003), 26–36.

[21] G. Kerkhoff, Multiple perceptual distortions and their modulation in patients with left visual neglect, *Neuropsychologia* **38** (2000), 73–86.

[22] G. Kerkhoff, I. Keller, V. Ritter and C. Marquardt, Repetitive optokinetic stimulation induces lasting recovery from visual neglect, *Restor Neurol Neurosci* (2006), in press.

[23] S. Kinomura, J. Larsson, B. Gulyas and P.E. Roland, Activation by attention of the human reticular formation and thalamic intralaminar nuclei, *Science* **271** (1996), 512–515.

[24] D. LaBerge and M.S. Buchsbaum, Positron emission tomographic measurements of pulvinar activity during an attention task, *Journal of Neuroscience* **10** (1990), 613–619.

[25] E. Ladavas, Is hemispatial deficit produced by right parietal lobe damage associated with retinal or gravitational coordinates? *Brain* **110** (1987), 67–80.

[26] F. Longoni, W. Sturm, S. Weis, C. Holtel, K. Specht, H. Herzog and K. Willmes, Functional reorganization after training of alertness in two patients with right hemisphere lesions, *Journal of Neuropsychology* **11** (2000), 250–261.

[27] D.J. Mort, P. Malhotra, S.K. Mannan, C. Rorden, A. Pambakian, C. Kennard and M. Husain, The anatomy of visual neglect, *Brain* **126** (2003), 1986–1997.

[28] F.M. Mottaghy, K. Willmes, B. Horwitz, H.-W. Müller, B.J. Krause and W. Sturm, Systems level modelling of a neuronal network subserving intrinsic alertness, *NeuroImage* **29** (2006), 225–233.

[29] S. Murtha, H. Chertkow, M. Beauregard, R. Dixon and A. Evans, Hypothesis about the role of the anterior cortex (ACC), *Human Brain Mapping* **4** (1996), 103–112.

[30] A.C. Nobre, G.N. Sebestyen, D.R. Gitelman, M.M. Mesulam, R.S.J. Frackowiak and C.D. Frith, Functional localization of the system for visuospatial attention using positron emission tomography, *Brain* **120** (1997), 515–533.

[31] P. Pantano, V. Di Piero, C. Fieschi, A. Judica, C. Guariglia and L. Pizzamiglio, Pattern of CBF in the rehabilitation of visuospatial neglect, *International Journal of Neuroscience* **66**(3–4) (1992), 153–161.

[32] J.V. Pardo, P.T. Fox and M.E. Raichle, Localization of a human system for sustained attention by positron emission tomography, *Nature* **349** (1991), 61–64.

[33] T. Paus, R.J. Zatorre, N. Hofle, Z. Caramanos, J. Gotman, M. Petrides and A.C. Evans, Time-changes in neural systems underlying attention and arousal during the performance of an auditory vigilance task, *Journal of Cognitive Neuroscience* **9** (1997), 392–408.

[34] D. Perani, G. Vallar, E. Paulesu, M. Alberon and F. Fazio, Left and right hemisphere contribution to recovery from neglect after right hemisphere damage, An [^{18}F]FDG PET study of two cases, *Neuropsychologia* **31** (1993), 115–125.

[35] S.R. Pierce and L.J. Buxbaum, Treatments of unilateral neglect, A review, *Archives of Physical Medicine and Rehabilitation* **83** (2002), 256–268.

[36] L. Pizzamiglio, D. Perani, S.F. Cappa, G. Vallar, S. Paolucci, F. Grassi, E. Paulesu and F. Fazio, Recovery of neglect after right

[37] A.M. Plohmann, L. Kappos, W. Ammann, A. Thordai, A. Wittwer, S. Huber, Y. Bellaiche and J. Lechner-Scott, Computer assisted retraining of attentional impairments in patients with multiple sclerosis, Journal of Neurology, *Neurosurgery and Psychiatry* **64** (1998), 455–462.

[38] M.I. Posner, The psychobiology of attention, in: *Handbook of Psychobiology*, M. Gazzaniga and C. Blakemore, eds, Academic Press, New York, 1975, pp. 441–480.

[39] M.I. Posner, *Chronometric explorations of mind*, Erlbaum, Hillsdale, 1978.

[40] M.I. Posner, A.W. Inhoff and F.J. Friedrich, Isolating attentional systems, A cognitive-anatomical analysis, *Psychobiology* **15** (1987), 107–121.

[41] M.I. Posner and S.E. Petersen, The attention system of the human brain, *Annual Review of Neuroscience* **13** (1990), 25–42.

[42] S.Z. Rapcsak, M. Verfaellie, W.S. Fleet and K.M. Heilman, Selective attention in hemispatial neglect, *Archives of Neurology* **46** (1989), 178–182.

[43] I.H. Robertson, The relationship between lateralised and non-lateralised attentional deficits in unilateral neglect, in: *Unilateral Neglect clinical and experimental studies*, I.H. Robertson and J.C. Marshall, eds, Lawrence Erlbaum, Hillsdale, 1993, pp. 257–275.

[44] I.H. Robertson, R. Tegnér, K. Tham, A. Lo and I. Nimmo-Smith, Sustained attention training for unilateral neglect, Theoretical and rehabilitation implications, *Journal of Clinical and Experimental Neuropsychologyogy* **17** (1995), 416–430.

[45] I.H. Robertson, T. Manly, N. Beschin, R. Daini, H. Haeske-Dewick, V. Homberg, M. Jehkonen, G. Pizzamiglio, A. Shiel and E. Weber, Auditory sustained attention is a marker of unilateral spatial neglect, *Neuropsychologia* **35** (1997), 1527–1532.

[46] I.H. Robertson, V. Ridgeway, E. Greenfield and A. Parr, Motor recovery after stroke depends on intact sustained attention, a 2-year follow-up study, *Neuropsychology* **11** (1997), 290–295.

[47] I.H. Robertson, J.B. Mattingley, C. Rorden and J. Driver, Phasic alerting of neglect patients overcomes their spatial deficit in visual awareness, *Nature* **395** (1998), 169–172.

[48] R.G. Robinson and J.T. Coyle, The differential effects of right versus left hemispheric cerebral infarction on catecholamines and behavior in the rat, *Brain Research* **188** (1980), 63–78.

[49] R.G. Robinson, Lateralized behavioral and neurochemical consequences of unilateral brain injury in rats, in: *Cerebral lateralization in nonhuman species*, S.G. Glick, ed., Academic Press, Orlando, 1985, pp. 135–156.

[50] H. Samuelsson, E. Hjelmquist, C. Jensen, S. Ekholm and C. Blomstrand, Nonlateralized attentional deficits, an important component behind persisting visuospatial Neglekt? *Journal of Clinical and Experimental Neuropsychology* **20** (1998), 73–88.

[51] G.L. Shulman, M. Corbetta, R.L. Buckner, M.E. Raichle, J.A. Fiez, F.M. Miezin and S.E. Petersen, Top-down modulation of early sensory cortex, *Cerebral Cortex* **7** (1997), 193–206.

[52] K.E. Stephan, J.C. Marshall, K.J. Friston, J.B. Rowe, A. Ritzl, K. Zilles and G.R. Fink, Lateralized cognitive processes and lateralized task control in the human brain, *Science* **301**(5631) (2003), 384–386.

[53] W. Sturm, W. Hartje, A. Orgaß and K. Willmes, Computer-assisted rehabilitation of attention disorders, in: *Development in the assessment and rehabilitation of brain damaged patients*, F. Stachowiak, ed., Narr, Tübingen, 1993.

[54] W. Sturm, K. Willmes, B. Orgaß and W. Hartje, Do specific attention deficits need specific training? *Neuropsychological Rehabilitation* **8** (1997), 81–103.

[55] W. Sturm, A. De Simone, B. Krause, K. Specht, V. Hesselmann, I. Rademacher, H. Herzog, L. Tellmann, H.W. Müller-Gärtner and K. Willmes, Functional anatomy of intrinsic alertness, evidence for a fronto-parietal-thalamic-brainstem network in the right hemisphere, *Neuropsychologia* **37** (1999), 797–805.

[56] W. Sturm, B. Fimm, A. Cantagallo, N. Cremel, P. North, A. Passadori, L. Pizzamiglio, M. Rousseaux, P. Zimmermann, G. Deloche and M. Leclercq, Computerised training of specific attention deficits in stroke and traumatic brain injured patients, a multicentric efficacy study, in: *Applied Neuropsychology of Attention*, M. Leclercq and P. Zimmermann, eds, Psychology Press, Hove, 2002.

[57] W. Sturm, F. Longoni, S. Weis, K. Specht, H. Herzog, R. Vohn, M. Thimm and K. Willmes, Functional reorganisation in patients with right hemisphere stroke after training of alertness, a longitudinal PET and fMRI study in eight cases, *Neuropsychologia* **42**(4) (2004), 434–450.

[58] W. Sturm, B. Schmenk, B. Fimm, K. Specht, S. Weis, A. Thron and K. Willmes, Spatial attention, more than intrinsic alerting? *Exp Brain Res*, in press.

[59] W. Sturm and K. Willmes, On the functional neuroanatomy of intrinsic and phasic alertness, *Neuroimage* **14** (2001), 76–84.

[60] J. Talairach and P. Tournoux, *Co-planar stereotactic atlas of the human brain*, Thieme Stuttgart, 1988.

[61] C.M. Thiel, K. Zilles and G.R. Fink, Cerebral correlates of alerting, orienting and reorienting of visuospatial attention, an event-related fMRI study, *NeuroImage* **21**(1) (2004), 318–328.

[62] M. Thimm, G.R. Fink, J. Küst, H. Karbe and W. Sturm, Impact of Alertness-Training on Spatial Neglect, A Behavioral and fMRI Study, *Neuropsychologia* **44** (2006), 1230–1246.

[63] G. Vallar, D. Perani, S.F. Cappa, C. Messa, G.L. Lenzi and F. Fazio, Recovery from aphasia and Neglekt after subcortical stroke, neuropsychological and cerebral perfusion study, *Journal of Neurology, Neurosurgery and Psychiatry* **51** (1988), 1269–1276.

[64] R. Vandenberghe, D.R. Gitelman, T.B. Parrish and M.M. Mesulam, Functional specificity of superior parietal mediation of spatial shifting, *Neuroimage* **14** (2001), 661–673.

[65] D. Wilkinson and P. Halligan, The relevance of behavioral measures for functional-imaging studies of cognition, *Nature Reviews Neuroscience* **5**(1) (2004), 67–73.

[66] B.A. Wilson, J. Cockburn and P. Halligan, *Behavioral Inattention Test*, Test Companyn, Titchfield, Thames Valley 1987.

[67] F.C. Wilson, T. Manly, D. Coyle and I.H. Robertson, The effect of contralesional limb activation training and sustained attention training for self-care programmes in unilateral spatial neglect, *Restorative Neurology and Neuroscience* **16** (2000), 1–4.

[68] M.G. Woldorff, P.T. Fox, M. Matzke, J.L. Lancester, S. Veeraswamy, F. Zamerripa, M. Seabolt, T. Glass, J.H. Gao, C.C. Martin, C.C. and P. Jarabek, Retinotopic organization of early visual spatial attention effects as revealed by PET and ERPs, *Human Brain Mapping* **5** (1997), 280–286.

[69] P. Zimmermann and B. Fimm, *Test Battery for Attention Performance (TAP)*, Psytest, Herzogenrath, 1997.

Using limb movements to improve spatial neglect: The role of functional electrical stimulation

Gail A. Eskes[a,b,]* and Beverly Butler[b]
[a]*Department of Psychiatry, Dalhousie University Halifax, Nova Scotia, Canada*
[b]*Department of Psychology, Dalhousie University Halifax, Nova Scotia, Canada*

Received 4 January 2006
Revised 14 March 2006
Accepted 22 June 2006

Abstract. *Purpose*: Spatial neglect is common after right-hemisphere stroke and has proven resilient to a number of therapeutic interventions. Both active and experimenter-induced passive movements of the left limb in left hemispace have been shown to ameliorate neglect in subsets of patients by improving performance on tasks requiring attention to the left side of space. However, the high incidence of contralesional hemiparesis and poor motor recovery in neglect makes active limb movement therapies applicable to only a small subset of patients. The purpose of our studies was to investigate the effects of passive movements of the left hand by functional electrical stimulation (FES), a common and portable motor rehabilitation technique, on performance in a visual scanning task.
Methods: The effect of FES-induced passive movement on target detection in a visual scanning task was compared to no movement and active movement conditions and also investigated in scanning tasks in both near and far space.
Results: Passive limb movement effects in neglect were variable across and within studies, reference spaces, and individuals, with a subset of positive responders differing from non-responders in regard to constructional deficits and lesion location.
Conclusions: The potential viability of FES as a therapy for neglect deserves further investigation and directions for future research in this area are discussed.

Keywords: Limb movement, active, passive, functional electrical stimulation (FES), neglect, stroke

1. The relevance of limb movements to rehabilitation of visuo-spatial neglect

Spatial neglect is defined as a difficulty in orienting, processing or responding to stimuli in the space contralateral to a brain lesion [24]. Neglect is more common after right hemisphere stroke (thus left-sided neglect is the focus of study of this article), and, depending upon how it is assessed, symptoms are present in up to 85% of patients in the acute phase and 69% in the early rehabilitation phase [12,25]. The presence of neglect after stroke is of clinical importance in that it is associated with poor recovery of everyday life tasks such as dressing, bathing, eating and mobility [3,22,30] leading to reduced independence and poor reintegration to the community [36,49]. Thus, identifying and applying effective strategies for the rehabilitation of neglect could have a major benefit by improving the health outcomes of stroke for patients. Unfortunately, attempts at establishing rehabilitation techniques for neglect have had limited success. A recent Cochrane Review [9] concluded that the effectiveness of cognitive rehabilitation strategies for neglect remains unproven and re-

*Corresponding author: Gail Eskes, Ph.D., Department of Psychiatry, Dalhousie University, Rm 4080 AJLB, 5909 Veterans Memorial Lane, Halifax, N.S. B3H 2E2, Canada. Tel.: +902 473 6825; Fax: +902 473 6511; E-mail: Gail.Eskes@Dal.Ca.

search on intervention strategies is needed. In terms of recommendations for further research, the review concluded that, "advances in thinking about dissociable types of neglect, and targeting these with theory-based rehabilitation strategies, must be the way forwards".

One focus of our laboratory has been the investigation of limb movement effects on subtypes of spatial neglect, originally based on Rizzolatti's premotor theory of spatial attention [39]. The premotor theory assumes that spatial attention is mediated by multiple independent circuits and that there is a close link between motor programming in a spatial framework and the facilitation of stimulus processing (attention) within that framework [39]. According to this theory, neglect can result from a lesion to one of several independent centers responsible for controlling movements of action and attention [40] and thus activation via motor programming may be predicted to affect spatial attention and improve neglect.

Modification of the spatial attentional deficits in neglect by motoric task demands was earlier demonstrated by Joanette et al. [27] who reported the improvement in left-sided neglect with a detection task that compared pointing with the left (contralesional) hand to pointing with the right hand. Early studies of line bisection and cancellation performance by Halligan and colleagues [19,20] also showed improvement in visual tasks with the use of the left hand compared to the right. The interaction of the attention and motor systems in neglect has since been highlighted by Robertson and colleagues in studies of limb activation (e.g., moving a finger or pushing a button on cue). Using mostly single case studies, they reported that active left limb movement in left hemi-space (i.e., left side of the body) significantly reduced neglect on visual scanning tasks compared to no movement, or right-sided movement by either the left or right hand [43–45]. Improvement in walking trajectory with left hand movements was also seen in a group of 6 neglect patients compared to controls, although not all patients showed improvement [46]. The positive effects do not appear to be dependent upon left-sided visual cueing, since left hand movements out of sight of the subject or projected to the right side via mirrors have the same beneficial effect [31,43]. Arousal effects of the left hand movement on the right hemisphere were also ruled out by the lack of effect of left hand movement on neglect when carried out on the right side of space in early studies [20, 43] and confirmed by later reports [17,33].

Other studies of one or a few cases with neglect have confirmed the positive effects of left limb activation (LA), as measured by a variety of neglect tests as well as functional activities, although there are often inconsistent findings among tests within the same study and within individuals [2,10,35,50]. This inconsistency may be due to differences in task sensitivity, fluctuations in attentional function or carry-over practice effects.

While the majority of the studies have used single subject designs, study of this technique in larger case series or by incorporation of this technique in clinical rehabilitation settings in conjunction with normal therapy procedures also has been investigated in a small number of group studies with mixed results. Cubelli, Paganelli, Achilli and Pedrizzi [14] attempted to replicate three studies reported by Robertson and North [43, 45] in a consecutive series of 10 patients with right hemisphere damage and left neglect. Group analyses indicated a positive effect of left limb movement in only one out of three studies with only one subject showing consistent effects of left hand movement in left hemispace over the three studies. Examination of clinical variables failed to distinguish between responder and non-responders. Limited effects were also seen in a randomized control trial ($n = 50$) in an acute rehabilitation unit comparing limb activation during conventional therapy with conventional therapy alone. Length of stay and one measure of neglect at 12 weeks were significantly improved, although other functional and perceptual measures did not reach significance [28]. Kalra et al. concluded that while these results suggested that LA training could have a positive influence on functional outcome and resource use, more investigation of the specificity of the effect on neglect was needed. Another outpatient group study ($n = 40$) of perceptual training with or without LA techniques by Robertson et al. [48] found that weekly 45-min sessions over 12 weeks led to significantly improved left-sided motor function lasting up to 18–24 months. As with the Kalra study, however, there was no significant effect on measures of neglect or functional independence. Thus, the findings from both single case and group studies are variable and inconsistent responses are seen, both across patients and measures, highlighting the need for further study of this technique with consideration of individual patient differences.

In terms of evaluating intervention effects, neglect is not a unitary phenomenon but appears to comprise different subtypes. One classification system for neglect is based on the differences in neglect presence or severity seen in different spatial coordinate systems: e.g., neglect for personal space (body frame) versus peripersonal space (reaching space) [5,6] or extra-personal space (far space, or locomotor space) [21]. The dissociability of neglect and existence of these spatial frames and their neural correlates has also been systematically studied and confirmed by Rizzolatti and colleagues in non-human primates [38,39].

The beneficial effects of limb movements also can extend to multiple spatial reference frames, at least in the short term. Robertson and North (1993) [42] found that motor activation on the left side improved target detection in both peripersonal (near) and extrapersonal (far) space in a single case study. Direct investigation of the interaction of these spatial coordinate systems was further undertaken by Robertson [47] in a multiple-baseline by function single subject design. This study examined the effect of left LA (using a "Neglect Alert Device") during normal therapy activities on neglect in functional tests of personal space (combing hair), near space (placing blocks on a baking tray) and far space (spatial bias when walking). The results showed a statistically significant improvement on neglect tests in all spatial coordinate systems during the training, but the effect was only maintained for the near space baking tray task during a 9-day follow-up non-training period. They suggested that LA influences all three areas of space (as was predicted theoretically) and differences in maintenance may have been related to task differences (e.g., difficulty or sensitivity). Alternatively, LA effects may only be obtained in near space, and further examination of this issue in tests matched for difficulty and sensitivity would be important. The dissociability of LA effects in different spatial frames was also reported in a second study by Maddicks et al. [32] who found that the benefits of LA were seen immediately for both near (picking up coins task) and far (naming shapes on a wall) space, but not for personal space (beard trimming task), and, unlike Robertson's study, were only maintained in far space upon further follow-up testing. These studies highlight the limited understanding of the mechanism(s) underlying the LA effect even in near space, suggesting that further examination of this issue is critical. At a minimum, these results suggest that including measures of all three areas of space would be important in the evaluation of any training technique for neglect.

In addition to active left limb movement, passive movement induced by an experimenter can also be effective in improving neglect, suggesting that the intentional motor programming aspects of the active procedure may not be necessary for the effect. While an earlier case study by Robertson and North [42] suggested passive movement was ineffective, Ladavas et al. [31] found that passive left limb movement in left space improved visual scanning on the left compared to the effects of passive movement in centre or right space, independent of visual cuing. It was suggested that the passive movement effect may be related to the proprioceptive spatial cueing within personal space that modulates related spatial frameworks in near space to decrease neglect.

The potential positive effect of passive limb movement on attention in neglect was of interest to us given the high incidence of hemiparesis associated with, and perhaps exacerbated by, the neglect syndrome [52]. As stroke patients with neglect frequently have limited upper limb recovery, development of an alternative, easy to use, and portable limb activation method would be beneficial in neglect rehabilitation. In addition, the contribution of sensory (kinesthetic/proprioception) information vs active motor programming to the LA effect deserved more investigation. Our first study was thus designed to replicate and extend findings of active and passive limb movement effects on neglect [15]. For passive movement, we used a common rehabilitation technique, functional electrical stimulation (FES), which is used to facilitate, enhance or generate a muscle contraction in hemiplegic limbs. FES is accomplished by electrically innervating intact peripheral motor nerves in a coordinated manner that produces movement and provides function [4,51]. The use of FES in stimulating passive movement was desirable since it is an already established and accepted rehabilitation technique that could be easily adapted in either hospital or home settings. The purpose of the first study was thus to examine whether passive movement as generated by the FES technique could also improve neglect as measured by visual scanning performance, in comparison to no movement and to active movement.

2. Functional electrical stimulation effects on spatial neglect

Nine individuals with right hemisphere stroke and left-sided spatial neglect were tested in Experiment I. Neglect severity ranged from mild (27/100 on the Sunnybrook Bedside Neglect Battery) [8] to severe (100/100). All participants were oriented, with no diffuse cognitive deficits. Time after stroke varied from acute (2 weeks) to chronic (13 years). Visual scanning performance was measured using letter/number targets equally distributed in random positions on left and right sides amongst nonsense distractors on a page. The participants orally reported all targets detected and the percentage of correctly identified targets was analyzed for the left and right sides of the page.

We compared visual scanning during no limb movement, passive left limb movement in left hemispace produced by FES (for details of the procedure, see [15]) and active left limb movement in left hemispace (button press to a tone cue every 8–12 sec randomly). For FES-induced passive movement, a passive movement was obtained by stimulation of the finger extensors of the left forearm, with the programming set to produce a regular finger movement every 10 seconds. Scanning performance was measured in 10 trials in each movement condition, with the order of movement conditions counterbalanced across participants.

Eight individuals were able to participate in the FES-induced passive limb movement condition. Six of eight participants showed an increase in visual scanning hits on the left side with a significant ($p < 0.05$) overall average improvement of 17.8% compared to the no movement condition. In contrast, no significant change in target detection was seen on the right side during passive movement of the left limb. Three individuals received active movement (two of which were in the PM condition as well). Similarly, in the active movement condition left-sided target detection increased in two of three participants ($p < 0.01$, $p < 0.06$), with an average of 17% compared to no movement, while right-sided target detection was not affected (Fig. 1).

The results of this study replicated previous findings on the ability of active left limb movement in left hemispace to reduce neglect, although the variability in response to this manipulation must be noted. Given the small numbers, it is difficult to draw any conclusions about which variables might predict response, although this is clearly an important topic for future research. The results also confirmed that FES, a common upper-limb rehabilitation technique used to induce passive left limb movement in left hemispace also has the ability to improve left-sided visual scanning in at least a subset (6/8) of neglect patients. Even with this larger group, we did not identify any clinical markers that might predict effects, since neglect severity or chronicity were not correlated with the positive effects. These passive effects are consistent with the report of Ladavas et al. [31] and, while not directly comparable to the Ladavas method, our results appeared equivalent in size compared to the Ladavas et al. technique. Together, these studies suggest that intentional motor programming is not required to improve attention to

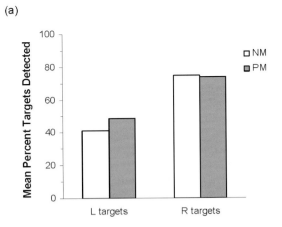

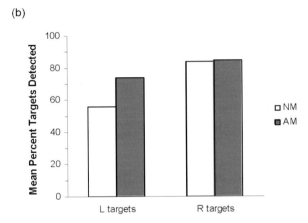

Fig. 1. Mean percent of targets detected on the left and right sides for the a) FES-induced passive movement (PM) and b) active movement (AM) conditions compared to the related no movement (NM) condition in Experiment I.

the left side in neglect. Thus, the passive effects may be mediated by sensory/proprioceptive input, which activates left-sided spatial representations for personal body space and interacts with spatial representations of peri-personal reaching space.

These findings were encouraging with regard to the use of FES as a potential rehabilitation tool for neglect. Given the variability in response, however, we decided to replicate this study with another group of patients with neglect and to also examine the generalizability of this effect to neglect in different spatial reference frames, both in near and far space. This examination of spatial frames was motivated by the case study by Robertson et al. [47] who found significant long-lasting effects of limb activation in near (peri-personal) space as measured by the baking tray task, but not in personal (hair combing task) or far space (walking through doorways). As Robertson et al. noted, one possible interpretation of the lack of long-lasting effect in all spatial domains may have been differences in task demands or difficulty, rather than lack of effect on the spatial frame of reference, per se. Thus, the use of matched tasks in each spatial domain would be important to follow up on this finding. In addition, Frassinetti et al. [16] had also reported a positive effect of mechanically-driven passive limb movements in both near and far space, when neglect was measured in different spaces by matched procedures using a cancellation task and a line bisection task. Thus, Experiment II was designed to examine the effects of FES-induced passive left limb movements, and active left limb movements compared to no movements in matched visual scanning tasks in near and far space.

3. Functional electrical stimulation effects on spatial neglect in near and far space

For this study, we tested three groups: 1) NEG consisted of seven males with unilateral lesions as confirmed by CT scans and meeting our neglect criteria (see below); 2) RHC contained seven males and three females with right hemisphere lesions confirmed by CT scans who did not meet neglect criteria; and 3) NC comprised ten healthy age-matched normal controls (five males, five females). Neglect was defined as performance at or below cutoff values on at least three of six conventional subtests of the standardized Behavioral Inattention Test [54]. All patients were oriented with no diffuse cognitive deficits. See Table 1 for a summary of demographic and clinical characteristics of the groups.

Visual scanning performance was tested using target detection sheets divided into eight imaginary columns with 6 targets (capital letters and numbers) per column. Approximately the same number of distractor symbols was also distributed across the sheet. Five trials were presented in near space (on the table 30 cm from the subject) and far space (projected onto a white wall, 250 cm from the subject), for each movement condition. The size of the stimuli was corrected to match on visual angle at each distance. The subjects were asked to read aloud all of the letters and numbers to avoid any confounding limb movements by the right hand and they were given 2 minutes to complete each trial.

Limb activation conditions included no movement, passive movement (induced by FES) and active movement (pushing a mouse button with the index finger when cued by a tone). FES-induced passive movement enervated the finger extensors in the left forearm and was begun before scanning and continued throughout the scanning trials. Five trials in each space/movement condition were administered, with order of blocks randomized. Number of targets detected was determined by scoring of audiotapes by scorers blind to the condition.

Binary logistic regression analyses of target detection (hits vs misses) were computed using the variables of space (peripersonal, extrapersonal), movement (no, passive, active), column (1–8), and the interactions involving space, movement and column entered into the regression. Logistic regression estimates the probability of detecting a target based on a non-linear function of the target's position in an x-y co-ordinate system and provides a measure of the slope of the performance gradient (for more description of this procedure, see [11]). A level of significance of $p < 0.05$ was adopted. Each group was analyzed separately.

Neglect group: Analyses of data from the no movement condition [11] revealed that the neglect group showed significant gradients of decreasing target detection from right to left on the stimulus page in both near and far space both in the group analyses and in all individual analyses. FES-induced passive left limb movement (PM) had no significant effect on these gradients of target detection in either near or far space in the group overall (Fig. 2), but variability in individual responses was evident among the seven neglect participants. Passive movement significantly improved left-sided performance (seen as a decrease in slope) for 3 individuals (#s1017, 1014 and 1018) in one or both testing spaces, and one individual (#1022) had a change in slope which indicated improved target detection performance only on the right side (Table 2 and Fig. 3). Negative effects only (increased slope) were seen in 2 other individuals (#s1016 and 1034) and one individual (#1019) was unaffected by PM in either space (Table 2). Only one individual (#1034) could participate in the active movement condition, with no significant improvement seen in performance.

Right hemisphere controls: Analyses of the RHC group under the no movement condition revealed no significant gradients of performance for either space overall, and individual analyses showed that 6/10 individuals had no gradient in their performance. Two individuals showed a significant rightward sloping gradient (i.e., performance worsened from left to right) in either near or far space under the no movement condi-

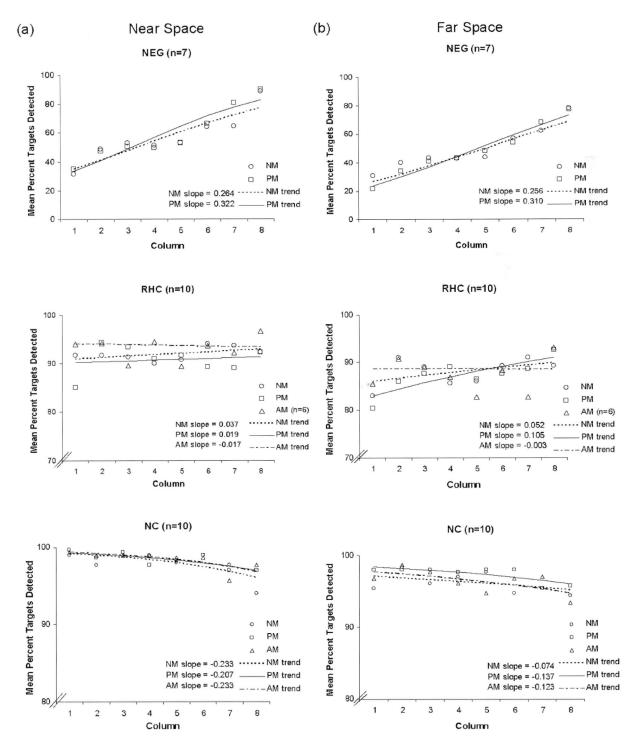

Fig. 2. Mean percent of targets detected per column in (a) near and (b) far space for each group under no movement (NM), FES-induced passive movement (PM) and active movement (AM) conditions. Groups were neglect (NEG), right-hemisphere control (RHC), and normal control (NC). Trend lines are based on predicted values from logistic regression analyses of target detection performance across columns in each co-ordinate space. Note the change in scale for the control groups in order to more clearly illustrate the trends.

Table 1
Summary of demographic, clinical and neuropsychological data for the normal control (NC), right hemisphere-lesion control (RHC) and neglect (NEG) groups in Experiment II. Neglect individuals are ordered according to response to passive movement (see text for details)

Subject	Age (years)	Education (years)	Post-stroke (days)	NAART (FSIQ)	NCSE (total)	BIT (total)	DSf (score)	DSb (score)	VOSP NL (/10)	VOSP PD (/20)
NC (mean)	57.9	15.8	N/A	109.28	75.2	144.6	8.2	7.5	9.4	19.9
RHC (mean)	55.4	12.1	57.7	102.41	72.1	140.6	7.8	5.2	8.9	17.5
NEG										
1017	70	11	76	97.38	71	135	8	5	4	15
1014	62	8	71	88.46	61	36	8	4	5	12
1018	71	7	144	88.8	57	103	7	2	6	17
1022	67	10	66	104.4	71	125	9	3	9	12
1034	47	12	239	115.3	77	130	9	8	5	12
1016	62	11	70	102.84	69	120	8	4	7	14
1019	54	8	89	85.68	61	46	8	2	2	13
NEG (mean)	**61.86**	**9.57**	**107.90**	**97.55**	**66.71**	**99.29**	**8.14**	**4.00**	**5.43**	**13.57**

NAART – North American Adult Reading Test, NCSE – Neurocognitive Screening Examination (Cognistat), BIT – Behavioural Inattention Test, DSf – Digit Span forward, DSb – Digit Span backward, VOSP NL – Visual Object and Space Perception Battery: Number Location, VOSP PD – Visual Object and Space Perception Battery: Position Discrimination.

Table 2
Target detection gradients in near and far space for individual neglect participants. Positive logistic regression slopes indicate decreasing target detection from right to left

Neglect subject	Near space		Far space	
	NM slope	PM slope	NM slope	PM slope
1017	0.1972	0.0699*	0.3861	0.0277*
1014	11.73	3.18*	2.77	0.7679*
1018	0.4201	0.2648*	0.3035	0.3586+
1022	0.2215	0.2987	0.2633	0.5693*
1034	0.2022	0.4503+	0.2484	0.5090+
1016	0.2225	0.2073	0.1409	0.2573+
1019	0.7589	0.8363	0.3768	0.1872

*Positive change in performance; +Negative change in performance.
NM = no movement condition; PM = passive movement condition.

tion. A further two RHC subjects exhibited significant leftward decreasing gradients similar to neglect participants even though their performance did not reach criteria for neglect in baseline testing (these dissociations are discussed more fully in [11]). Overall, no significant effects of either passive or active left limb movements were identified for the group (Fig. 2). For passive movement, individual analyses showed 8/10 individuals conformed to this non-significant effect. Of interest, however, were positive responses to passive movement seen in the two RHC subjects whose performance had shown a rightward decreasing gradient in the no movement condition. With passive movement both of these individuals showed a significant improvement in the affected (right-sided) space; one in near (#1035) and one in far (#1000) space (i.e., better performance on the right side; Fig. 4). Active movement also eliminated the rightward decreasing slope in one individual (#1035) in near space.

Normal controls: In the no movement condition the normal control group performance showed a significant decreasing gradient in the rightward direction (i.e., decreasing slope from left to right) for near space and the same trend (although not significant) in far space. Eight and five individuals showed a trend for this slope in near and far space, respectively (although only one slope reached significance). Neither passive nor active movement had a significant effect on performance overall (Fig. 2), and this negative finding was seen in individual analyses in 8/10 individuals. One NC individual with a rightward sloping gradient did show improvement in performance with both active and passive movement (i.e., target detection was improved on the right side; NC#8 in Fig. 4). In contrast, active movement resulted in an increased rightward sloping gradient (decreased performance on the right) in another NC individual.

In summary, FES-induced passive movement again produced a positive effect on neglect in Experiment II, at least in a subset of 4/7 individuals, while having negative ($n = 2$) or no ($n = 1$) effect in others. In a preliminary effort to identify factors that might distinguish the individuals with a positive effect from those showing negative or no effects, baseline neuropsychological test results (Table 1) and stroke localization information (from CT scans) were inspected. Positive responding individuals scored more poorly on the construction subtest of the Cognistat, consistent with right parietal damage (mean of 0.5 vs 1.7, positive responders vs others, respectively) and were more likely to have right subcortical-frontal systems damage, particularly in the caudate and putamen/globus pallidus (Table 3).

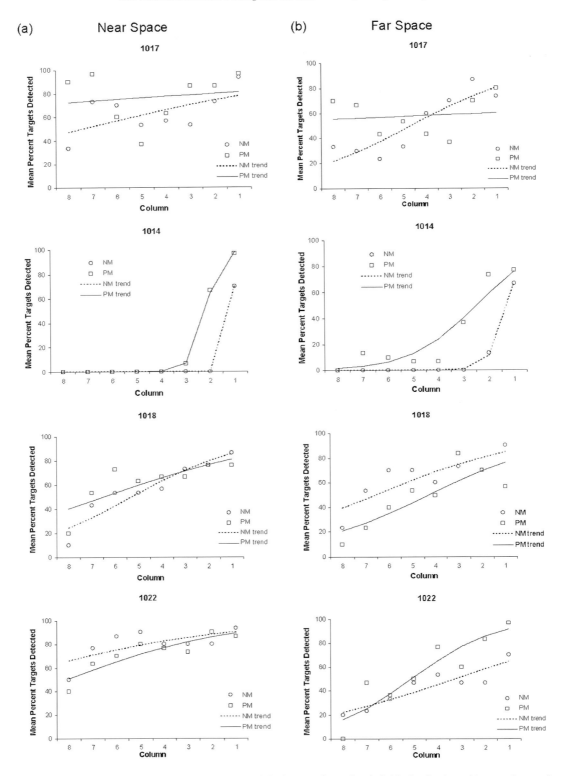

Fig. 3. Mean percent of targets detected per column in (a) near and (b) far space for neglect individuals who showed improved target detection in the FES-induced passive movement (PM) condition. Slope values and significance levels are seen in Table 2. Details of analyses as in Fig. 2.

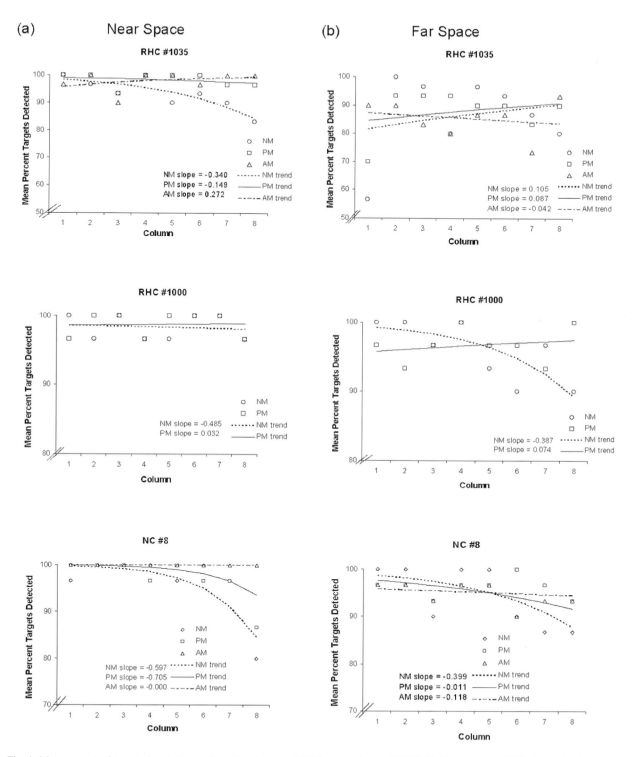

Fig. 4. Mean percent of targets detected per column in (a) near and (b) far space for two RHC individuals and one NC individual who showed improved target detection under passive movement (PM) and active movement (AM) conditions. Details of analyses as in Fig. 2. Note the differences in scale in order to more clearly illustrate the trends.

Table 3
Lesion localization for the neglect group

Neglect subject	Frontal		Temporal		Parietal			Subcortical			
	inf	sup	inf	sup	inf	Sup	post	IC	CN	LN	Th
1017*	+	+		+	+		+	+	+	+	
1014*	+		+	+	+	+	+	+	+	+	
1018*	+	+		+	+	+	+	+	+	+	+
1022*	+		+	+	+		+	+	+	+	
1034				+	+	+	+				
1016	+			+	+	+	+			+	
1019						+	+	+			

+Indicates damage in this area.
*Indicates positive responder to FES-induced passive movement.
inf – inferior, sup – superior, post – posterior, IC – internal capsule, CN – caudate nucleus, LN – lentiform nucleus (putamen and globus pallidus), Th – thalamus.

FES-induced passive or active movement effects in the two control groups were infrequent, but some findings were notable. Specifically, three individuals (1 NC and 2 RHC) with rightward sloping gradients in their scanning performance showed increased performance with either passive or active movement, suggesting that left limb movements can improve right-sided target detection as well, when performance is not at ceiling. Negative effects of limb movements were rare in controls and active movement produced a rightward sloping gradient (i.e., decreased performance on the right side) in only one NC.

4. Role of functional electrical stimulation in rehabilitation of spatial neglect

The above studies were designed to replicate and extend the findings of passive and active limb movement effects on visual scanning performance in individuals with right hemisphere damage and spatial neglect. Passive movement was induced by a common rehabilitation technique, Functional Electrical Stimulation (FES) used to facilitate and generate limb movements in a hemiplegic limb during physiotherapy. FES-induced passive movement of the left limb improved left-sided visual scanning performance in 6/8 individuals in Experiment I and eliminated the leftward decreasing gradients of performance indicative of neglect in 4/7 individuals with spatial neglect in Experiment II. These effects were seen in both near and far space, although not necessarily in the same individuals. Active movement had a similar positive effect on left-sided performance (2/3 showed improvement in Experiment I), but the number of individuals with spatial neglect able to produce active movements was very small (4/16 participants in the two experiments).

The positive effects of passive movement in both studies on neglect are consistent with the findings reported by Ladavas et al. [31] and Frassineti et al. [16], who used direct manipulation of the finger or limb by the experimenter to produce the movement. Ladavas et al. found that passive movement of the left finger on the left side significantly improved detection performance for left objects compared to left finger movement on the right side and this pattern was seen in 16/20 patients in their group. Similarly, Frassinetti et al. reported that passive left arm movements from the elbow in left hemi-space improved performance on both line bisection and object cancellation using either verbal or manual responses, with most or all patients (7–8/8) showing the effect. In addition, no differences in passive movement effects in near and far space were observed [16].

We used FES to produce finger movements similar to active finger movements that were reported to improve neglect in earlier studies (e.g., [43,45]). While direct comparison of the strength of our effects with those of Ladavas and colleagues is difficult, given the differences in patients, tasks and analysis methods, the more consistent response of patients to the larger arm movements suggests that a passive finger movement may be a weaker stimulus in terms of the amelioration of neglect. Given the positive effects obtained by this simple movement, investigation of different "doses" of FES-induced finger movements, either by lengthening of the time the device is worn, or by manipulating the amount and extent of stimulation provided would be warranted. In fact, the smaller number of subjects showing the positive effect in Experiment II (4/7) compared to Experiment I (6/8) may be related to the reduction in length of testing per condition during which passive movement was provided (10 trials vs 5 trials in Experiment I vs II respectively). Alternatively, differences in impaired proprioceptive function, lesion location or other relevant variables not yet identified may have contributed to the inconsistency of the effect.

The advantage of FES as a treatment technique is that it can be a safe, easily administered and portable method for inducing limb movements in individuals who would not normally be able to produce active movements for the purposes of treating neglect. Another advantage is the positive effect of FES in rehabilitating stroke-induced hemiplegia per se. A meta-analysis of controlled studies of functional electrical stimulation of upper and lower limbs concluded that FES promotes recovery of muscle strength that would likely be of clinical significance in post-stroke rehabilitation [18]. In addition, a 6-week treatment study involving daily use of a non-invasive neuroprosthetic neuromuscular stimulation system by sub-acute CVA patients with either no or partial active voluntary movement of the fingers and wrist, reported improvements over control participants in spasticity, active movement, and functional measures [37].

In addition to potential clinical value, findings from studies of passive movement effects on neglect also may provide increased understanding of the basic mechanisms underlying limb movement effects on spatial attention. A number of mechanisms have been proposed for the effects of active movement. According to the premotor model [41] neglect is a deficit of spatial representation derived from damage to cortical and subcortical circuits that underlie multiple spatial representations that interact to form a spatial reference system within which goal-directed motor movements are organized. According to this model, left limb movements produce activation of a personal spatial representation which interacts with the near peri-personal spatial coordinates in order to draw attention to the left side of space [44]. It has also been suggested that left limb movement effects may be derived from activation of the damaged right hemisphere and thus enhancement of its proposed role in attention to the left side [29]. The lack of effect of left limb movements carried out in the right side of space is difficult to reconcile with this view, however [17,20,43].

The positive effects of passive movement on neglect suggest that intentional motor programming is not necessary for any model of the LA effect, and proprioceptive cuing related to finger/limb position may be able to enhance the impaired spatial representation of the left side as well as active movement. Whether the size of the passive effect would be similar to full active movement is still unresolved. Further studies to compare the contribution of kinesthetic and proprioceptive cuing on spatial attention are in progress. In addition, the effects of passive and active movement on right-sided target detection in the control groups also suggests that the LA effect may extend to right-sided processing as well, perhaps also reflecting some low-level contribution of arousal when performance is not at maximum. Previous studies with neglect subjects have discounted the role of arousal in the LA effect, given negative results with right-sided movement [17,20,33,43]. Active or passive limb movement may generate a level of arousal that is below threshold for neglect subjects, while still improving performance in control subjects without neglect. This hypothesis could be tested by including a right-sided movement condition.

Another goal of our research was to examine the response of different subtypes of neglect with the passive movement response. In Experiment II, the neglect group showed both near and far neglect overall, and no differences between near and far space in terms of the passive movement effect. This lack of difference is similar to the findings of Frassinetti et al. [16] who found no difference in passive arm movement effects on line bisection and visual scanning between near and far space in their group of 8 subjects with neglect. However, our analyses of individual neglect subjects revealed that the null space effect was due to an inconsistent pattern of limb movement efficacy in the spatial reference frames across, and sometimes within individuals. Potential individual differences in space effects were not reported by Frassinetti.

Differences in neuroanatomical findings between responders and non-responders did emerge, with responders showing a greater tendency to have subcortical (particularly caudate)-frontal systems damage. This association between subcortical-frontal damage and response to passive movement may suggest that neglect in these individuals was exacerbated by, or even a direct result of, damage in this area and passive movement acted to activate and enhance the function of these damaged circuits, perhaps via intact areas mediating proprioceptive feedback from the passive movement [1,34]. Neglect due to subcortical-frontal damage has been associated with difficulties in initiating motor reaches to the left side by the unaffected limb, as opposed to neglect of a perceptual nature [13,23], although other techniques have yielded contradictory findings [26]. In fact, an investigation of the frequency of perceptual vs response biases in a large group of individuals with neglect using the modified Landmark test indicated that while both types of bias are often seen in the same individual, subcortical damage was more likely to be associated with response biases, while frontal damage was associated more frequently with perceptual bias [7]. While it is tempting to speculate that our responders with subcortical damage would have shown a response bias on the Landmark test (in addition perhaps to a perceptual bias due to other sites of damage), confirmation of the specificity of limb movement effects for individuals with neglect associated with subcortical damage and response bias must await further investigation.

5. Summary

FES-induced passive left limb movements appear a viable possibility for rehabilitation of at least a subset of individuals with spatial neglect. The variability in response to limb activation in neglect provides impetus for further examination of the neurobehavioural mechanisms of these effects and continued research on the application of limb movements in therapeutic and everyday functional contexts. Based on evidence from imaging studies showing some similar, but weaker brain activation patterns during passive compared to active limb movements [34,53], further investigation of patterns of brain activation and movement effects on neglect comparing different active and passive movement techniques (i.e., FES, mechanical motorized devices) and degrees of movement is warranted. In addition, systematic activation of affected right-hemisphere pathways by specific rehabilitation processes (i.e., attentional or perceptual vs proprioceptive or kinesthetic components) is critical to obtain information on the effectiveness of these measures individually or in combination when targeted toward different subsets of individuals.

Acknowledgements

We thank the individuals with stroke and their caregivers for their participation and help, particularly Dr. Ed Harrison and Ms. Alison McDonald for assistance with the initiation and conduct of these studies, and Dr. Robert Vandorpe for help with the lesion localization analyses. This research was supported by funds from the Heart & Stroke Foundation of Nova Scotia, and the QEII Health Science Research Fund. GE was supported in part by the Nova Scotia Department of Health Designated Mental Health Research Fund; BB by an NSERC Predoctoral Fellowship and an Isaak Walton Killam Memorial scholarship during the conduct of these studies.

References

[1] F. Alary, C. Simoes, V. Jousmaki, N. Forss and R. Hari, Cortical activation associated with passive movements of the human index finger: An MEG study, *Neuroimage* **15** (2002), 691–696.

[2] M.J. Bailey, M.J. Riddoch and P. Crome, Treatment of visual neglect in elderly patients with stroke: A single-subject series using either a scanning and cueing strategy or a left-limb activation strategy, *Physical Therapy* **82** (2002), 782–797.

[3] D.H. Barer, The influence of visual and tactile inattention on predictions for recovery from acute stroke, *Quarterly Journal of Medicine* **74** (1990), 21–32.

[4] L.A. Benton, L.L. Baker, B.R. Bowman and R.L. Waters, Functional Electrical Stimulation: A Practical Clinical Guide, 2nd edn., Ranchos Los Amigos, Downey, CA, 1981.

[5] N. Beschin and I.H. Robertson, Personal versus extrapersonal neglect: A group study of their dissociation using a reliable clinical test, *Cortex* **33** (1997), 379–384.

[6] E. Bisiach, D. Perani, G. Vallar and A. Berti, Unilateral neglect: Personal and extra-personal, *Neuropsychologia* **24** (1986), 759–767.

[7] E. Bisiach, R. Ricci, M. Lualidi and M.R. Colombo, Perceptual and response bias in unilateral neglect: Two modified versions of the Milner Landmark test, *Brain and Cognition* **37** (1998), 369–386.

[8] S.E. Black, B. Vu, D. Martin and J. Szalai, Evaluation of a bedside battery for hemispatial neglect in acute stroke, *Journal of Clinical and Experimental Psychology* **12** (1990), 102.

[9] A. Bowen, N.B. Lincoln and M. Dewey, Cognitive rehabilitation for spatial neglect following stroke (Cochrane Review), in: *The Cochrane Library*, Issue 3, Update Software, Oxford, 2002.

[10] T. Brunila, N. Lincoln, A. Lindell, O. Tenovuo and H. Hamalainen, Experiences of combined visual training and arm activation in the rehabilitation of unilateral visual neglect: A clinical study, *Neuropsychological Rehabilitation* **12** (2002), 27–40.

[11] B.C. Butler, G.A. Eskes and R.A. Vandorpe, Gradients of detection in neglect: comparison of peripersonal and extrapersonal space, *Neuropsychologia* **42** (2004), 346–358.

[12] L.R. Cherney, A.S. Halper, C.M. Kwasnica, R.L. Harvey and M. Zhang, Recovery of functional status after right hemisphere stroke: Relationship with unilateral neglect, *Archives of Physical Medicine and Rehabilitation* **82** (2001), 322–328.

[13] H.B. Coslett, D. Bowers, E. Fitzpatrick, B. Haws and K. Heilman, Directional hypokinesia and hemispatial inattention in neglect, *Brain* **113** (1990), 475–486.

[14] R. Cubelli, N. Paganelli, D. Achilli and S. Pedrizzi, Is one hand always better than two? A replication study, *Neurocase* **5** (1999), 143–151.

[15] G.A. Eskes, B. Butler, A. McDonald, E.R. Harrison and S.J. Phillips, Limb activation effects in hemi-spatial neglect, *Archives of Physical Medicine and Rehabilitation* **84** (2003), 323–328.

[16] F. Frassinetti, M. Rossi and E. Ladavas, Passive limb movements improve visual neglect, *Neuropsychologia* **39** (2001), 725–733.

[17] G. Gainotti, R. Perri and A. Cappa, Left hand movements and right hemisphere activation in unilateral spatial neglect: a test of the interhemispheric imbalance hypothesis, *Neuropsychologia* **40** (2002), 1350–1355.

[18] M. Glanz, S. Klawansky, W. Stason, C. Berkey and T.C. Chalmers, Functional electrostimulation in poststroke rehabil-

itation: A meta-analysis of the randomized controlled trials, *Archives of Physical Medicine and Rehabilitation* **77** (1996), 549–553.
[19] P.W. Halligan and J.C. Marshall, Laterality of motor response in visuo-sptial neglect: A case study, *Neuropsychologia* **27** (1989), 1301–1307.
[20] P.W. Halligan, L. Manning and J.C. Marshall, Hemispheric activation vs spatio-motor cueing in visual neglect: a case study, *Neuropsychologia* **29** (1991), 165–176.
[21] P.W. Halligan and J.C. Marshall, Left neglect for near but not far space in man, *Nature* **350** (1991), 498–500.
[22] P.W. Halligan and J.C. Marshall, The history and clinical presentation of neglect, *Lawrence Erlbaum Associates, Hove* (1993), 351.
[23] K.M. Heilman, D. Bowers, B. Coslett, H. Whelan and R.T. Watson, Directional hypokinesia: Prolonged reaction times for leftward movements in patients with right hemisphere lesions and neglect, *Neurology* **35** (1985), 855–859.
[24] K.M. Heilman, D. Bowers, E. Valenstein and R.T. Watson, Hemispace and Hemispatial Neglect, in: *Neurophysiological and neuropsychological aspects of spatial neglect*, M. Jeannerod, ed., Elsevier Science Publishers B.V., North-Holland, 1987, pp. 115–150.
[25] D.B. Hier, J. Mondlock and L.R. Caplan, Behavioral abnormalities after right hemisphere stroke, *Neurology* **33** (1983), 337–344.
[26] M. Husain, M.J.B., C. Rorden, C. Kennard and J. Driver, Distinguishing sensory and motor biases in parietal and frontal neglect, *Brain* **123** (2000), 1643–1659.
[27] Y. Joanette, M. Brouchon, L. Gautheir and M. Samson, Pointing with left vs right hand in left visual field neglect, *Neuropsychologia* **24** (1986), 391–396.
[28] L. Kalra, I. Perez, S. Gupta and M. Wittink, The influence of visual neglect on stroke rehabilitation, *Stroke* **28** (1997), 1386–1391.
[29] M. Kinsbourne, Mechanisms of unilateral neglect, in: *Neurophysiological and Neuropsychological Aspects of Spatial Neglect*, M. Jeannerod, ed., Elsevier Science Publishers B.V., North-Holland, 1987, pp. 69–85.
[30] G. Kinsella and B. Ford, Acute recovery patterns in stroke patients, *Medical Journal of Australia* **2** (1980), 663–666.
[31] E. Ladavas, A. Berti, E. Ruozzi and F. Barboni, Neglect as a deficit determined by an imbalance between multiple spatial representations, *Experimental Brain Research* **116** (1997), 493–500.
[32] R. Maddicks, S. Marzillier and G. Parker, Rehabilitation of unilateral neglect in the acute recovery stage: The efficacy of limb activation therapy, *Neuropsychological Rehabilitation* **13** (2003), 391–408.
[33] J.B. Mattingley, I.H. Robertson and J. Driver, Modulation of covert visual attention by hand movement: Evidence from parietal extinction after right-hemisphere damage, *Neurocase* **4** (1998), 245–253.
[34] T. Mima, N. Sadato, S. Yazawa, T. Hanakawa, H. Fukuyama, Y. Yonekura and H. Shibasaki, Brain structures related to active and passive finger movements in man, *Brain* **122** (1999), 1989–1997.
[35] B. O'Neill and T.M. McMillan, The efficacy of contralesional limb activation in rehabilitation of unilateral hemiplegia and visual neglect: A baseline-intervention study, *Neuropsychological Rehabilitation* **14** (2004), 437–447.
[36] S. Paolucci, G. Antonucci, L.E. Gialloreti, M. Traballesi, S. Lubich, L. Pratesi and L. Palombi, Predicting stroke inpatient rehabilitation outcome: The prominent role of neuropsychological disorders, *European Neurology* **36** (1996), 385–390.
[37] H. Ring and N. Rosenthal, Controlled study of neuroprosthetic functional electrical stimulation in subacute poststroke rehabilitation, *Journal of Rehabilitation Medicine* **37** (2005), 32–36.
[38] G. Rizzolatti, M. Gentilucci and M. Matelli, Selective spatial attention: One center, one circuit, or many circuits? in: *Attention and Performance*, (Vol. 11), M.I. Posner and O.S.M. Marin, eds, Lawrence Erlbaum Associates, Hillsdale, New Jersey, 1985, pp. 251–265.
[39] G. Rizzolatti and R. Camarda, eds, Neurophysiological and Neuropsychological Aspects of Spatial Neglect, Neural circuits for spatial attention and unilateral neglect, Elsevier Science Publishers B.V., North-Holland, 1987, 289–313.
[40] G. Rizzolatti and V. Gallese, Mechanisms and theories of spatial neglect, in: *Handbook of Neuropsychology*, (Vol. 1), F. Boller and J. Grafman, eds, Elsevier Science Publisher, B.V., 1988, pp. 223–246.
[41] G. Rizzolatti and A. Berti, Neglect as a neural representation deficit, *Revue Neurologique (Paris)* **146** (1990), 626–634.
[42] I. Robertson and N. North, Active and passive activation of left limbs: Influence on visual and sensory neglect, *Neuropsychologia* **31** (1993), 293–300.
[43] I.H. Robertson and N. North, Spatio-motor cueing in unilateral left neglect: The role of hemispace, hand and motor activation, *Neuropsychologia* **30** (1992), 553–563.
[44] I.H. Robertson, N.T. North and C. Geggie, Spatio-motor cueing in unilateral left neglect: Three case studies of its therapeutic effects, *Journal of Neurology, Neurosurgery and Psychiatry* **55** (1992), 799–805.
[45] I.H. Robertson and N.T. North, One hand is better than two: Motor extinction of left hand advantage in unilateral neglect, *Neuropsychologia* **32** (1994), 1–11.
[46] I.H. Robertson, R. Tegner, S.J. Goodrich and C. Wilson, Walking trajectory and hand movements in unilateral left neglect: A vestibular hypothesis, *Neuropsychologia* **32** (1994), 1495–1502.
[47] I.H. Robertson, K. Hogg and T.M. McMillan, Rehabilitation of unilateral neglect: Improving function by contralesional limb activation, *Neuropsychological Rehabilitation* **8** (1998), 19–29.
[48] I.H. Robertson, T.M. McMillan, E. MacLeod, J. Edgeworth and D. Brock, Rehabilitation by limb activation training reduces left-sided motor impairment in unilateral neglect patients: A single-blind randomised control trial, *Neuropsychological Rehabilitation* **12** (2002), 439–454.
[49] L. Rose, D.M. Bakal, T.S. Fung, P. Farn and L.E. Weaver, Tactile extinction and functional status after stroke – A preliminary investigation, *Stroke* **25** (1994), 1973–1976.
[50] C. Samuel, A. Louis-Dreyfus, R. Kaschel, E. Makiela, M. Troubat, N. Anselmi, V. Cannizzo and P. Azouvi, Rehabilitation of very severe unilateral neglect by visuo-spatio-motor cueing: Two single case studies, *Neuropsychological Rehabilitation* **10** (2000), 385–399.
[51] B. Singer, Functional electrical stimulation of the extremities in the neurological patients: A review, *Australian Journal of Physiotherapy* **33** (1987), 33–41.
[52] R. Sterzi, G. Bottini, M.G. Celani, E. Righetti, M. Lamassa, S. Ricci and G. Vallar, Hemianopia, hemianaesthesia, and hemiplegia after right and left hemisphere damage. A hemispheric difference, *Journal of Neurology, Neurosurgery, and Psychiatry* **56** (1993), 308–310.

[53] C. Weiller, M. Juptner, S. Fellows, M. Rijntjes, G. Leonhardt, S. Kiebel, S. Muller, H.C. Diener and A.F. Thilmann, Brain representation of passive and active movements, *NeuroImage* **4** (1996), 105–110.

[54] B. Wilson, J. Cockburn and P. Halligan, Development of a behavioral test of visuospatial neglect, *Archives of Physical Medicine and Rehabilitation* **68** (1987), 98–102.

Future directions for research and treatment

The need for randomised treatment studies in neglect research

N.B. Lincoln[a,*] and A. Bowen[b]
[a]Institute of Work Health and Organisations, University of Nottingham, UK
[b]School of Psychological Sciences, University of Manchester, UK

Received 15 October 2005
Revised 27 December 2005
Accepted 3 February 2006

Abstract. *Purpose*: The aim was to review the methodological quality of trials to evaluate rehabilitation for spatial neglect and to determine the overall effectiveness of interventions.
Methods: A systematic literature review and meta-analysis were conducted of trials completed by 2005. Trials identified were independently assessed for methodological quality by two reviewers. Outcomes were analysed as the standardised mean difference and 95% confidence intervals with random effects models.
Results: 25 trials of neglect rehabilitation were identified, 12 randomised controlled trials and 13 controlled clinical trials. The methodological quality was generally poor with only 4 trials achieving an A rating, i.e. low risk of selection bias. The immediate effect of cognitive rehabilitation on disability was small, 0.26 [−0.16, 0.67] and neither this nor the persisting effect 0.61 [−0.42, 1.63] was statistically significant. The most frequently used standardised neglect test (number of single letters correctly cancelled) favoured the experimental group 0.58 [0.10, 1.05] but was not significant. When cancellation errors were measured there was a small immediate effect favouring the experimental group, of borderline statistical significance, −0.65 [−1.28, −0.01] $p = 0.05$, and a significant persisting effect −0.76 [−1.39, −0.13] $p = 0.02$. Cognitive rehabilitation also significantly improved immediate ($p = 001$) and persisting ($p = 0.02$) line bisection performance but these findings are based on only four and one study respectively.
Conclusions: The quality of trials identified was poor. Analysis of randomised controlled trials showed some evidence of an effect of intervention on measures of impairment. There was no evidence to support the effects of intervention on measures of disability. Further trials must use methods that reduce bias, have adequate statistical power, and include valid disability outcome measures.

Keywords: Neglect, inattention, meta-analysis, review

1. Introduction

The rehabilitation of spatial neglect is well established and there are examples of effective interventions with individuals [4,15,19,20]. However for a treatment to be widely adopted in clinical practice it needs to be shown to generalise from individual cases to the target clinical population. Because no two people are the same and conditions such as neglect are so heterogeneous single case designs, useful for proof of concept, cannot provide the evidence of generalisation that group studies provide. Rehabilitation staff rely on evidence derived from randomised controlled trials (RCT). In an RCT every individual has an equal chance of being allocated to either group, usually but not necessarily a therapy group and a control group. The random allocation process increases the likelihood that the groups

*Corresponding author: Professor N.B. Lincoln, Institute of Work, Health and Organisations, University of Nottingham, Science and Technology Park, Nottingham, NG7 2RQ, UK. Tel.: +44 0115 9515315; E-mail: nadina.lincoln@nottingham.ac.uk.

are balanced at baseline. Properly conducted RCTs are the only type of study that can determine whether improvements seen after rehabilitation can be attributed to the rehabilitation rather than to other strong contenders, such as spontaneous recovery or placebo effects. Well conducted RCTs also eliminate the false positive findings that can result from selection bias, causing an imbalance between groups at baseline.

Despite these advantages, there remains a dearth of methodologically sound RCTs of the rehabilitation of spatial neglect. A less robust alternative is to consider controlled clinical trials (CCT) in which two groups receiving different interventions are compared but with no randomisation to groups. In 2002 we published a systematic review of the evidence from RCTs and CCTs [3]. The aim of the present study was to update this review to determine the overall effectiveness of cognitive rehabilitation strategies for neglect.

The methodological quality of the trials determines the conclusions we can draw and the confidence we can have in their findings. There are now published guidelines to enable researchers to design studies in a way which minimises bias and maximises the robustness of the findings [12,16]. The key standards to be achieved relate to randomisation, allocation concealment, 'blinded' assessment of outcomes and standardised, reliable, valid measures of outcome. Randomisation should be done using a method that is free from bias and open to verification by an independent observer. While coin tossing is random, it cannot subsequently be verified. The preferred method is a computer generated random allocation sequence held by an independent randomisation centre and a study monitoring body which can check on adherence to the randomisation procedure. Many clinical trials units provide this service, the allocation of patients is not in the control of the researchers who know the patients, and therefore minimises the chance of selection bias. Randomisation should be independent of the people doing recruitment, providing intervention or assessing outcome.

Once patients are allocated to groups, no changes should be made to the allocation. All participants should be followed up, independently of whether they complete the treatment, for an intention to treat analysis [12]. The only exception to follow up should be patients who withdraw consent, but any loss to follow-up should be clear from the study description. A CONSORT diagram [16] is a useful way of summarising these events and is required for publication in several high quality journals. Excluding participants who have further strokes for example renders the trial unrepresentative of clinical practice, as stroke patients will have further strokes. Since adherence to treatment is likely to be a key factor in treatment effectiveness, excluding patients who find treatment unacceptable gives an unrealistic picture of clinical effectiveness. Those dropping out are likely to be a highly selective subgroup i.e. those for whom the treatment is not proving helpful. Untoward chance events are likely to affect participants in both intervention and control groups and therefore if the sample size is adequate such events should be balanced out between the groups.

Outcomes should be assessed by an observer who is unaware of the group allocation of patients. In rehabilitation studies this may be difficult to achieve but guidelines are provided [29]. Most rehabilitation studies can only be conducted single blind, with outcome assessors unaware of the intervention delivered. It is rarely possible to conceal the intervention from the patient or from the person providing the intervention. Outcome measures need to be standardised with established reliability and validity. Developing measures specifically for a study is not considered good practice unless there is no acceptable published measure available and adequate development work has been carried out.

The effectiveness of rehabilitation for spatial neglect is an important issue as many patients have neglect following a stroke. These people tend to progress less well with rehabilitation and it affects long term outcome in independence in activities of daily living and quality of life [15,19,20]. These narrative reviews have summarised the studies on a range of rehabilitation strategies. The strategies can broadly be divided into two major approaches, 'top down', in which patients are being trained to compensate for the spatial neglect, and 'bottom up' strategies in which the underlying controlling factors responsible for the occurrence of spatial neglect are modified. The 'top down' strategies are characterised by scanning training programmes, in which patients were trained to scan visual space to compensate for their failure to attend to one side [10,34]. Scanning training programmes have been shown to reduce impairment [3] but few studies assessed whether treatment effects generalised to daily life. Poor generalisation may be resolved by training patients on daily life tasks [33] but despite the intuitive appeal of targeting real activities, this approach may be limited due to the range of activities requiring training [15]. One major limitation is that it requires patients to be aware of their deficit and to voluntarily maintain orientation of attention to the neglected side.

'Bottom up' strategies are characterised by sensory stimulation, to re-map the representation of space.

These have included optokinetic stimulation [22], neck muscle vibration [28] and transcutaneous electrodermal stimulation [27]. Other techniques which involve the manipulation of visual input are eye patching [2], hemi-spatial goggles [38], wearing prisms [26] or prism adaptation training [9,25]. Although patients have benefited on measures of impairment, the effectiveness of the techniques seems to vary [15] and improvement in functional outcomes have not been demonstrated [26]. The advantage of prism adaptation and hemi-spatial goggles is that they are non-invasive, require minimum supervision and do not require the voluntary orientation of attention to the neglected side.

Research has demonstrated that techniques, based on both 'bottom up' and 'top down' strategies, seem to reduce neglect in treated patients as compared with controls. Effects seem to be small and of short duration. However given that many of the trials contain very small samples it is possible that treatment effects are being missed. A Cochrane review and meta-analysis of trials [3] showed evidence for the effectiveness of treatments on impairment measures. However at that time there were too few studies to determine the effects on functional abilities or for examining long term outcomes. Since then the number of trials has increased. The present review was conducted in conjunction with an update of the Cochrane review. For the latter, which will shortly be published online (www.thecochranelibrary.com) we decided to reduce the risk of selection bias by only including RCTs and excluding the previously included CCTs. For the purposes of the present paper we aimed to examine the methodological quality of all trials of neglect rehabilitation and to make recommendations for the design of future studies. In addition the aim was to analyse the effects of intervention on functional outcomes and to assess persisting effects of intervention.

2. Method

We sought all controlled trials in which cognitive rehabilitation was compared to a control treatment for spatial neglect following stroke. Cognitive rehabilitation was broadly defined to include therapy activities designed to directly reduce the level of cognitive deficits or the resulting disability. Drug treatments were not included. Outcomes were classified according to whether they assessed impairment or activity and participation. Standardised measures of impairment included target cancellation, line bisection and figure copying. Outcomes on measures of activity and participation included measures of independence in activities of daily living (Barthel Index, Functional Independence Measure) and questionnaire measures of the effects of neglect on daily life [1,31,39]. The length of follow up to examine persisting effects after the end of the rehabilitation was also considered

This review was based on the search strategy developed for the Cochrane Stroke Group (www.dcn.ed.ac.uk/csrg). Their specialised trials register was searched by the Review Group Coordinator. In addition, the reviewers searched electronic databases, the National Research Register (July 2005), screened reference lists and used SCISEARCH of the three citation index databases, Science Citation Index (SCI), Social Sciences Citation Index (SSCI) and Arts and Humanities Citation Index (A&HCI) for citation tracking of relevant included studies. The search terms were those of the Cochrane review [3].

Two reviewers independently selected trials using four inclusion criteria (types of trials, participants, interventions and outcome measures) and independently assessed the methodological quality. Differences were resolved by discussion. Study characteristics and outcomes were abstracted. Where these data were not available or unclear from the reports then this was sought and/or confirmed by correspondence with the first author of the publication. Where a crossover design was used [18,28] only data from the first treatment period were considered. Trials in which the same patients were included were only entered once.

All trials identified were reviewed on the extent they met the criteria for high quality research trials [12,16] and classified into categories, listed below, according to the methodological quality. These were based on guidelines for Cochrane reviews [12].

A RCT with concealment of allocation

B/C RCT with unclear (B) or inadequate (C) concealment of allocation

The results from the RCTs were analysed to compare a rehabilitation approach with any other control. Outcomes were treated as continuous and mean and standard deviation data were requested or calculated. Outcomes were analysed as the standardised mean difference and 95% confidence intervals. Random effects models were used.

3. Results

25 trials of neglect rehabilitation were identified, 12 RCTs [5–8,13,23,24,26,27,34,35,38] and 13 CCTs [2,

Table 1
Methodological characteristics of studies identified

Trial	Main type of intervention	Rand	Conc	Indep	Outcome Impairment	Outcome Participation	Blind	n	Follow Up	Category
7	Scanning and cueing	✓	✓	X	✓	✓	✓	42	X	A
13	Limb activation/motor cueing	✓	✓	✓	✓	✓	✓	50	X	A
23	Computerised scanning and feedback	✓	✓	X	✓	✓	X	30	6 m	A
24	Limb activation	✓	✓	✓	✓	✓	✓	36	18–24 m	A
5	Scanning and oral reading	✓	X	X	✓	✓	X	4	X	B/C
6	Visual scanning	✓	X	X	✓	✓	X	12	6 w	B/C
8	Feedback of eye movements	✓	X	X	✓	✓	✓	18	8 w	B/C
26	Prisms	✓	X	X	✓	✓	X	39	X	B/C
27	Scanning with cueing	✓	X	X	✓	✓	✓	20	X	B/C
34	Scanning training	✓	X	X	✓	X	X	25	X	B/C
35	Head movement, scanning and feedback	✓	X	X	✓	✓	X	22	2 m	B/C
38	Hemi-blinding goggles	✓	X	X	✓	X	✓	8	X	B/C
2	Eye patching	X	X	X	X	✓	✓	15	3 m	D
18	Scanning	X	X	X	✓	✓	✓	23	X	D
22	Optokinetic stimulation	X	X	X	✓	✓	✓	22	X	D
9	Prism adaptation	X	X	X	✓	✓	X	13	5 w	E
10	Perceptual remediation	X	X	X	✓	✓	X	77	4 m	E
11	Rod lifting	X	X	X	✓	✓	X	14	1 m	E
14	Bed orientation	X	X	X	X	✓	X	20	X	E
17	Scanning	X	X	X	X	✓	X	31	X	E
25	Prisms	X	X	X	✓	X	X	12	2 h	E
28	Neck vibration	X	X	X	✓	✓	X	20	2 m	E
30	Video feedback	X	X	X	✓	X	X	14	3 h	E
33	Computerised tracking and obstacle course	X	X	X	X	✓	X	40	X	E
37	Scanning and spatial assembly	X	X	X	✓	X	X	18	1 w	E

Rand – Randomised Con – Concealed allocation Indep- independent person conducting randomisation.
✓ reported X not reported/not clear h hours, w weeks, m months.
A RCT with concealment of allocation and 'blind' assessment of outcome.
B/C RCT with unclear (B) or inadequate (C) concealment of allocation, and unclear or no 'blind' assessment of outcome.
D CCT with 'blind' assessment of outcome.
E CCT with unclear or no 'blind' assessment of outcome.

9–11,14,17,18,22,25,28,30,33,37]. Two trials included a mixture of randomised and non-randomised patients [28,38]. In one case [38] the authors provided the randomised data so that those cases could be analysed with the other RCTs. Trials are summarised in Table 1.

The method of randomisation was rarely specified in sufficient detail. Of the 12 RCTs, six [7,8,13,23,24,38] described the randomisation process and four [7,13,23,24] achieved adequate allocation concealment (category A). One attempted concealment [8] but this was not considered adequate and seven were judged unclear or inadequate [5,6,26,27,34,35,38]. In the non-randomised trials allocation was by date of admission [11,17,33], alternate [2,22], consecutive batches [25,30], by ward or bed [9,10,14,18], not specified [37] or modified [28]. Few studies adequately described how, or even whether, they had attempted to conceal allocation.

Blinded assessment of outcome was reported in 6 of the 12 RCT's [7,8,13,24,27,38] and 3 of 13 CCT's [2,18,22]. The remainder of the trials did not report who conducted the assessments and whether the assessors were blinded or not. Most (21 out of 25) studies measured outcome on impairment measures of neglect, such as cancellation, line bisection and text reading. Several recent studies [5,8,9,11,23,24] used the Behavioural Inattention Test [36], which was analysed either as a total score, as a summary of the behavioural subtests or as individual subtests. Three used questionnaire measures [11,22,28] of the consequences of neglect in daily life. Others (10 out of 25) used generic measures of independence in activities of daily living, such as the Barthel Index [7,13,14,22,27], Frenchay Activities Index [23] and Functional Independence Measure [35].

Outcomes were usually assessed at the end of treatment to determine whether there has been an effect of the intervention but only 5 RCTs and 8 CCTs provided a longer term follow up to determine whether any treatment effects persisted beyond the end of the intervention. Few trials reported losses to follow-up. All category A trials provided this information but for others it was not clear whether no losses to follow-up had occurred or whether researchers excluded those who

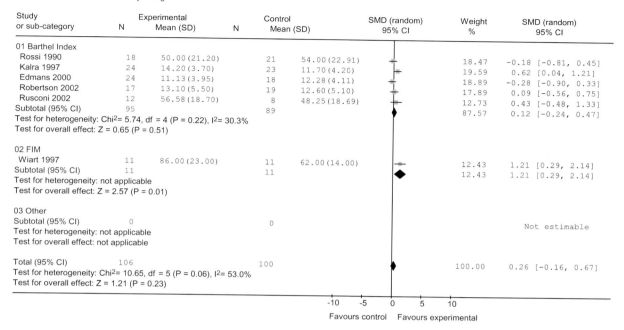

Fig. 1. Short-term effects of cognitive rehabilitation on independence in activities of daily living.

failed to complete follow-up. To reduce selection bias outcomes were only analysed for the 306 participants from the 12 RCTs. Six studies reported a measure of disability immediately after the end of rehabilitation or on discharge, six with the Barthel Index [7,13,24,26,27] and one with the Functional Independence Measure [35]. One study used the Frenchay Activities Index [23] but the data were not available for this review. Results are shown in Fig. 1.

The overall effect for the six studies (206 participants) measuring immediate effect on disability was small, with a wide confidence interval that included zero 0.26 [−0.16, 0.67] $p = 0.23$ and was not statistically significant. Results are shown in Fig. 1. The persistence of effects on disability over time was only assessed in two studies [24,35]. There was no overall evidence for a persisting effect on ADL functioning from these two studies 0.61 [−0.42, 1.63] $p = 0.24$.

The number of targets correctly cancelled was measured using four types of targets single letter, double letter, line and shape. Outcomes for only one of these targets significantly favoured the experimental group: double letter cancellation 1.8 [0.85, 2.76] $p = 0.0002$ (one B/C rated study [34]). Four studies with 103 participants used the number of errors cancelling targets [6,23,26,36] and showed a small effect favouring the experimental group, which was of borderline statistical significance, −0.65 [−1.28, −0.01] $p = 0.05$. Results are shown in Fig. 2. Only one [23] was A rated. Four studies reporting line bisection performance [26,27,36,38] suggested a favourable outcome for the experimental group −0.84 [−1.36, −0.33], $p = 0.001$. However, none of these studies were A rated. Results are shown in Fig. 3. There was no evidence ($p = 0.35$) of an overall effect on the three studies using the BIT behavioural subtest summary score [5,8,23]. Therefore, there was evidence that cognitive rehabilitation improved immediate performance on standardised tests of neglect although this varied depending on the test used. Outcome favoured the experimental group on one of the four cancellation measures and line bisection. There was no evidence in favour of either group on single letter, line or shape cancellation targets or the BIT behavioural subtest score.

The results on whether beneficial effects on neglect assessments persisted at follow-up were limited to four studies [5,8,23,35]. Three studies [5,23,35] on 52 participants showed a persisting effect favouring the experimental group −0.76 [−1.39, −0.13] $p = 0.02$ on cancellation number of errors. Only one B/C rated study [35] provided data on persisting effects on line bisection but these favoured the experimental group,

Review: Cognitive rehabilitation for spatial neglect following stroke - 2005 update temp title. (Version 06)
Comparison: 01 Cognitive rehabilitation versus any control: immediate effects
Outcome: 03 Cancellation - numbers of errors

Study or sub-category	N	Experimental Mean (SD)	N	Control Mean (SD)	Weight %	SMD (random) 95% CI
Cottam 1987	6	28.50 (28.20)	6	34.00 (10.80)	18.47	-0.24 [-1.38, 0.90]
Robertson 1990	17	43.40 (30.40)	13	43.20 (28.30)	28.66	0.01 [-0.72, 0.73]
Rossi 1990	18	2.40 (4.24)	21	9.80 (9.16)	30.20	-0.99 [-1.66, -0.32]
Wiart 1997	11	4.00 (4.00)	11	12.00 (7.00)	22.66	-1.35 [-2.29, -0.41]
Total (95% CI)	52		51		100.00	-0.65 [-1.28, -0.01]

Test for heterogeneity: Chi² = 6.78, df = 3 (P = 0.08), I² = 55.7%
Test for overall effect: Z = 2.00 (P = 0.05)

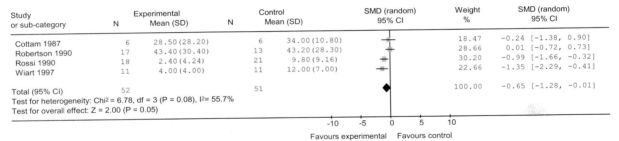

Fig. 2. Short-term effects of cognitive rehabilitation on letter cancellation.

Review: Cognitive rehabilitation for spatial neglect following stroke - 2005 update temp title. (Version 06)
Comparison: 01 Cognitive rehabilitation versus any control: immediate effects
Outcome: 04 Line bisection - error scores/right deviation

Study or sub-category	N	Experimental Mean (SD)	N	Control Mean (SD)	Weight %	SMD (random) 95% CI
Rossi 1990	18	0.68 (0.85)	21	2.20 (2.29)	40.48	-0.84 [-1.50, -0.18]
Wiart 1997	11	17.00 (14.00)	11	45.00 (25.00)	23.95	-1.33 [-2.27, -0.39]
Rusconi 2002	12	4.27 (8.94)	8	17.87 (18.90)	23.48	-0.95 [-1.90, 0.00]
Zeloni 2002	4	37.50 (35.20)	4	26.30 (22.25)	12.08	0.33 [-1.07, 1.74]
Total (95% CI)	45		44		100.00	-0.84 [-1.36, -0.33]

Test for heterogeneity: Chi² = 3.76, df = 3 (P = 0.29), I² = 20.1%
Test for overall effect: Z = 3.20 (P = 0.001)

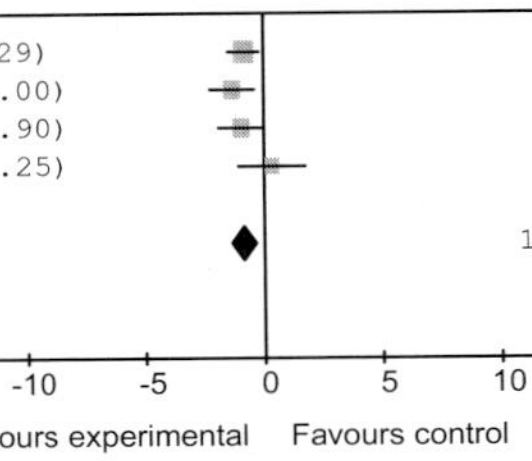

Fig. 3. Short-term effects of cognitive rehabilitation on line bisection.

-1.09 [-2.0, -0.18], $p = 0.02$. Two studies [8,23] of 31 participants did not find a persisting effect favouring the experimental group on the BIT behavioural subtest summary score $p = 0.87$.

4. Discussion

Randomisation to intervention and control groups is essential in research to evaluate the effects of treatment but fewer than half the trials identified used random allocation. Few RCTs specified the methods used for randomisation and few used adequate concealment. In addition, once carried out this was not always adhered to. The principle of randomisation is that it leaves the participants in the groups due to chance to prevent selection bias. Although post-randomisation changes to group membership may balance the groups on variables that can easily be identified (e.g. age, gender), it may introduce selection bias on other variables not measured. Similarly, matching defeats the purpose of randomisation. While groups may be similar on the variables used for matching, there may be selection bias on other characteristic not measured. Once groups are established it is important that a complete follow-up is attempted. The lack of information on attrition is important as an intervention that produces a high level of non-participation will not be generally effective and excluding these people from the analysis leads to a false positive result.

Several CCTs compared patients on different wards or hospitals. The disadvantage is that there may be systematic differences between groups independently of the treatment for neglect being offered, such as differences in admission and discharge policies, staff and in other components of the rehabilitation package. Such performance biases [12] may make evaluation of the intervention for neglect irrelevant. Allocation cannot be concealed when it is determined by ward/hospital admission. Researchers recruiting participants may be influenced if they know that the next patient will be a control or by knowledge of the intervention given to the last person.

Few trials reported blind assessment of outcome. Some attempted to reduce observer bias by including functional outcomes assessed by staff/carers. However it was unclear whether these were simply independent of the treatment being offered or were unaware of the treatment offered. Expectations are likely to differ if observers know a treatment has been given and this may bias results. It is rarely possible to conceal the intervention from the patient. However greater attempts could be made to deliver a sham or attention placebo intervention. These controls would correct for the novelty effect of new equipment and make others providing routine rehabilitation less aware of the intervention allocation of the participants.

Sample sizes were generally very small. Few studies mentioned conducting a power calculation to determine the sample size needed to detect a clinically significant difference between groups. Given the practical difficulties of conducting trials of rehabilitation for neglect, meta-analysis of several small studies provides an ideal opportunity to examine treatment effects in a larger group of participants. However the trials have to be appropriately designed before such analyses are warranted. Therefore we only included RCTs not CCTs in the updated Cochrane review and meta-analysis. We also conducted separate sensitivity analyses of only the A rated RCTs to examine whether those with B/C ratings inflate the effect size.

Studies generally provided good, detailed and comprehensive descriptions of baseline characteristics of participants. This would enable subgroups to be defined who benefited and who did not benefit from treatment, once the number of trials suitable for inclusion in meta – analysis becomes large enough. Individual patient meta-analysis is increasingly being used to define subgroups on the baseline characteristics and can detect treatment effects when individual studies are small [32].

Meta – analysis also requires that a common outcome is measured although the actual measurement tool used may vary between studies. Many used the Behavioural Inattention Test (BIT) [36] which does provide a common measure of both impairment (conventional tests) and a more ecologically relevant measure (behavioural subtests). Some trials also assessed outcomes on measures of functional abilities, such as the Barthel Index. However, scales developed specifically to assess the functional effects of neglect [1,31,39] may prove to be more sensitive. Since the aim of treatment of neglect is to improve rehabilitation outcomes, future trials must include measures of functional abilities. In the original Cochrane review [3] few trials included assessment of functional outcomes. In the 2005 update the proportion had increased but still only six of the 12 RCTs did so and only two assessed whether it persisted beyond the end of treatment. There needs to be a consensus about the 'best' measures and those designing trials need to include these in future in order to facilitate meta-analysis. For clinical purposes it is clearly essential that the benefits outlast the period of intervention, therefore outcomes need to be assessed after the end of treatment. Although this occurred, in some cases the time interval was inadequately short i.e. hours or days.

Overall the results suggest that cognitive rehabilitation shows promise and warrants robust investigation of clinical and cost effectiveness. A range of different rehabilitation interventions exist and although we do not yet have enough evidence to choose between them, we can say that collectively they improve outcome on some measures of impairment and some of these effects persisted after the end of intervention. There was no evidence to support or refute the effect of the interventions on independence in activities of daily living, either at the end of treatment or on follow-up, however this may be because previous studies have been too small and lacked the statistical power to show an impact on gross measures of disability. Improvements in the methodological quality of future trials are required and have been outlined in this paper.

Acknowledgements

We would like to thank Brenda Thomas and Clare Starmer for their help with literature searching and the study authors for providing unpublished data and answering queries on their papers.

References

[1] P. Azouvi, F. Marehal, C. Samuel et al., Functional consequences and awareness of unilateral neglect: Study of an evaluation scale, *Neuropsychological Rehabilitation* **6** (1996), 133–150.
[2] J.M. Beis, J.M. Andre, A. Baumgarten and B. Challier, Eye patching in unilateral spatial neglect: Efficacy of two methods, *Archives of Physical Medicine and Rehabilitation* **80** (1999), 71–76.
[3] A. Bowen, N.B. Lincoln and M. Dewey, *Cognitive rehabilitation for spatial neglect following stroke (Cochrane Review)*, In: The Cochrane Library, 2002; Issue 2. Oxford: Update Software.
[4] A. Bowen and R. Wenman, The rehabilitation of unilateral spatial neglect: a review of the evidence, *Reviews in Clinical Gerontology* **12** (2002), 357–373.
[5] L.R. Cherney, A.S. Halper and D. Papachronis, Two approaches to treating unilateral neglect after right hemisphere stroke: a preliminary investigation, *Topics in Stroke Rehabilitation* **9** (2003), 22–34.

[6] G. Cottam, *Visual scanning training for right hemisphere stroke patients exhibiting spatial neglect*, Dissertation. University of Mississippi, 1987.

[7] J.A. Edmans, J. Webster and N.B. Lincoln, A comparison of two approaches in the treatment of perceptual problems after stroke, *Clinical Rehabilitation* **14** (2000), 230–243.

[8] Y. Fanthome, N.B. Lincoln, A.E.R. Drummond and M.F. Walker, The treatment of visual neglect using feedback of eye movements: a pilot study, *Disability and Rehabilitation* **17** (1995), 413–417.

[9] F. Frassinetti, V. Angeli, F. Meneghello, S. Avanzi and E. Làdavas, Long-lasting amelioration of visuospatial neglect by prism adaptation, *Brain* **125** (2002), 608–623.

[10] W.A. Gordon, M.R. Hibbard, S. Egelko, L. Diller, M. Shaver, A. Lieberman and K. Ragnarsson, Perceptual remediation in patients with right brain damage: a comprehensive program, *Archives of Physical Medicine and Rehabilitation* **66** (1985), 353–359.

[11] M. Harvey, B. Hood, A. North and I.H. Robertson, The effects of visuomotor feedback training on the recovery of hemispatial neglect symptoms: assessment of a 2-week and follow-up intervention, *Neuropsychologia* **41** (2003), 886–893.

[12] J.P.T. Higgins and S. Green, Editors, Cochrane Handbook for Systematic Reviews of Interventions 4.2.5, http://www.cochrane.org/resources/handbook, 2005.

[13] L. Kalra, I. Perez, S. Gupta and M. Wittink, The influence of visual neglect on stroke rehabilitation, *Stroke* **28** (1997), 1386–1391.

[14] J. Loverro and M. Reding, Bed orientation and rehabilitation for patients with stroke and hemianopsia or visual neglect, *Journal of Neurological Rehabilitation* **2** (1988), 147–150.

[15] T. Manly, Cognitive rehabilitation for unilateral neglect: Review, *Neuropsychological Rehabilitation* **12** (2002), 289–310.

[16] D. Moher, K.F. Schulz and D.S.G. Altman for the CONSORT group, The CONSORT statement: revised recommendations for improving the quality of reports of parallel-group randomised trials, *Lancet* **357** (2001), 1191–1194.

[17] J.P. Neimeier, The lighthouse strategy: use of visual imagery to treat visual inattention in stroke patients, *Brain Injury* **12** (1998), 399–406.

[18] S. Paolucci, G. Antonucci, M.G. Grasso and L. Pizzamiglio, The role of unilateral spatial neglect in rehabilitation of right brain-damaged ischemic stroke patients: A matched comparison, *Archives of Physical Medicine and Rehabilitation* **82** (2001), 743–749.

[19] A. Parton, P. Malhotra and M. Husain, Hemispatial neglect, *J. Neurol. Neurosurg. Psychiatry* **75** (2004), 13–21.

[20] S.R. Pierce and L.J. Buxbaum, Treatments of unilateral neglect: A review, *Archives of Physical Medicine and Rehabilitation* **83** (2002), 256–268.

[21] L. Pizzamiglio, R. Frasca, C. Guariglia, C. Inoccia and G. Antonucci, Effect of optokinetic stimulation in patients with visual neglect, *Cortex* **26** (1990), 535–540.

[22] L. Pizzamiglio, L. Fasotti, M. Jehkonen, G. Antonucci, L. Magnotti, D. Boelen and S. Asa, The use of optokinetic stimulation in rehabilitation of the hemineglect disorder, *Cortex* **40** (2004), 441–450.

[23] I.H. Robertson, J.M. Gray, B. Pentland and L.J. Waite, Microcomputer-based rehabilitation for unilateral visual neglect: a randomised controlled trial, *Archives of Physical Medicine and Rehabilitation* **71** (1990), 663–668.

[24] I.H. Robertson, T.M. McMillan, E. McLeod, J. Edgeworth and D. Brock, Rehabilitation of unilateral neglect by limb activation: A randomised single blind controlled trial, *Neuropsychological Rehabilitation* **12** (2002), 439–454.

[25] Y. Rossetti, G. Rode, L. Pisella, A. Farné, L. Li, D. Boisson and M.-T. Perenin, Prism adaptation to a rightward optical deviation rehabilitates left hemispatial neglect, *Nature* **395** (1998), 166–169.

[26] P.W. Rossi, S. Kheyfets and M. Reding, Fresnel prisms improve visual perception in stroke patients with homonymous hemianopia or unilateral visual neglect, *Neurology* **40** (1990), 1597–1599.

[27] M.L. Rusconi, C. Meinecke, P. Sbrissa and B. Bernardini, Different cognitive trainings in the rehabilitation of visuospatial neglect, *Europa Medicophysica* **38** (2002), 159–166.

[28] I. Schindler, G. Kerkhoff, H.-O. Karnath, I. Keller and G. Goldenberg, Neck muscle vibration induces lasting recovery in spatial neglect, *Journal of Neurology, Neurosurgery and Psychiatry* **73** (2002), 412–419.

[29] P.C. Siemonsma and M.F. Walker, Practical guidelines for independent assessment in randomized controlled trials (RCTs) of rehabilitation, *Clinical Rehabilitation* **11** (1997), 273–279.

[30] K. Tham and R. Tegner, Video feedback in the rehabilitation of patients with unilateral neglect, *Archives of Physical Medicine and Rehabilitation* **78** (1997), 410–413.

[31] D. Towle and N.B. Lincoln, Development of a questionnaire for detecting everyday problems in stroke patients with unilateral visual neglect, *Clinical Rehabilitation* **5** (1996), 135–140.

[32] M.F. Walker, J. Leonardi-Bee, P. Bath, P. Langhorne, M. Dewey, S. Corr, A. Drummond, L. Gilbertson, J.R.F. Gladman, L. Jongbloed, P. Logan and C. Parker, Individual patient data meta-analysis of randomized controlled trials of community occupational therapy for stroke patients, *Stroke* **35** (2004), 2226–2232.

[33] J.S. Webster, P.T. McFarland, L.J. Rapport, B. Morrill, L.A. Roades and P.S. Abadee, Computer-assisted training for improving wheelchair mobility in unilateral neglect patients, *Archives of Physical Medicine and Rehabilitation* **82** (2001), 769–775.

[34] J. Weinberg, L. Diller, W.A. Gordon, L. Gerstman, A. Liebermann, P. Lakin, G. Hodges and O. Ezrachi, Visual scanning training effect on reading related tasks in acquired right brain damage, *Archives of Physical Medicine and Rehabilitation* **58** (1977), 479–486.

[35] L. Wiart, A. Bon Saint Come, X. Debelleix, H. Petit, P.A. Joseph, J.M. Mazaux and M. Barat, Unilateral neglect syndrome rehabilitation by trunk rotation and scanning training, *Archives of Physical Medicine and Rehabilitation* **78** (1997), 424–429.

[36] B.A. Wilson, J. Cockburn and P.W. Halligan, *Behavioural inattention test*, Bury St Edmunds: Thames Valley Test Company, 1987.

[37] G.C. Young, D. Collins and M. Hren, Effects of pairing scanning training with block design training in the remediation of perceptual problems in left hemiplegics, *Journal of Clinical Neuropsychology* **5** (1983), 201–212.

[38] G. Zeloni, A. Farnè and M. Baccini, Viewing less to see better *J Neurol, Neurosurg Psychaitry* **73** (2002), 195–198.

[39] P. Zoccolotti, G. Antonucci and A. Judica, Psychometric characteristics of two semi-structured scales for the functional evaluation of hemi-inattention in extra-personal and personal space, *Neuropsychological Rehabilitation* **2** (1992), 179–191.

Prism adaptation first among equals in alleviating left neglect: A review

Jacques Luauté[a,b,c,d,*], Peter Halligan[e], Gilles Rode[a,b,c,d], Sophie Jacquin-Courtois[a,b,c,d] and Dominique Boisson[a,b,c,d]

[a] *Hospices Civils de Lyon, Hôpital Henry Gabrielle, Service de Rééducation Neurologique, Saint Genis Laval, F-69230, France*
[b] *INSERM, U534, Espace et Action, Bron, F-69500, France*
[c] *Université Claude Bernard Lyon 1, Faculté de Médecine, Lyon, F-69000, France*
[d] *Institut Fédératif des Neurosciences de Lyon (IFNL), Hôpital Neurologique, Lyon, France*
[e] *School of Psychology, Cardiff University, Cardiff, UK*

Received 1 April 2006
Revised 13 June 2006
Accepted 22 June 2006

Abstract. *Purpose:* The current paper was designed to provide a critical overview on the different methods proposed for the rehabilitation of left spatial neglect.
Methods: On the basis of a previous systematic review of the literature, we analyzed all articles available aiming at reducing left spatial neglect which included a long term functional assessment.
Results: The aim of most early rehabilitation approaches, such as visuo-scanning training, was to re-orient visual scanning toward the neglected side. This review confirmed the utility of this method for rehabilitation purposes. More recent – theory driven – procedures, also based on a training approach, include limb activation, mental imagery training and video-feedback training. Although there is ground for optimism, the functional effectiveness of these methods still relies on few single-case studies. Newer methods have tried to stimulate automatic orientation of gaze or attention towards neglected space in a bottom-up fashion. Sensory stimulations can remove most of the classical signs of left neglect but their effects are short-lived. Such stimulations are not functionally relevant for rehabilitation except for trunk rotation or repeated neck muscle vibrations if they are associated with an extensive training program. A more promising intervention is prism adaptation given the growing evidence of relatively long-term functional gains from comparatively short term usage.
Conclusion: Overall, there is now evidence for several clinically relevant long-term benefits in the case of visual scanning training, mental imagery training, video feedback training, neck muscle vibration and trunk rotation if associated with visual scanning training and prism adaptation. However, the amount of evidence is still limited to a small number of relevant published articles and it is mandatory to continue the research in this field. In this review, the possible routes for new rehabilitation procedures are discussed on the basis of the actual knowledge regarding the neuro-cognitive mechanisms underlying the therapeutic effect of prism adaptation.

Keywords: Left neglect, stroke, rehabilitation, prism adaptation, review

1. Introduction

Patients with right cerebral hemisphere lesions often show a reduced tendency to respond to stimuli and to search actively for them in the left part of space [1].

---

*Corresponding author: Dr. Jacques Luauté, Hôpital Henry Gabrielle, 20, route de Vourles, 69230 Saint Genis-Laval, France. Fax: +33 4 78 86 50 30; E-mail: jacques.luaute@chu-lyon.fr.

This condition, described as left neglect, is frequently associated with contralesional motor or somato-sensory deficit. In addition, left neglect provides for poor motor and functional recovery [2–4]. Spatial neglect occurs in about 25–30% of all stroke patients [5] and for a high proportion of them, the disorder can be chronic [6]. For these reasons, left neglect represents a challenging problem for rehabilitation. It is not surprising that over the past 60 years, many different attempts to alleviate this impairment have been developed; but the question remains as to how effective these treatments are, given the heterogeneity of the population and spontaneous recovery. Furthermore, in a rehabilitation perspective, it is mandatory to take into account functional outcomes and the chronicity of the effect.

The purpose of this study was to analyze the current literature in order to provide a critical review of the methods available for the rehabilitation of left neglect. Twenty one articles [7–27] were selected on the base of a systematic search (for more details concerning the methodology see [28]). In the following section, the current evidence of the different methods analyzed in these articles is reported with regard to their clinical effectiveness. A summary of these data is provided in the Table 1. These results also give the opportunity to discuss the mechanisms by which such interventions may foster recovery with special emphasis on the putative neural mechanism by which prism adaptation modulate left spatial neglect.

1.1. Visual scanning training

In the early 1970's Diller and Co-workers investigated the use of various strategies to compensate for the right side deviation of the gaze [29]. The idea was to favour a re-orientation of visual scanning toward the neglected side by means of a top-down training program based on explicit instruction. From a practical point of view, the training programme was progressive, based on the principles of "anchoring, pacing, density and feedback". Anchors to the left was frequently ensured by visual cues such as a red line located in the left part of the page that the patient was asked to look at before beginning the exercise (e.g. [23]). In order to enhance visual exploration to the left, a scanning board was some times used (e.g. [27]).

Two randomized control trials showed (on the base of partial data) a long lasting improvement, over 6 months after the end of the procedure, on functional skills such as reading and writing [23,27]. In a single-case study with multiple baseline and follow-up assessments, Pizzamiglio et al. (1992) [12] showed evidence for the generalization of visuo-scanning training to other activities of daily living (utilizing commonly used object; description of figures, environment; serving tea; card sorting). Improvement of wheelchair navigation was shown by Webster et al. (1984) [22]. However, other authors claimed that a generalization to functional skills was not systematic unless the duration of the training program lasted more than a month and that the training material was very similar to the test material [30–32]. According to the studies analyzed in the current review, it seems that the beneficial effect was maintained after the rehabilitation terminated. However, only partial data were reported in these studies and it is also possible that training influenced the rate of learning compensatory strategies but not the final level of performances.

Collectively, there is now good evidence for the functional utility of this classical rehabilitation method, currently still used by many in occupational therapy.

1.2. Limb activation

In keeping with the results of Halligan et al. [33] and the need to make use of existing perceptual cues present on the left, Robertson and North [34] used the patient's own left arm as a cue to improve left neglect. Using single-case reports, latter studies showed that active left limb movements in the left hemi-space significantly reduced neglect, compared with no movement, movements performed with the right hand and movements of the left hand performed in the right hemi-space [35]. These results subsequently inspired the development of the limb activation rehabilitation technique. In clinical practice, the patient is required to initiate movements with his/her left paretic limb in the left part of the space. Robertson et al. [14] developed a specific apparatus to elicit limb activation: the Neglect Alert Device (NAD). This device emits a loud buzzing noise and a red light if the switch is not pressed within a predetermined time interval. The device is placed in the left part of the space and the patient is required to press the switch with his impaired left arm to turn off the buzzer during a variety of situations.

In our review two randomized control trials [11, 15] and four single-case studies with appropriate design [14,17,25,26] were analyzed. All the single-case studies showed that limb activation produced significant long term gains in several ADL areas such as reading, walking strategy, dressing, cleaning, feeding and meal preparation.

Results of the two RCT are less clear-cut in the sense that Robertson et al. (2002) [15], showed a significant improvement of motor functions in the group treated by limb activation but failed to show significant generalization on functional skills as assessed by 3 scales (Barthel index, Bergego's scale and the behavioural BIT). Kalra et al. (1997) [11] reported a significant reduction in median length of hospital stay (42 versus 66 days) in the group of patients receiving spatio-motor cueing and a trend toward Barthel Index improvement.

Altogether, single-case studies showed interesting results; however the functional effectiveness of limb activation still remains to be demonstrated in randomized controlled trials. It is possible that limb activation may be effective in some conditions but this could depends on the duration of the procedure and also depend on the version of limb activation employed (visuo-motor cueing, spatio-motor cueing or neglect alert device). It is also likely that limb activation is more conductive for some patients than others. Moreover, an important constraint that limits the use of this intervention for many stroke patients is the requirement that patients must have recovered minimal contralateral limb movement.

1.3. Mental imagery training

These techniques, currently used in sport competition, are directly inspired by the representational theory of left spatial neglect [36]. The purpose is to restore space representation by enhancing or training mental imagery through a top-down mechanism. In one single-case study, Smania et al. [19] used visual and movement imagery exercises to enhance left space representation [19]. In this study, improvement of the Zocolloti's semi-structured scale was reported in two patients. The effect persisted over 6 months after the end of the training.

The observation that the use of an elongated stick could produce a virtual extension of "body space" (presumably the result of remapping of far space as near space [37]) led to the development of a more specific technique: space remapping training. The principle here was to generalize the effect into and toward the neglected left space. Castiello et al. (2004) [38] used this method in a clinical trial in which patients with left neglect were instructed to reach and grasp a real object in right space while simultaneously observing the grasping of a virtual object by a virtual hand in the left space. Results of this study revealed significant improvement in grasping accuracy for the left side of the space following specific training. More studies are however needed to confirm these promising results.

1.4. Feedback training

Since left visuo-spatial neglect is often associated with anosognosia (lack of appropriate awareness for a neurological/neuropsychological deficit and also a recognized contributor of poor outcome), some researchers have suggested the need to alleviate anosognosia before an effective training procedure can be implemented [39]. In keeping with this hypothesis, specific feedback training procedures were developed involving a bottom-up mechanism to produce the feedback (i.e. aiming to restore self awareness) and a top-down mechanism to compensate for neglect behaviour.

Soderback et al. [20] video-recorded their 4 patients in order to provide a feedback of their neglect behaviour, in a cooking task, before employing a learning strategy in order to help patients to improve their performance [20]. In this single case-study, a long term beneficial effect was reported for the four patients. Tham et al. [21], administered a guided interview during which the patient's neglect behaviour was pointed out to him/to her in order to increase self-awareness [21]. After the training period, the four patients included in this study, improved their skills on a cooking task and on the motor and process skills (AMPS) scale. Like mental imagery training, these results need to be confirmed by larger series and if possible randomized controlled trials.

However, as argued by Harvey et al. (2003) [40], all these approaches require the patients to voluntary initiate and maintain attention to the left side, a demanding task in its own right and one that many patients find difficult to apply in everyday life.

1.5. Sensory stimulations

Other approaches to neglect rehabilitation involved the idea of enhancing automatic orientation toward the left space, without the requirement of language mediated attentive learning. Vestibular stimulation, optokinetic stimulation (OPK), neck muscle vibration (NMV), trunk rotation (TR) proved to alleviate most of the classic symptoms of left neglect (for a review see [41,42]). These effects provide clear evidence of how simple bottom-up mechanisms can overcome high level cognitive deficits. Hence it seems likely that these stimulations work by affecting the activity of cortical networks responsible for calibrating spatial coordinate's frames. Functional imaging studies in healthy subjects showing contralateral cortical activation after vestibular stimulation support this hypothesis [43].

Table 1
Studies designed to alleviate left neglect with long term functional outcome assessment

Articles' Ref.	Interventions	Design	Patients (n=)	Duration	Outcome	Results
Weinberg et al., 1977 [23]	VST	RCT	25	4 w	Reading; Copying	Improv > 1 yr*
Young et al., 1983 [27]	VST	RCT	18	4 w	Reading; Copying	Improv > 6 mth*
Pizzamiglio et al., 1992 [12]	VST	Single case MB	13	8 w	Reading; Zoccolotti	Improv > 5 mth*
Webster et al., 1984 [22]	VST	Single case MB	3	4 w	WC navig.	Improv > 1 yr
Worthington, 1996 [26]	LA	Single case MB	1	10 w	Reading	Improv > 18 mth
Kalra et al., 1997 [11]	LA	RCT	25	12 w	BI	No improv
					Hospital duration	Reduction
Robertson et al., 1998 [14]	LA (NAD)	Single case MB	1	18 d	Combing; Navig.; BTT	Improv > 9 d
Samuel et al., 2000 [17]	LA (SMc)	Single case MB	2	8 w	Bergego	Improv > 1 mth
Wilson et al., 2000 [25]	LA	Single case MB	1	10 d	Self care routines	Improv > 10 d
Robertson et al., 2002 [15]	LA	RCT	17	12 w	BI; Bergego; B-BIT	No improv
					motor function	Improv of motor function > 2 yr
Brunila et al., 2002 [7]	LA + VST	Single case MB	4	3 w	Reading	Improv > 3 w
Smania et al., 1997 [19]	Mental imagery	Single case MB	2	8 w	Zocolloti	Improv > 6 mth
Soderback et al., 1992 [20]	Feedback	Single case MB	4	26 d	Cooking task	Improv > 2 mth
Tham et al., 2001 [21]	Feedback	Single case MB	4	4 w	AMPS (reading, writing, cooking, garden); BTT	Improv > 9 w
Wiart et al., 1997 [24]	TR + VST	RCT	11	4 w	FIM	Improv > 1 mth*
Schindler et al., 2002 [18]	NMV + VST	Cross-over	10	3 w	Reading; personal care spatial orientation	Improv > 2 mth
Pizzamiglio et al. 2004 [13]	OPK	RCT	11	6 w	BI	No improv
Frassinetti et al., 2002 [9]	Prism adaptation	CT	7	2 w (10 sess)	Reading; B-BIT	Improv > 5 w
Farne et al., 2002 [8]	Prism adaptation	Single case MB	6	1 sess	Reading	Improv > 1 d
Jacquin-Courtois et al., In press [10]	Prism adaptation	Single case MB	1	1 sess	WC navig.	Improv > 96 h
Rode et al. In press by 2006 [16]	Prism adaptation	Single case MB	1	1 sess	Writing	Improv > 48 h

Footnotes and abbreviations:
Interventions: VST: Visual scanning training; *LA*: Limb activation; *SMc*: Spatio-motor cueing; *NAD:* Neglect alert device; *TR:* Trunk rotation; *NMV:* Neck muscle vibration; *OPK:* Optokinetic stimulation.

Design: RCT: Randomized control trial; *MB:* multiple baseline; *CT:* control trial.
Patients: n = number of patients in the experimental group.
Duration refers to the duration of the procedure: w : week(s); d : day(s); *sess:* session.
Outcome: B-BIT: Behavioural BIT [85]; *Zoccolotti:* Zoccolotti' semi structure scale [86]; *WC navig.:* Wheelchair navigation; *BI:* Barthel index [87]; *Bergego:* Bergego's functional scale [88]; *FIM:* functional independence measure [89]; *BTT:* Baking tray task; *AMPS:* Assessment of motor and process skills [90].
Results: Improv: Improvement; *yr:* year; *mth:* month(s); *w* : week(s); *d* : day(s); *h* : hour(s). *: partial data.
Circulatory diagrams with two types of segmentations: vertical segmentation for the different functional topics (Roman numbers) and horizontal segmentation for the levels of evidence (Arabian numbers):

Functional topics:

N°	Functional outcomes	N°	Functional outcomes
I	Spatial orientation	XIV	Problem solving
II	Feeding	XV	Memory
III	Dressing	XVI	Utilising commonly used object
IV	Grooming	XVII	Description of figures, environment
V	Cleaning	XVIII	Serving tea
VI	Transfers	XIX	Card sorting
VII	Posture	XX	Map navigation
VIII	Walking strategy	XXI	Picture scanning
IX	Stairs climbing	XXII	Sentence copying
X	Wheelchair navigation	XXIII	Reading and setting time
XI	Reading	XXIV	Telephone dialling
XII	Writing	XXV	Handling money
XIII	Social interaction	XXVI	Cooking

I–V: Bergego's functional scale.
II–IX: Barthel index.
II–XV: Functional independence measure
XVI–XIX: Zocollotti semi-structured scale
XX–XXV: Behavioural BIT
▓ Improvement
▒ No improvement

Arabian numbers: levels of evidence adapted from Ball et al. (2001) [91]:
1: level 1 (randomized control trial).
2–3: level 2 (cohort studies) and level 3 (case-control, cross-over and single-case studies with multiple base line assessment).
4: level 4 (other types of studies).

However, the remediation is usually short-lived and thus is not functionally relevant for rehabilitation. A sustained functional gain was only found in two studies: (i) Wiart et al. (1997) [24], found (on the base of partial data issued from a randomized control trial) a long term (>1 month) functional improvement on the functional independence measure (FIM) after a training programme combining trunk rotation and visual scanning solicitation (ii) Schindler et al. (2002) [18] reported, in a cross-over trial, a long-lasting improvement of reading, personal care and spatial orientation using a combined treatment – repeated neck muscle vibration stimulations and visual exploration training – compared with the standard treatment (only visual exploration training). The association of a standard visual scanning training and OPK stimulation was also followed by a beneficial effect [13]; however, the group comparison showed that OPK did not provide additional effect. Altogether, the combination of trunk rotation with visual scanning training or repeated NMV with visual scanning training appears to facilitate the recovery of patients with left neglect.

1.6. Prism adaptation

Recently, a promising intervention – prism adaptation – was described by Rossetti et al. (1998) [44]. This took advantage of the effect of the well known phenomenon of visuo-motor adaptation. Prism adaptation has been widely used since the end of the nineteenth century as a paradigm to demonstrate visuo-motor short-term plasticity [45]. Exposure to prisms produces a lateral shift of the visual field so that the visual target appears at a displaced position. Adaptation to such an optical induced shift critically requires a set of successive perceptual-motor pointing movements. While the initial movements tend to approximate to the virtual position of the target, subsequent pointing movements ensure that the pointing error rapidly decreases so that subjects can readily point towards the real target position [46]. This initial error reduction comprises a "strategic component" of the reaction to prisms and does not necessarily produce adaptation at this stage [47]. To obtain robust compensatory aftereffects, following removal of prisms, further pointing movements are required. These reinforce the sensory motor adaptation and are considered characteristic of the "real or true" adaptive component of the adaptation [48]. The after-effects result from a compensatory shift in manual straight-ahead pointing in a direction opposite to the original visual shift produced by prisms. Rossetti et al. [44] proposed that right prism adaptation with leftward negative after-effects (using the intact right hand) improved left neglect symptoms. A significant reduction of left neglect was demonstrated across a variety of different standard tests following a brief period (3–5 minutes) of prism adaptation [44].

There are now several articles that showed a long-lasting generalization of the effect across different measures including wheelchair navigation [10], reading [8] and spatial dysgraphia [16] after a single prism adaptation session. Furthermore, a long-lasting amelioration using the behavioural measures of the BIT was reported following a twice-daily adaptation program during a period of two weeks [9].

Hence, although relatively new, prism adaptation is an exciting method which has shown relatively long-term functional gains from comparatively short-term usage. To clearly establish the functional benefits of prism adaptation, a large-scale RCT is currently in progress.

2. Discussion and conclusion

Overall, there is now growing evidence for several clinically relevant long term benefits (4–6 weeks) for a number of treatment methods currently available. These include visual scanning training (VST), limb activation, mental imagery training, feedback training, neck muscle vibration (NMV) and Trunk rotation – if associated with VST – and prism adaptation.

From a theoretical point of view, these results give the opportunity to discuss rehabilitation-induced plastic reorganization of lesioned brain system. As previously argued, conventional methods, such as VST and feedback training, are essentially based on a top-down approach involving attentional and language processes spared by the lesion. Mental imagery training also involves the training of high level functions but in this case, the idea is to restore the impaired cognitive function. Hence, according to the model proposed by Code (2001) [49], VST and feedback training would be considered as involving a behavioural and cognitive compensatory mechanism whereas mental imagery training would be considered as involving a cognitive restorative mechanism.

The rationale underlying Limb activation is based on activating a poorly attended body schema by making voluntary initiated contra-lesional limb movements in the left side of the space which in turn activates corresponding areas of extra-personal space [50]. More generally, it can be hypothesized that rehabilitation techniques which stimulate neural circuits non-impaired but functionally connected with the lesion might favour recovery. Indeed, neuro-plasticity following brain damage could share common mechanisms with normal Hebbian learning mechanisms [51]. In this Hebbian learning connectionist model, it is argued that strengthening of synaptic connections occurs when pre and post-synaptic neurons are coactive: "cells that fire together, wire together". Limb activation also seems to take advantage of an inter-hemispheric inhibitory process given that Robertson and North (1994) [52] showed that the beneficial effects of single left limb activation in left hemi-space could be eliminated if the right limb was simultaneously moved.

Sensory stimulations can temporarily remediate hemi-spatial neglect, including the most cognitive aspects of this condition, which provide clear evidence for a bottom-up mechanism. These interventions are also characterized by their specific directional effect both in terms of the side of the stimulation and also in terms of the side of the brain affected by the stimulation. Hence, sensory stimulations probably modulate lateralized spatial cognition processes via a bottom-up mechanism [41]. However, a functional gain was reported only when lateralized neck muscle vibration and lateralized trunk rotation were associated with classical VST [18,24]. These results tend to confirm the hypothesis proposed by Husain and Rorden [53] that it might be noteworthy to combine an intervention based on non-lateralized attentional processes and a lateralized stimulation.

Concerning prism adaptation, the specificity of the effect on left spatial neglect has been investigated in two experiments (unpublished work) [54]. In the first one, five stroke patients with left neglect were exposed to **left** prisms in order to assess the lateral specificity of prism adaptation. A battery of five neuropsychological tests (line bisection, line cancellation, figure copying, drawing a daisy from memory and a reading task) were performed before, immediately after adaptation and 2 hours later. Analysis of variance (ANOVA) was performed to compare the mean score of the 5 patients, on each neuropsychological test, across sessions. Contrary to right prism adaptation, no significant effect was observed after a single session of left prism adaptation. Hence this experiment favours a specific effect of prism adaptation on left spatial neglect in terms of the direction of prisms: only right prisms can improve neglect. Interestingly, the cognitive effects of prism, in non-brain damaged subjects, are also supported by an asymmetrical pattern of performance on line bisection judgment tasks, depending on the direction of prisms [55, 56]. Contrary to right brain damaged patients with left neglect, only adaptation to left-deviating prisms induced a rightward bias in normals. These asymmetric results may reflect the inherent asymmetry of the brain's structural organisation related to space cognition. On the bases of these latter studies and considering that the right parietal cortex seems to be specifically involved in line bisection judgment tasks [57,58], it could be hypothesized that the right parietal lobe would be critically sensitive to prism adaptation at least for those tasks involving explicit linear judgements [56].

In the second experiment, we searched if the therapeutic effect of this technique could rely on the error signal generated by the first pointing movements performed through prisms. Five different patients with left neglect following stroke performed a series of 50 pointing movements toward visual targets whose locations was shifted to the right (10°) immediately after the onset of movement, thus reproducing the error signal produced by prismatic goggles that produce a 10° rightward shift of the visual wide-field (cf. [44]). Experimental paradigm, neuropsychological tests and statistical analysis were comparable to the first experiment. Results showed no significant difference between sessions, which argues against a role of error signal and support the hypothesis that only **adaptation** to rightward prisms – i.e. visuo-motor realignment – can ameliorate left spatial neglect.

Improvement of numerous neglect-related manifestations such as visual exploration toward the left hemispace [59], postural balance [60], contralesional somato-sensory perception [61–63], temporal order judgment [64], visuo-verbal tasks [8], mental representation [65–67] as well as the generalization to functional tasks [8–10,16], suggest that this low-level sensory-motor intervention modulates cortical areas in a bottom-up fashion [68].

The neural substrate underlying the therapeutic effect of this method remains to be fully elucidated. One possibility is that prism adaptation reduces left spatial neglect by facilitating the recruitment of intact brain areas responsible for controlling normal visuo-spatial output by way of short-term sensori-motor plasticity. Such an account would predict the implication of at least three brain structures: (i) the cerebellum which is known to be implicated in visually directed movements [69] and eye-hand coordination [70]. The involvement of the cerebellum is also supported by lesion-studies in both monkey [71] and man [48,72,73]. (ii) The posterior parietal cortex (PPC) is also clearly implicated in sensori-motor and multi-sensory integration [74]. Moreover, the only functional imaging study using prism adaptation in normal subjects showed that the PPC, contralateral to the hand used for adaptation was clearly activated [75]. It should be noted that in this latter study, the optical deviation was reversed (left to right) every five trials to maintain the subject in a state of on-going adaptation. This suggests that the PPC probably participates in the "strategic corrections" after visuo-motor transformation induced by prisms but not necessarily in sensori-motor realignment. Pisella et al., (2004) [76] recently confirmed this hypothesis by showing that a patient with a bilateral parietal region was fully able to adapt to an optical deviation. (iii) Finally, the ventral pre-motor cortex (PMv) seems also to be involved in short-term sensori-motor plasticity. It has been shown in monkeys that this region plays an important role in visually guided movements [77] and in spatial visual information processing [78]. Furthermore, Kurata and Hoshi (1999) [79] showed that the monkeys loose their ability to adapt to wedge prisms after muscimol injection into the PMv.

However, as indicated by Danckert and Ferber [80], the gap might be important between what we know about sensori-motor plasticity in normal subjects and what happens in brain damaged neglect patients. In a recent functional imaging study, we investigated the anatomical substrates underlying the beneficial effect of prism adaptation in five patients with left spatial neglect following right stroke [81]. We used a co-variation analysis to examine linear changes over sessions as a function of neglect improvement. The network of significant brain regions associated with improvement of left neglect performance produced by prism adaptation included the right cerebellum, left thalamus, left temporal cortex, right frontal cortex and right parietal cortex. These results suggest that prism adaptation actively modulates cerebral areas implicated in visuo-motor plasticity albeit now relying on intact cerebello-cerebral connections. This study also highlighted a potential role for the temporal cortex in neglect improvement after prism adaptation. This was not expected but the recent implication of this region in spatial cognition could explain this activation. Indeed, it has been recently shown that the right temporal lobe is damaged significantly more often in patients with left neglect than in patients with right brain damage without neglect [82]. Moreover, recovery of spatial deficit attention seems to depend on the reactivation of this region [83].

These results also illustrate the complexity to investigate how a given intervention can modulate brain plasticity in the domain of neurological rehabilitation. From the perspective of functional imaging techniques, plasticity can be defined as the reorganization of distributed brain activity that accompanies an intervention. Hence, the first step is to know the neural network associated with this intervention in normal subjects. Then, in these intervention studies, the post effect session is by definition the second session. Therefore an order effect cannot be ruled out in a classical factorial design comparing brain activity before and after the intervention. To get around this irrelevant order effect, a covariation analysis has to be performed to search for specific brain areas associated with the beneficial effect of the intervention. Finally, spontaneous recovery must be taken into account by appropriate designs using for instance multiple baseline assessment of the condition.

The combined knowledge of brain lesion location and the network of brain areas activated by an intervention could serve to choose more appropriately rehabilitation techniques for a given patient. Moreover, these informations could serve to enhance the recovery of spatial neglect by "theory-driven" combination of several interventions. Following this idea, the combination of a classical VST program and prism adaptation could represent a good example given that the first one is a top down intervention involving language and memory processes whereas the other is a bottom-up intervention involving sensory-motor plasticity. Alternatively, it is possible that combining two methods which share a common network of activation enhances the beneficial effect. The association of prism adaptation and limb activation is in line with this hypothesis. Indeed, both methods depend on active motor procedures and highlight the role of action in neglect rehabilitation [84].

References

[1] E. Bisiach, Unilateral neglect and related disorders, in: *Handbook of Clinical and Experimental Neuropsychology*, F. Denes and L. Pizzamiglio, eds, Hove: Psychology Press, 1999.

[2] D. Boisson and A. Vighetto, La négligence spatiale. De l'évaluation clinique aux possibilités thérapeutiques, *Ann Réadapt Méd Phys* **32** (1989), 539–562.

[3] G. Denes, C. Semenza, E. Stoppa and A. Lis, Unilateral spatial neglect and recovery from hemiplegia: a follow-up study, *Brain* **105** (1982), 543–552.

[4] M. Jehkonen, J.P. Ahonen, P. Dastidar, A.M. Koivisto, P. Laippala, J. Vilkki and G. Molnar, Visual neglect as a predictor of functional outcome one year after stroke, *Acta Neurol Scand* **101** (2000), 195–201.

[5] P. Appelros, G.M. Karlsson, A. Seiger and I. Nydevik, Neglect and anosognosia after first-ever stroke: incidence and relationship to disability, *J Rehabil Med* **34** (2002), 215–220.

[6] H. Samuelsson, C. Jensen, S. Ekholm, H. Naver and C. Blomstrand, Anatomical and neurological correlates of acute and chronic visuospatial neglect following right hemisphere stroke, *Cortex* **33** (1997), 271–285.

[7] T. Brunila, N. Lincoln, A. Lindell, O. Tenovuo and H. Hämäläinen, Experiences of combined visual training and arm activation in the rehabilitation of unilateral visual neglect: A clinical study, *Neuropsychological-rehabilitation* **12** (2002), 27–40.

[8] A. Farne, Y. Rossetti, S. Toniolo and E. Ladavas, Ameliorating neglect with prism adaptation: visuo-manual and visuo-verbal measures, *Neuropsychologia* **40** (2002), 718–729.

[9] F. Frassinetti, V. Angeli, F. Meneghello, S. Avanzi and E. Ladavas, Long-lasting amelioration of visuospatial neglect by prism adaptation, *Brain* **125** (2002), 608–623.

[10] S. Jacquin-Courtois, G. Rode, D. Boisson and Y. Rossetti, Wheel-chair driving improvement following visuo-manual prism adaptation, *Cortex*, in press, (2006).

[11] L. Kalra, I. Perez, S. Gupta and M. Wittink, The influence of visual neglect on stroke rehabilitation, *Stroke* **28** (1997) 1386–1391.

[12] L. Pizzamiglio, G. Antonucci, A. Judica, P. Montenero, C. Razzano and P. Zoccolotti, Cognitive rehabilitation of the hemineglect disorder in chronic patients with unilateral right brain damage, *J Clin Exp Neuropsychol* **14** (1992), 901–923.

[13] L. Pizzamiglio, L. Fasotti, M. Jehkonen, G. Antonucci, L. Magnotti, D. Boelen and S. Asa, The use of optokinetic stimulation in rehabilitation of the hemineglect disorder, *Cortex* **40** (2004), 441–450.

[14] I.H. Robertson, K. Hogg and T.M. Mac Millan, Rehabilitation of Unilateral Neglect: Improving Function by Contralesional Limb Activation, *Neuropsychological Rehabilitation* **8** (1998), 19–29.

[15] I.H. Robertson, T.M. Mac Millan, E. Mac Leod, J. Edgeworth and D. Brock, Rehabilitation by limb activation training reduces left-sided motor impairment in unilateral neglect patients: A single-blind randomised control trial, *Neuropsychological Rehabilitation* **12** (2002), 439–454.

[16] G. Rode, L. Pisella, L. Marsal, S. Mercier, Y. Rossetti and D. Boisson, Prism Adaptation Improves Spatial Dysgraphia Following Right Brain Damage, *Neuropsychologia* **44** (2006), 2427–2433.

[17] C. Samuel, A. Louis-Dreyfus, R. Kaschel, E. Makiela, M. Troubat, N. Anselmi, V. Cannizzo and P. Azouvi, Rehabilitation of very severe unilateral neglect by visuo-spatio-motor cueing: Two single case studies, *Neuropschological Rehabilitation* **10** (2000), 385–399.

[18] I. Schindler, G. Kerkhoff, H.O. Karnath, I. Keller and G. Goldenberg, Neck muscle vibration induces lasting recovery in spatial neglect, *J Neurol Neurosurg Psychiatry* **73** (2002), 412–419.

[19] N. Smania, F. Bazoli, D. Piva and G. Guidetti, Visuomotor imagery and rehabilitation of neglect, *Arch Phys Med Rehabil* **78** (1997), 430–436.

[20] I. Soderback, I. Bengtsson, E. Ginsburg and J. Ekholm, Video feedback in occupational therapy: its effects in patients with neglect syndrome, *Arch Phys Med Rehabil* **73** (1992), 1140–1146.

[21] K. Tham, E. Ginsburg, A.G. Fisher and R. Tegner, Training to improve awareness of disabilities in clients with unilateral neglect, *Am J Occup Ther* **55** (2001), 46–54.

[22] J.S. Webster, S. Jones, P. Blanton, R. Gross, G.F. Beissel and J. Wofford, Visual Scaning Training With Stroke Patients, *Behavior Therapy* **15** (1984), 129–143.

[23] J. Weinberg, L. Diller, W.A. Gordon, L.J. Gerstman, A. Lieberman, P. Lakin, G. Hodges and O. Ezrachi, Visual scanning training effect on reading-related tasks in acquired right brain damage, *Arch Phys Med Rehabil* **58** (1977), 479–486.

[24] L. Wiart, A.B. Come, X. Debelleix, H. Petit, P.A. Joseph, J.M. Mazaux and M. Barat, Unilateral neglect syndrome rehabilitation by trunk rotation and scanning training, *Arch Phys Med Rehabil* **78** (1997), 424–429.

[25] F.C. Wilson, T. Manly, D. Coyle and I.H. Robertson, The effect of contralesional limb activation training and sustained attention training for self-care programmes in unilateral spatial neglect, *Restor Neurol Neurosci* **16** (2000), 1–4.

[26] A.D. Worthington, Cueing Strategies in Neglect Dyslexia, *Neuropschological Rehabilitation* **6** (1996), 1–17.

[27] G.C. Young, D. Collins and M. Hren, Effect of pairing scanning training with block design training in the remediation of perceptual problems in left hemiplegics, *J Clin Neuropsychol* **5** (1983), 201–212.

[28] J. Luauté, P. Halligan, Y. Rossetti, G. Rode and D. Boisson, Visuo-spatial Neglect; a systematic review of current interventions and their effectiveness, *Neuroscience and Biobehavioral Reviews*, in press, (2006).

[29] L. Diller and J. Weinberg, Hemi-Inattention in Rehabilitation: The Evolution of a Rational Remediation Program (Weinstein Edn). Raven Press, New York, 1977, 63–82.

[30] W.D. Gouvier, B. Bua, P. Blanton and J. Urey, Behavioral changes following visual scaninng training: observation of five cases, *J Clin Exp Neuropsychol* **9** (1987), 74–80.

[31] R.C. Wagenaar, P.C. Van Wieringen, J.B. Netelenbos, O.G. Meijer and D.J. Kuik, The transfer of scanning training effects in visual inattention after stroke: five single-case studies, *Disabil Rehabil* **14** (1992), 51–60.

[32] Y. Fanthome, N.B. Lincoln, A. Drummond and M.F. Walker, The treatment of visual neglect using feedback of eye movements: a pilot study, *Disabil Rehabil* **17** (1995), 413–417.

[33] P.W. Halligan, L. Manning and J.C. Marshall, Hemispheric activation vs spatio-motor cueing in visual neglect: a case study, *Neuropsychologia* **29** (1991), 165–176.

[34] I.H. Robertson and N.T. North, Spatiomotor cueing in unilateral neglect: the role of hemispace, hand and motor activation, *Neuropsychologia* **30** (1992), 553–563.

[35] I.H. Robertson, N.T. North and C. Geggie, Spatiomotor cueing in unilateral left neglect: three case studies of its therapeutic effect, *J Neurol Neurosurg Psychiatry* **55** (1992), 799–805.

[36] E. Bisiach, C. Luzzatti and D. Perani, Unilateral neglect, representational schema and consciousness, *Brain* **102** (1979), 609–618.

[37] A. Farne and E. Ladavas, Dynamic size-change of hand peripersonal space following tool use, *Neuroreport* **11** (2000), 1645–1649.

[38] U. Castiello, D. Lusher, C. Burton, S. Glover and P. Disler, Improving left hemispatial neglect using virtual reality, *Neurology* **62** (2004), 1958–1962.

[39] S.M. McGlynn and D.L. Schacter, Unawareness of deficits in neuropsychological syndromes, *J Clin Exp Neuropsychol* **11** (1989), 143–205.

[40] M. Harvey, B. Hood, A. North and I.H. Robertson, The effects of visuomotor feedback training on the recovery of hemispatial neglect symptoms: assessment of a 2-week and follow-up intervention, *Neuropsychologia* **41** (2003), 886–893.

[41] G. Vallar, C. Guariglia and M.L. Rusconi, Modulation of the Neglect Syndrome by Sensory Stimulation. In Parietal Lobe Contributions to Orientation in 3D space Springer, 1997.

[42] Y. Rossetti and G. Rode, Reducing spatial neglect by visual and other sensory manipulations: non-cognitive (physiological) routes to the rehabilitation of a cognitive disorder, in: *The cognitive and neural bases of spatial neglect*, H.O. Karnath, A.D. Milner and G. Vallar, eds, 2002.

[43] O. Fasold, M. von Brevern, M. Kuhberg, C.J. Ploner, A. Villringer, T. Lempert and R. Wenzel, Human vestibular cortex as identified with caloric stimulation in functional magnetic resonance imaging, *Neuroimage* **17** (2002), 1384–1393.

[44] Y. Rossetti, G. Rode, L. Pisella, A. Farne, L. Li, D. Boisson and M.T. Perenin, Prism adaptation to a rightward optical deviation rehabilitates left hemispatial neglect, *Nature* **395** (1998), 166–169.

[45] G.M. Redding, Y. Rossetti and B. Wallace, Applications of Prism Adaptation: A Tutorial in Theory and Method, *Neuroscience and Biobehavioral Reviews* **29** (2005), 431–444.

[46] Y. Rossetti, K. Koga and T. Mano, Prismatic displacement of vision induces transient changes in the timing of eye-hand coordination, *Percept Psychophys* **54** (1993), 355–364.

[47] G. M. Redding and B. Wallace, Adaptive spatial alignment and strategic perceptual-motor control, *J Exp Psychol Hum Percept Perform* **22** (1996), 379–394.

[48] M.J. Weiner, M. Hallett and H.H. Funkenstein, Adaptation to lateral displacement of vision in patients with lesions of the central nervous system, *Neurology* **33** (1983), 766–772.

[49] C. Code, Multifactorial processes in recovery from aphasia: developing the foundations for a multileveled framework, *Brain Lang* **77** (2001), 25–44.

[50] I.H. Robertson and N.T. North, Active and passive stimulation of left limbs: influence on visual and sensory neglect, *Neuropsychologia* **31** (1993), 293–300.

[51] I.H. Robertson and J.M. Murre, Rehabilitation of brain damage: brain plasticity and principles of guided recovery, *Psychol Bull* **125** (1999), 544–575.

[52] I.H. Robertson and N.T. North, One hand is better than two: motor extinction of left hand advantage in unilateral neglect, *Neuropsychologia* **32** (1994), 1–11.

[53] M. Husain and C. Rorden, Non-spatially lateralized mechanisms in hemispatial neglect, *Nat Rev Neurosci* **4** (2003), 26–36.

[54] J. Luaute, S. Jacquin-Courtois, G. Rode, Y. Rossetti, and D. Boisson, Amélioration de l'héminégligence après adaptation prismatique: effet consécutif à l'erreur de signal et/ou à la plasticité cérébrale? Société de Neuropsychologie de Langue Française.Paris, *Oral communication* (1999).

[55] C. Colent, L. Pisella, C. Bernieri, G. Rode and Y. Rossetti, Cognitive bias induced by visuo-motor adaptation to prisms: a simulation of unilateral neglect in normal individuals? *Neuroreport* **11** (2000), 1899–1902.

[56] C. Michel, L. Pisella, P.W. Halligan, J. Luauté, G. Rode and Y. Rossetti, Simulating unilateral neglect using prism adaptation: Implication for theory, *Neuropsychologia* **41** (2003), 25–39.

[57] B. Fierro, F. Brighina, M. Oliveri, A. Piazza, B. La, V.D. Buffa and E. Bisiach, Contralateral neglect induced by right posterior parietal rTMS in healthy subjects, *Neuroreport* **11** (2000), 1519–1521.

[58] G.R. Fink, J.C. Marshall, N.J. Shah, P.H. Weiss, P.W. Halligan, M. Grosse-Ruyken, K. Ziemons, K. Zilles and H.J. Freund, Line bisection judgments implicate right parietal cortex and cerebellum as assessed by fMRI, *Neurology* **54** (2000), 1324–1331.

[59] S. Ferber, J. Danckert, M. Joanisse, H.C. Goltz and M.A. Goodale, Eye movements tell only half the story, *Neurology* **60** (2003), 1826–1829.

[60] C. Tilikete, G. Rode, Y. Rossetti, J. Pichon, L. Li and D. Boisson, Prism adaptation to rightward optical deviation improves postural imbalance in left-hemiparetic patients, *Curr Biol* **11** (2001), 524–528.

[61] R.D. McIntosh, Y. Rossetti and A.D. Milner, Prism adaptation improves chronic visual and haptic neglect: a single case study, *Cortex* **38** (2002), 309–320.

[62] A. Maravita, J. McNeil, P. Malhotra, R. Greenwood, M. Husain and J. Driver, Prism adaptation can improve contralesional tactile perception in neglect, *Neurology* **60** (2003), 1829–1831.

[63] H.C. Dijkerman, M. Webeling, J.M. ter Wal, E. Groet and M.J. Van Zandvoort, A long-lasting improvement of somatosensory function after prism adaptation, a case study, *Neuropsychologia* **42** (2004), 1697–1702.

[64] N. Berberovic, L. Pisella, A.P. Morris and J.B. Mattingley, Prismatic adaptation reduces biased temporal order judgements in spatial neglect, *Neuroreport* **15** (2004), 1199–1204.

[65] G. Rode, Y. Rossetti, L. Li and D. Boisson, Improvement of mental imagery after prism exposure in neglect: a case study, *Behav Neurol* **11** (1998), 251–258.

[66] G. Rode, Y. Rossetti and D. Boisson, Prism adaptation improves representational neglect, *Neuropsychologia* **39** (2001), 1250–1254.

[67] Y. Rossetti, Jacquin-Courtois, G. Rode, H. Ota, C. Michel and D. Boisson, Does action make the link between number and space representation? Visuo-manual adaptation improves number bisection in unilateral neglect, *Psychol Sci* **15** (2004), 426–430.

[68] G. Rode, L. Pisella, Y. Rossetti, A. Farne and D. Boisson, Bottom-up transfer of sensory-motor plasticity to recovery of spatial cognition: visuomotor adaptation and spatial neglect, *Prog Brain Res* **142** (2003), 273–287.

[69] J.F. Stein, Role of the cerebellum in the visual guidance of movement, *Nature* **323** (1986), 217–221.

[70] R.C. Miall, H. Imamizu and S. Miyauchi, Activation of the cerebellum in co-ordinated eye and hand tracking movements: an fMRI study, *Exp Brain Res* **135** (2000), 22–33.

[71] J.S. Baizer, I. Kralj-Hans and M. Glickstein, Cerebellar lesions and prism adaptation in macaque monkeys, *J Neurophysiol* **81** (1999), 1960–1965.

[72] T.A. Martin, J.G. Keating, H.P. Goodkin, A.J. Bastian and W.T. Thach, Throwing while looking through prisms. I. Focal olivocerebellar lesions impair adaptation, *Brain* **119** (1996), 1183–1198.

[73] L. Pisella, Y. Rossetti, C. Michel, G. Rode, D. Boisson, D. Pélisson and C. Tilikete, Ipsidirectional impairment of prism adaptation after unilateral lesion of anterior cerebellum, *Neurology* **12** (2005), 150–152.

[74] J. Xing and R.A. Andersen, Models of the posterior parietal cortex which perform multimodal integration and represent space in several coordinate frames, *J Cogn Neurosci* **12** (2000), 601–614.

[75] D.M. Clower, J.M. Hoffman, J.R. Votaw, T.L. Faber, R.P. Woods and G.E. Alexander, Role of posterior parietal cortex in the recalibration of visually guided reaching, *Nature* **383** (1996), 618–621.

[76] L. Pisella, C. Michel, H. Grea, C. Tilikete, A. Vighetto and Y. Rossetti, Preserved prism adaptation in bilateral optic ataxia: strategic versus adaptive reaction to prisms, *Exp Brain Res* **156** (2004), 399–408.

[77] H. Mushiake, Y. Tanatsugu and J. Tanji, Neuronal activity in the ventral part of premotor cortex during target-reach movement is modulated by direction of gaze, *J Neurophysiol* **78** (1997), 567–571.

[78] M.S. Graziano, X.T. Hu and C.G. Gross, Visuospatial properties of ventral premotor cortex, *J Neurophysiol* **77** (1997), 2268–2292.

[79] K. Kurata and E. Hoshi, Reacquisition deficits in prism adaptation after muscimol microinjection into the ventral premotor cortex of monkeys, *J Neurophysiol* **81** (1999), 1927–1938.

[80] J. Danckert and S. Ferber, Revisiting unilateral neglect, *Neuropsychologia* **44** (2006), 987–1006.

[81] J. Luauté, C. Michel, G. Rode, L. Pisella, S. Jacquin-Courtois, N. Costes, F. Cotton, D. LeBars, D. Boisson, P. Halligan and Y. Rossetti, Functional anatomy of the therapeutic effects of prism adaptation on left neglect, *Neurology* **66** (2006), 1859–1867.

[82] H.O. Karnath, B.M. Fruhmann, W. Kuker and C. Rorden, The Anatomy of Spatial Neglect based on Voxelwise Statistical Analysis: A Study of 140 Patients, *Cereb Cortex* **14** (2004), 1164–1172.

[83] M. Corbetta, M.J. Kincade, C. Lewis, A.Z. Snyder and A. Sapir, Neural basis and recovery of spatial attention deficits in spatial neglect, *Nat Neurosci* **8** (2005), 1603–1610.

[84] G. Rode, Y. Rossetti, M. Badan and D. Boisson, Role of rehabilitation in hemineglect syndromes, *Rev Neurol* **157** (2001), 497–505.

[85] B. Wilson, J. Cockburn and P. Halligan, Development of a behavioral test of visuospatial neglect, *Arch Phys Med Rehabil* **68** (1987), 98–102.

[86] P. Zoccolotti, G. Antonucci and A. Judica, Psychometric characteristics of two semi-structured scales for the functional evaluation of hemi-inattention in extra-personal and personal space, *Neurpsychological Rehabilitation* **2** (1992), 179–191.

[87] F.I. Mahoney and D.W. Barthel, Functional evaluation: the Barthel index, *Md State Med J* **14** (1965), 61–65.

[88] P. Azouvi, F. Marchal, C. Samuel, L. Morin, C. Renard, A. Louis-Dreyfus, C. Jokic, L. Wiart, P. Pradat-Diehl, G. Deloche and C. Bergego, Functional Consequences and Awareness of Unilateral Neglect: Study of an Evaluation Scale, *Neuropschological-rehabilitation* **6** (1996), 133–150.

[89] C.V. Granger, B.B. Hamilton, R.A. Keith, M. Zielezny and F.S. Sherwin, Advances in functional assessment for medical rehabilitation, *Topics in Geriatric Rehabilitation* **1** (1986), 59–74.

[90] A.G. Fischer, Assessment of motor and process skills (3rd ed.), 1999.

[91] C. Ball, D. Sackett, B. Phillips, B. Haynes, S. Straus and M. Dawes, Oxford Centre for Evidence-based Medicine Levels of Evidence, 2001, Internet Communication, http://www.cebm-net/levels_of_evidence.asp.

Simulating unilateral neglect in normals: Myth or reality?

Carine Michel
INSERM ERIT-M 207, Université de Bourgogne, BP 27877, F-21078 Dijon, France
Tel.: +33 0 3 80 39 90 06; Fax: +33 0 3 80 39 67 02; E-mail: carine.michel@u-bourgogne.fr

Received 23 December 2005
Revised 1 March 2006
Accepted 22 June 2006

Abstract. Hemispatial neglect is a neurological deficit of perception, attention, representation, and/or performing actions within the left-sided space. The condition also produces many functional debilitating effects on everyday life, and is associated with poor functional recovery and inability to benefit from treatment. Numerous methods of rehabilitation (sensory stimulations or active training) have been proposed to alleviate neglect condition. It has been recently shown that visuo-manual adaptation to rightward optical shift leads to profound and enduring improvements of neglect symptoms. Based on the different methods commonly used in the rehabilitation of neglect, several techniques have been employed to simulate neglect symptoms in healthy subjects with a view to better understand the physiopathology of neglect. The present paper reviews studies of neglect-like behaviour in healthy individuals and in particular the use of prism adaptation as a procedure for simulating various symptoms of clinical neglect in normals. Neglect-like symptoms following prism adaptation offer insights as to the mechanisms of spatial neglect and provide an understanding of the interaction between low level sensorimotor processes and spatial cognition. Implications for the functional mechanisms and the anatomical substrates of prism adaptation are discussed in terms of inter-sensory plasticity and sensorimotor coordination and the way these may affect higher-level representations of space.

Keywords: Simulation of neglect, healthy subjects, prism adaptation, space representation, plasticity

The standard definition of neglect since the 1970s is unambiguous in maintaining that the disorder cannot be attributed to either primary sensory or motor defects [54]. From a neuropsychological perspective, it is now generally accepted that neglect is a heterogeneous disorder whose different symptoms can be explained in terms of damage to (at least) one of three different cognitive mechanisms mediating attention (e.g. [53]), intention [120] and/or space representation [10]. Despite dissociations this heterogeneous condition is more frequent, longer lasting and more severe after right brain damage than after equivalent lesions of the left hemisphere [13,117]. Several directional specific improvements in neglect have already been reported by sensory stimulations or active training (see [107,118] for reviews). More recently, in a series of elegant studies Rossetti and co-workers [93,104,106] have shown that visuo-manual adaptation to rightward optical shift produces profound and enduring improvements of neglect symptoms. Prism adaptation acts on spatial cognition and is responsible for extra-ordinary transfer of adaptation to many visual, tactile, motor and cognitive domains [73,115, reviews 105,107]. Therefore this revue focuses on prism adaptation as a robust procedure for simulating neglect in normals. Neglect-like symptoms in normals offer potential novel insights into the mechanisms of spatial neglect and a fundamental understanding of the interaction between low level sensorimotor processes and spatial cognition. In the light of the recent results, the present review hopes to provide some tentative hypotheses concerning the neuronal substrate of prism adaptation.

1. Simulating neglect in healthy subjects

Based on previous techniques to rehabilitate neglect, several techniques have been used to transiently produce neglect-like behaviour in healthy subjects. Usually attempts to produce neglect in normals is based on the assumption that the right side of the human brain is specialised for visuo-spatial functions [28,41, see for review 6]. On line bisection (where the subject is required to estimate the centre of a line), brain asymmetry in favour of the right hemisphere visuospatial function is considered responsible for 'pseudoneglect' manifestations such as reliable leftward estimation of the centre of the line. This leftward bias was initially reported by Bowers and Heilman [14] and subsequently by many others since [15,87, for review and meta-analysis see 60]. In the same way, brain asymmetry in favour of the right hemisphere is revealed when the sensorimotor system is altered in neglect condition after right hemisphere lesion. Neglect performance on line bisection is characterized by a rightward bias (e.g. [10, 47]). Numerous line bisection studies in normals have shown that less right hemisphere activation (or more left hemisphere activation) during the line bisection task, reduces pseudoneglect until it becomes a mild rightward neglect-like bias. For instance, leftward bisection bias decreases when the right hand (versus left hand) is used [18,44,60,109], when exploration of the line to be bisected favours the right part with right-to-left scanning [18,24,98], when attention is oriented to the right extremity of the line with spatial [51,87,97], or with spatio-motor [48] cueing and with appropriate variation of luminance contrast [16]. Even visual illusions can produce rightward bias in perceptual estimation of the line centre [23,42,77,111]. In the same way, right hemisphere involvement appears to decreases when lines are located in right hemispace [71,78,87,97] or when short line lengths are used such that rightward crossover bias is seen [67,78]. However, the hypothesis of a right hemisphere disengagement is not obvious in the latter condition. Furthermore performances on line bisection in the elderly also argue in favour of the disengagement of right hemisphere in some neglect-like behaviours. Indeed, because of differential ageing of the right hemisphere [81,102] or reduced hemispheric asymmetry with ageing (HAROLD model for Hemispheric Asymmetry Reduction in OLDs adults) [19,34, 99], studies of the elderly show a rightward bias on line bisection [43]. Additional arguments include the disruption of cerebral activity with transcranial magnetic stimulation or by sensory manipulations. For instance, the use of repetitive transcranial magnetic stimulation over right frontal and right posterior parietal cortices produces rightward neglect-like bias in line bisection [17,39,40] whereas stimulation of left hemisphere induces no discernable effect. Neglect-like deficits of visual attention may be also induced by rTMS targeting the right parietal cortex [114]. Also, sensory manipulations such as neck-proprioceptive (vibration of neck muscles) or vestibular (injection of iced water into the ear) stimulations may affect the distributed network involved in constructing an egocentric reference and therefore produce neglect-like behaviour in healthy subjects [3,62,63]. Collectively, neglect-like behaviour in healthy subjects seems to depend on the modulation of right hemisphere involvement during the target task. Neglect-like behaviour appears only when artefacts responsible for attentional shift, illusory or rTMS are used *during* the task execution which makes the simulation of visual neglect strongly dependent on the experimental condition. Furthermore, sensory stimulation (neck muscle vibration, caloric vestibular stimulation [61], or optokinetic stimulation [76]) produces fairly *symmetrical* effects. Although attempts to simulate neglect have to be interpreted with caution, they nevertheless provide some insights into the inherent asymmetrical bias in the organization of the normal brain. The following section will consider the link between the cerebral plasticity of sensorimotor coordination and the brain organization for space representation. The disruption on the normal brain asymmetry by producing albeit temporary cerebral plasticity is relevant to understanding both the *directional* improvement of neglect symptoms and simulation of neglect-like behaviour in healthy subjects *after* prism adaptation procedure.

2. Close link between sensorimotor coordination and space representation

The neuropsychological processes underlying space perception and the integration of sensory inputs in providing for internal space representation has been a central scientific and philosophic issue in cognitive sciences for many centuries. Above all considerations spatial environment may be viewed as useful space for actions. Space representation could be considered as the mental representation of the environment topographically structured, mapped across the brain and relatively accurate of the physic reality [9]. Although sensory integration has been reported at birth (e.g. [68,80]), development of a space referential depends upon experience – namely motor activity throughout childhood which allows correspondence to development between sensory experience and motor activity. According to Piaget [92], motor activity gives rise to the development of sensorimotor coordination. Goal directed behaviour plays a crucial role in the coherence of relations between perception of each sensory modality and action. Famous experiments of sensory deprivation at the early stage of post-natal life in kittens conducted by Held and Hein [57] prove a clear demonstration of the unifying integrative role of action between different sensory modalities. Owing to the continuous reinforcement by motor experience, spatial relations between external physical and internal representation become stable. Subsequent sensorimotor plasticity provides for appropriate motor response allowing progressive adjustment of motor control during physiological changes (e.g. in the elderly), pathological conditions (central or peripheral damage of central nervous system) or in reaction to experimental perturbation (hypogravity or optical perturbation of the optical field...). When constant disturbance is applied to the sensorimotor system by deviation of the optical field for instance, the progressive motor adjustment corresponds to an adaptation of the sensorimotor conflict. This adaptation is not possible when disruption of the optical displacement is variable [56]. Since the development of the internal structured space representation in childhood is largely based on the coherence between sensory modalities and motor action, it is necessary to raise the question of whether manipulation of sensorimotor coordination during adulthood may alter subsequent space representation. Furthermore, it has been already shown that space representation is particularly sensitive to adaptation of sensorimotor conflict in brain-damaged patients [106]. Could effects of sensorimotor adaptation also affect space representation in healthy adults as in brain-damaged patients? For this to take place would require presumably the involvement of functional parts of the intact brain. Research using prism adaptation paradigms that demonstrate the link between sensorimotor coordination plasticity and space representation in healthy subjects will be discussed in the following section.

3. Neglect-like behaviour in healthy subjects following prism adaptation (Table 1)

3.1. First simulation of neglect in line bisection

The first attempted simulation of visual neglect using prism adaptation was shown employing the line bisection task [27]. The abundance of experimental conditions associated with line bisection task offers an insight into mechanisms implied in neglect condition. Line bisection is an invaluable tool to gain a better understanding of the functional processes involved when responding to different stimulus presentations (e.g. spatial location, line length, spatial cueing). The recent evidence showing that various symptoms of visual neglect can be improved following short adaptation periods to a 10 right prismatic shift of the visual field [106, 107] challenges the traditional distinction in clinical literature between low level sensorimotor deficits and those assumed to involve higher level/cognitive systems. The results obtained by Colent et al. [27] provided the first report of a cognitive effect (i.e. higher level) of prism adaptation in healthy subjects and appears to be a faithful simulation of main characteristics of neglect: e.g. the directional bias in line bisection, its rightward specificity and the predominance of perceptual effects. Whereas perceptual and motor factors are involved in line bisection tasks [72,87], prism adaptation is responsible for a stronger perceptual than motor bias [27,82] as shown in neglect patients [5,50,88]. This contrast is particularly interesting when one considers that prism adaptation requires active motor behaviour to be developed, all of which would predict a predominantly motor effect. The following description attempts to provide an illustration of neglect simulation in healthy individuals and provides a deeper understanding of the cognitive after-effects of prism adaptation and their relationship with the well-established sensorimotor after-effects.

3.2. Following investigations in line bisection task

First extension of results in line bisection was obtained for both different line lengths and different line locations [82]. When after-effects are explored for different line lengths, rightward bias is greater when lines are longer [82] with a predominance of perceptual bias as previously shown [27]. Following prism adaptation, rightward neglect-like bias in normal subjects increases with line length, -a well know characteristic of clinical neglect performance [10,47]. When the extent of the spatial bias following prism adaptation is explored by varying the relative hemispatial location of the lines across body midline (to the left, to the right and in front of the subject's body midline) there is a significant rightward shift both in manual and in perceptual bisection tasks but not for right-sided lines. This result can be interpreted as an illustration of neglect-like

Table 1
Neglect-like symptoms induced by prism adaptation in healthy subjects

Studies	Space representations	Characteristics of neglect-like behaviour
[27]	Peripersonal space	Rightward bias in perceptual line bisection
[82]	Peripersonal space	Rightward bias depends on line length and line location
[46]	Peripersonal space	Rightward bias in the determination of the centre of a haptically and visual explored circle
[7]	Extrapersonal space	Rightward bias in perceptual line bisection
[85]	Extrapersonal space	Asymmetrical rightward bias in locomotor reaching task
[83]	Body scheme	Rightward postural shift
[21]	Space of numbers	Bias toward large numbers in number bisection
[38]	Peripersonal space	Rightward shift of eye movements during chimeric faces task
[84]		Simulation of the neglect's lack of awareness for the sensorimotor conflict responsible for greater and longer-lasting sensorimotor after-effects

behaviour for two main reasons. First, due to the increase of the motor contribution for left locations, the effects of prism adaptation not only induce a perceptual bias but also a pre-motor bias producing the leftward hypokinesia [31,53]. This pre-motor facilitation may reduce progressively as a function of leftward location in space as seen in some neglect patients [87]. Second, the use of the three spatial locations results in an enlargement of the horizontal extent of attention. As seen in many neglect patients [74], the requirement to allocate attention over space within an experimental session is likely to increase the spatial span of attention responsible for smaller bias in central locations than that previously shown for single central location [27]. Thus several of the main characteristics of neglect are qualitatively simulated in healthy subjects following prism adaptation on the standard clinical line bisection task.

3.3. Prism adaptation affects a supramodal space of representation

To establish whether cognitive after-effects are limited to cognitive spatial tasks involving visuo-manual coordination, cross-modal effects have also been explored using the innovatory centre estimation of circle. This task was primarily proposed by McIntosh for the assessment of neglect [79]. This method involves locating the centre of a haptically explored circle which avoids the adoption of counting strategies to solve problems of spatial cognition and forces subjects to rely on the haptically sourced spatial representations of the stimulus. In the study by Girardi et al. [46], healthy subjects were requested to estimate the centre of a haptically or visually explored circle, before and after a period of adaptation to leftward displacing prisms. Prism adaptation produced a significant rightward shift of the performance on both tasks. These results extend neglect expression to haptic modality and thereby strengthen the evidence for a cross-modal effect of this procedure. Although prism adaptation typically depends upon a visual displacement, it can nonetheless affect performance of spatial tasks where no visual information is provided or required. The effect of prism adaptation appears to take place at a supramodal level of space representation. Theses results underline the role of prism adaptation on right hemisphere functions (see Section 4) and reinforce the homology between effects of prism adaptation on spatial cognition and neglect-like behaviour.

3.4. Space representations affected by prism adaptation

Given the large number of reports describing space representations affected by prism adaptation in neglect patients (for review see [105]), one obvious question is whether cognitive after-effects in healthy subjects are restricted to representation of peripersonal space where development of visuo-manual adaptation takes place. The following sections provide some examples of illustrations for spaces whose representation can be affected by prism adaptation.

– *Extrapersonal space:*

To explore whether cognitive after-effects of prism adaptation in healthy subjects extend over peripersonal space, Berberovic and Mattingley [7] used a line bisection paradigm in extrapersonal space (i.e. beyond the immediate manual pointing space within visuo-manual adaptation takes place). In extrapersonal space adaptation to left-deviating prisms produces a rightward shift in the bisection judgements for lines, demonstrating the involvement of cognitive after-effects in the representation of extrapersonal space. This finding extends the cognitive after-effects of visuo-manual adaptation to extrapersonal space. The potential transfer of adaptation to tasks typically considered 'sensorimotor' due to the low involvement of cognitive strategies was also shown for far space. A recent study [85] using an experimental paradigm based on locomotor reaching task to a memorized target placed 7 meters away from the subjects showed that visuo-manual adaptation transferred to locomotor reaching with a rightward asymmetrical bias after adaptation to a leftward visual shift. This asymmetry may be explained by a cognitive additional component to sensorimotor after-effects especially when subjects are adapted to a leftward deviation. This additional asymmetrical component could be attributed to after-effects on spatial cognition as it was already proposed in line bisection task [7,27,82]. Therefore there may be an over-representation of the rightward lateral distance to cover which gives rise to a rightward misperception of the straight-head visual target. The rightward locomotor bias after prism adaptation may be qualitatively compared to the rightward locomotor bias observed in neglect patients [8,101].

– Body scheme and numbers representation:

The cerebral plasticity involved during prism adaptation may not only affect higher-level representations of extrapersonal space but it may also act on the internal body space representation. It has been shown that after-effects of a visuo-manual adaptation to a leftward optical shift could induce a rightward bias in postural control in normal subjects [83]. This result lends supports to the idea that prism adaptation may influence the space representation of inner postural body scheme. Such diversity of cognitive after-effects in healthy subjects motivates further enquiry to establish whether prism adaptation may affect higher cognitive functions of a non-spatial nature: the enigmatic representation of space numbers. The mental representation of the numbers is organized from left to right. Small numbers are associated with the left space and large numbers with the right space [2,32]. Calabria and colleagues [21] investigated effects of prism adaptation on number bisection where the mental number line had an assumed canonical orientation from left to right. Using the analogy from previous results with physical line bisection [7,27,82] subjects were required to estimate the centre of an interval defined by two numbers. After visuo-manual prism adaptation, subjects estimations were systematically biased towards larger numbers, i.e. towards numbers represented more to the right on the mental number line. This effect was proportional to the interval size and was more pronounced when an increasing order of presentation was used. These results are consistent with neglect misestimation for the centre of a line number [123] and offer additional evidence that not only brain-damaged patients [108] but also healthy controls can be affected by prism adaptation in a task that is not explicitly spatial. Calabria and co-workers conclude that sensorimotor interactions may play a crucial role in the organization of the relationship between space and number representation.

In summary the above results suggest that the performances of healthy subjects using prism adaptation may be considered to be a good approximation to neglect-like behaviour. Because of the numerous space representations modified by prism adaptation, it may be suggested that prism adaptation affects a supramodal level of spatial representations. Representational hypotheses of prism adaptation seem to rightly provide some accounts to explain the large diversity of neglect simulation and may correspond with an under-representation of the left part of space and an over-representation of the right side of space as reported in neglect (e.g. [11,12,49, 86,116]). Taken together with the evidence that various symptoms of visual neglect can be improved following prism adaptation, the neglect-like behaviour in normals reinforces the representational hypothesis of neglect and consequently challenges the traditional distinction in the standard clinical neuropsychological definition between low level sensorimotor deficits and those assumed to involve cognitive systems. Furthermore, it is worth underlying here that neglect-like behaviour cannot be simply attributed to ocular change following prism exposure for three main reasons. First, cognitive after-effects are not restricted to visual modality but have been shown in haptic task [46] and in postural evaluation without vision [83]. Second, visuo-manual prism adaptation is responsible for visual after-effect in the direction of the optical deviation (e.g. [119]). When optical deviation is shifted to the left, the gaze is consequently directed to the left during and after prism exposure. Because representational performance [96] and more precisely line bisection performance depends on the gaze direction [18,24] and more generally on spatial attention (e.g. [52,87]), it could have been expected that leftward optical deviation leads to a leftward estimation of the line centre contrary to rightward bias really shown [7,27,82]. However a visual shift in the direction opposite to the visual shift was shown both in healthy subjects (rightward shift after adaptation to a leftward visual shift) [38] and in neglect patients (leftward shift after adaptation to a rightward visual shift) [1,33]. This unexpected visual shift (see [64,66] for reviews) cannot be explained in terms of sensorimotor after-effects due to eye muscle potentiation [35] or to visual recalibration [29,30] but rather to reorganization of visuo-spatial functions following prism adaptation. Third,

Table 2
Anatomical substrate for prism adaptation. Functional involvement of each structure during adaptation processes is presented. Cerebellum is crucial for adaptive realignment whereas cortical structures are involved in strategic recalibration, and intentional/perceptual and representational after-effects

Neuroanatomical Substrate	Contribution in prism adaptation processes	Period in adaptation processes	References
1- Cerebellum 2- Lateral part 3- Anterior part	Adaptive realignment (1,2,3)	During and following prism exposure (1,2,3)	1- [e.g. 4, 75, 121] 2- [113] 3- [95]
Thalamus	Relay between cerebellum and cerebral cortex	Prism exposure Following prism exposure?	[26]
Associative motor areas	1-Strategic recalibration (error signal) 2- Intentional after-effects (hypokinesia)	1- Prism exposure 2- Following prism exposure	1- [65] 2- [82, 105]
Posterior parietal cortex	1- Superior lobule (strategic recalibration) 2- Inferior lobule (awareness of optical deviation) 3- Inferior lobule (representational after-effects)	1- Prism exposure 2- Prism exposure 3- Following prism exposure	1- [e.g. 25, 58, 94] 2- [20, 105, 107] 3- [e.g. 7, 27, 46, 82, 105, 106, 107]
Somato-sensory areas, associative visual areas	Perceptual after-effects	During and following prism exposure	[89, 110, 112]

dissociations have been shown between eye movement exploration and improvement of neglect condition [33, 37] and between the pattern of eye movements and perceptual judgements in healthy subjects following prism exposure [38]. These results underline the dissociation between cognitive and visual after-effects. In the same way, recent findings aimed at assessing change in spatial attention following prism adaptation failed to propose the redistribution of selective spatial attention in normals as in neglect patients [90]. Taken together these results cannot attribute cognitive after-effects of prism adaptation to visual or selective spatial attentional shifts following prism exposure.

3.5. Simulation of the apparent neglect deficit of awareness for the visual deviation

Neglect patients react in a peculiar way to the prism adaptation procedure. Namely, they exhibit a striking lack of awareness for the spatial distortion presumed to be occurring during prism adaptation procedure [105]. Indeed, patients do not appear overtly (no spontaneous nor directed comments) detect the visual perturbation whereas healthy subjects show a surprise reaction. Furthermore neglect patients show no skin conductance modification when prisms are unexpectedly introduced in the course of a pointing task [20]. On the other hand, they also show greater and longer-lasting sensorimotor as well as cognitive after-effects (see [105, 107] for reviews). Whereas prism after-effects do not exceed several minutes in normal subjects (e.g. [122]), after-effects reported in neglect patients can last over at least two hours [106], one day [36], or even four days [93]. In a recently submitted paper intended to clarify the contribution of awareness of the optical shift for the development of prism adaptation, an experimental reduction of the awareness of the optical shift was proposed in healthy subjects to mimic the reduction of awareness of neglect patients [84]. When subjects were unaware of the visual deviation during prism exposure because of its progressive stepwise increase from 2 degrees to 10 degrees, there were larger and longer-lasting direct after-effects (assessed by open-loop pointing task). Furthermore after-effects transferred to the non-exposed hand for the visual and auditory pointing tasks. Taken together with the clinical results, this finding reinforces the assumption that the strong power of strategies to reduce pointing error in the short term may reduce the error signals required for true adaptation (realignment) to develop.

4. Features of prism adaptation to simulate neglect-like behaviour in normals and neuroanatomical substrate (Fig. 1 and Table 2)

It could be questioned whether the cognitive bias observed through different visuo-spatial tasks is specific to the development of prism adaptation or whether it can be observed following passive prism exposure regardless of sensorimotor after-effects. It has been clearly established that active movements during prism exposure (compared with passive exposure without any movement) are essential to the development of sensorimotor and cognitive after-effects [82]. However, the question remains open whether there is a proportional link between the amplitude of cognitive after-effects and the amplitude of sensorimotor after-effects as suggested by studies in neglect patients [106]. Considering that in healthy subjects the classical procedure of prism adap-

a) In neglect patients

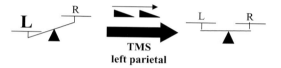

b) In healthy subjects

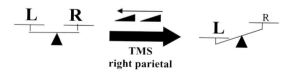

Fig. 1. Effects of prism adaptation on interhemispheric balance at parietal level. The size of the 'L' corresponds to the level of activation of the left hemisphere and the size of the 'R' to the level of activation of the right hemisphere. The optical deviation used to prism adaptation is symbolised by two triangles topped by an arrow. a) Effect of prism adaptation in neglect patients. In right brain-damaged patients, adaptation to a rightward visual shift balances interhemispheric parietal function to improve neglect symptoms as it was transiently shown with the use of rTMS over the left parietal cortex (e.g. [91]). b) Effect of prism adaptation in healthy subjects. Adaptation to a leftward visual shift disrupts interhemispheric balance to the detriment of the right hemisphere which is responsible for neglect-like behaviour as it was transiently shown with the use of rTMS over the right parietal cortex [17,39,40].

tation is responsible for cognitive after-effects qualitatively similar to neglect symptoms, it would be interesting to investigate whether the scope of the simulation of neglect (as the amplitude of line bisection bias for instance) directly depends on the amplitude of sensorimotor after-effects.

In addition to active pointing movements during prism exposure, the direction of the optical deviation is crucial to act on interhemispheric balance for representational parietal functions. According to the direction of the optical deviation, prism adaptation simulates neglect behaviour in normals or alleviates neglect condition. Leftward optical deviation during prism exposure leads to neglect-like behaviour [27] whereas rightward optical deviation gives rise to improvement of neglect symptoms [106] (Fig. 1). The question remains as to how the plasticity of inter-sensory and sensorimotor coordination affects higher-level cognitive representations of space. Whereas the anatomical substrate involved in prism adaptation has not been firmly established yet, a hypothesis can be proposed on the basis of the data currently available in the literature. The main candidates likely to explain differential sensitivity of prism adaptation on hemispheric balance are the cerebellum, the posterior parietal cortex and the frontal cortex. A crucial involvement in adaptive realignment process is attributed to the cerebellum because of its important role in the integration of the motor output (efference) and of the visual error resulting from this output (visual reafference) [55]. Brain lesions localized in the cerebellum and in afferent olivo-ponto-cerebellar system prevent development of adaptation as measured by after-effects both in humans and non-human primates [4,45,75,95,113,121, for review see 59]. Lateral cerebellum would be more precisely involved in adaptive processes as shown by a muscimol inactivation study [113] and more recently by a lateralized lesion of the anterior cerebellar cortex in humans which prevents the adaptation for ipsidirectional visual shift [95]. The latter result underlines the visual lateralization of the cerebellum in addition to the well-known motor lateralization. Connections between the cerebellum and the cerebral cortex are also important for adaptation. Indeed, frontal brain lesions in humans [22] and lesions of the premotor ventral cortex controlateral to the direction of the error signal prevent the development of adaptation in monkeys [65]. The error signal from premotor cortex to the cerebellum may be crucial to the development of adaptation. Recent functional imaging data support this functional cerebrocerebellar organization. Indeed, Luauté and collaborators showed [69, 70] in a PET study, the involvement of the right cerebellar hemisphere together with the left cerebral hemisphere in the beneficial effect of adaptation to rightward prisms in neglect patients. Collectively, it might assume a contribution of the left anterior cerebellum when healthy subjects adapt to a leftward optical deviation to simulate neglect-like symptoms.

This anatomical substrate for adaptive realignment responsible for sensorimotor after-effects may differ from the anatomical structure involved in strategic recalibration mainly responsible for error reduction during prism exposure. The superior posterior parietal cortex seems to be an appropriate candidate for strategic calibration during prism exposure. Indeed, the superior parietal cortex has been shown to be involved in strategic corrections of pointing movements during visual perturbations when optical devices involve strong strategic component (e.g. [58,100]). A brain imaging study tended also to confirm that the superior posterior parietal cortex is involved in the strategic aspect of prism adaptation especially when optical deviation is reversed (left or right) every five trials to maintain the subject in a state of on-going adaptation [25]. Furthermore, recent neuropsychological study shows that the adaptive component would be mainly supported by the cerebellum whereas the strategic component would rely on the superior parietal cortex [94]. As further evidence, patients with lesions of the parietal cortex are fully able to adapt to optical deviation by showing even greater after-effects than healthy subjects [94, 106]. In addition, patients with unilateral neglect exhibit extra-ordinary transfer of adaptation to many visual, motor and cognitive domains (e.g. [103,108, reviews 105,107]). Taken together with the experimental reduction of awareness of the optical shift in healthy subjects [84], there seems to be a functional balance between the strategic parietal recalibration and adaptive cerebellar realignment. When the strategic component is reduced either by cerebral damage [94,106] or by experimental reduction of the explicit knowledge of the optical deviation [84], the cerebellar plasticity might be reinforced, as if cerebellar plasticity might be under parietal control. Considering parietal involvement in strategic recalibration during prism exposure and representational after-effects in neglect patients and in healthy individuals, we may envisage a sequential involvement of parietal cortex in prism adaptation. The superior parietal cortex may act during prism exposure for strategic recalibration whereas the inferior parietal cortex may be considered as a secondary site of plasticity (of the cerebellum) responsible for cognitive after-effects. As mentioned above [82,106], cognitive after-effects strictly depend on the development of prism adaptation. The posterior parietal cortex is not the single substrate of cortical plasticity following prism adaptation. The visual areas [89,112] and parieto-frontal network [110] are also concerned. Collectively motor improvement in neglect patient with decreased reaction time to reach and grasp an object in the left hemispace [105] and increased motor contribution for the left hemispace in simulation of neglect in normals [82] emphasize the contribution of premotor cortex in cerebral plasticity following prism adaptation. All these results lead to better understand how the cerebral plasticity involved in prism adaptation may produce neglect-like behaviour in healthy individuals. Cerebellar plasticity may indirectly affect hemispheric balance for posterior parietal cortex, associative motor areas and associative visual areas via the thalamus [26] (see Table 2). In this way leftward optical deviation during prism exposure in healthy subjects may primarily involve left anterior cerebellum whose plasticity act in cortical level. Therefore plasticity processes may lead to a disruption of the interhemispheric balance to the detriment of the right hemisphere which is responsible for neglect-like behaviour.

5. Conclusion

Previous research strategies to simulate neglect-like behaviour in healthy subjects have primarily focused on physiological manoeuvres altering the balance of sensory inputs between left-sided and right-sided parts of the body and on weakening of the right hemisphere activation by attention or intentional processes. These manipulations emphasize the contribution of interhemispheric imbalance in the occurrence of the clinical manifestations of neglect. However these methods may have to be considered with caution because they produce transient symmetrical effect. Furthermore, these manipulations are responsible for neglect-like behaviour strongly restricted to experimental conditions. Recent significant and enduring improvements of neglect by visuo-manual adaptation to optical shift have provided the basis for new approaches in the simulation of neglect-like behaviour in normals. Simulation of neglect by prism adaptation not only extends on many levels of space representation eliciting mild neglect behaviour in numerous sensitive neuropsychological tests but also requires neither sensory stimulation nor attentional/intention artefact during behavioural assessment. In the light of the data currently available in the literature and of recent TEP study in neglect patients [69, 70], adaptation to a leftward visual shift in healthy subjects might involve plasticity of the left cerebellum to weaken activity of the right hemisphere. The disruption of the normal brain asymmetry seems to be the central process both shared by prism adaptation and other experimental procedures (sensory stimulations, shift of attention, rTMS...) to simulate neglect-like behaviour. Collectively these results are well compatible with the possibility to simulate mild neglect behaviour in normals. These recent but nevertheless promising approaches of cerebral organization by simulation of neglect may offer some insights into neurophysiological processes and the understanding of neglect.

Acknowledgements

I wish greatly to thank Pr. Y. Rossetti and his team for their helpful discussions on the present topic and Pr. T. Pozzo, C. Papaxanthis and E. Thomas for their positive criticism of the manuscript. This work was supported by the University of Bourgogne.

References

[1] V. Angeli, M.G. Benassi and E. Ladavas, Recovery of oculomotor bias in neglect patients after prism adaptation, *Neuropsychologia* **42** (2004), 1223–1234.

[2] D. Bächtold, M. Baumüller and P. Brugger, Stimulus-response compatibility in representational space, *Neuropsychologia* **36** (1998), 731–735.

[3] D. Bächtold, T. Baumann, P.S. Sandor, M. Kristos, M. Regard and P. Brugger, Spatial- and verbal-memory improvement by cold-waer caloric stimulation in healthy subjects, *Exp Brain Res* **136** (2001), 128–132.

[4] J.S. Baizer and M. Glickstein, Proceedings: Role of cerebellum in prism adaptation, *J Physiol* **236** (1974), 34P–35P.

[5] P. Bartolomeo, P. D'Erme, R. Perri and G. Gainotti, Perception and action in hemispatial neglect, *Neuropsychologia* **36** (1998), 227–237.

[6] A. Benton and D. Tranel, Visuoperceptual, Visuospatial, and visuoconstructive disorders, in: *Clinical Neuropsychology*, K.M. Heilman and E. Valensteinn, eds, Oxford University Press, New York, 1993, pp. 165–213.

[7] N. Berberovic and J.B. Mattingley, Effects of prismatic adaptation on judgements of spatial extent in peripersonal and extrapersonal space, *Neuropsychologia* **41** (2003), 493–503.

[8] A. Berti, N. Smania, M. Rabuffetti, M. Ferrarin, L. Spinazzola, A. D'Amico, E. Ongaro and A. Allport, Coding of far and near space during walking in neglect patients, *Neuropsychology* **16** (2002), 390–399.

[9] E. Bisiach, C. Luzzatti and D. Perani, Unilateral neglect, representational schema and consciousness, *Brain* **102** (1979), 609–618.

[10] E. Bisiach, C. Bulgarelli, R. Sterzi and G. Vallar, Line bisection and cognitive plasticity of unilateral neglect of space, *Brain Cogn* **2** (1983), 32–38.

[11] E. Bisiach, L. Pizzamiglio and D. Nico, Antonucci, Beyond unilateral neglect, *Brain* **119** (1996), 851–857.

[12] E. Bisiach, R. Ricci, G. Berruti, R. Genero, R. Pepi and T. Fumelli, Two-dimensional distortion of space representation in unilateral neglect: perceptual and response-related factors, *Neuropsychologia* **37** (1999), 1491–1498.

[13] A. Bowen, K. McKenna and R.C. Tallis, Reasons for variability in the reported rate of occurrence of unilateral spatial neglect after stroke, *Stroke* **30** (1999), 1196–1202.

[14] D. Bowers and K.M. Heilman, Pseudoneglect: effects of hemispace on a tactile line bisection task, *Neuropsychologia* **18** (1980), 491–498.

[15] J.L. Bradshaw, N.C. Nettleton, G. Nathan and L. Wilson, Bisecting rods and lines: effects of horizontal and vertical posture on left-side underestimation by normal subjects, *Neuropsychologia* **23** (1985), 421–425.

[16] J.L. Bradshaw, G. Nathan, N.C. Nettleton, L. Wilson and J. Pierson, Why is there a left side underestimation in rod bisection? *Neuropsychologia* **25** (1987), 735–738.

[17] F. Brighina, E. Bisiach, A. Piazza, M. Oliveri, V. La Bua, O. Daniele and B. Fierro, Perceptual and response bias in visuospatial neglect due to frontal and parietal repetitive transcranial magnetic stimulation in normal subjects, *Neuroreport* **13** (2002), 2571–2575.

[18] E.E. Brodie and L.E. Pettigrew, Is left always right? Directional deviations in visual line bisection as a function of hand and initial scanning direction, *Neuropsychologia* **34** (1996), 467–470.

[19] R. Cabeza, S.M. Daselaar, F. Dolcos, S.E. Prince, M. Budde and L. Nyberg, Task-independent and task-specific age effects on brain activity during working memory, visual attention and episodic retrieval, *Cereb Cortex* **14** (2004), 364–375.

[20] M. Calabria, C. Michel, J. Honoré, A. Guillaume, L. Pisella, J. Luauté, G. Rode, D. Boisson and Y. Rossetti, Prism adaptation and the lack of awareness in spatial neglect. Proceeding of the First Congress of the European Neuropsychological Societies 18th–20th, Modena, Italy, 2004, 222.

[21] M. Calabria, S. Jacquin-Courtois, C. Michel, S. Göbel, A. Farne and Y. Rossetti, Prism adaptation distorts the mental number line: A dynamical link between sensorimotor control and number representation, submitted.

[22] A.G. Canavan, R.E. Passingham, C.D. Marsden, N. Quinn, M. Wyke and C.E. Polkey, Prism adaptation and other tasks involving spatial abilities in patients with Parkinson's disease, patients with frontal lobe lesions and patients with unilateral temporal lobectomies, *Neuropsychologia* **28** (1990), 969–984.

[23] S. Chieffi, Effects of stimulus asymmetry on line bisection, *Neurology* **47** (1996), 1004–1008.

[24] S. Chokron, P. Bartolomeo, M.T. Perenin, G. Helft and M. Imbert, Scanning direction and line bisection: a study of normal subjects and unilateral neglect patients with opposite reading habits, *Brain Res Cogn Brain Res* **7** (1998), 173–178.

[25] D.M. Clower, J.M. Hoffman, J.R. Votaw, T.L. Faber, R.P. Woods and G.E. Alexander, Role of posterior parietal cortex in the recalibration of visually guided reaching, *Nature* **383** (1996), 618–621.

[26] D.M. Clower, R.A. West, J.C. Lynch and P.L. Strick, The inferior parietal lobule is the target of output from the superior colliculus, hippocampus, and cerebellum, *J Neurosci* **21** (2001), 6283–6291.

[27] C. Colent, L. Pisella, C. Bernieri, G. Rode and Y. Rossetti, Cognitive bias induced by visuo-motor adaptation to prisms: a simulation of unilateral neglect in normal individuals? *Neuroreport* **11** (2000), 1899–1902.

[28] M. Corbetta and G.L. Shulman, Control of goal-directed and stimulus-driven attention in the brain, *Nat Rev Neurosci* **3** (2002), 201–215.

[29] B. Craske, A current view of the processes and mechanisms of prism adaptation, in: *Aspects of neuronal plasticity*, F. Vital-Durand and M. Jeannerod, eds, 1975, pp. 125–138.

[30] B. Craske and M. Crawshaw, Oculomotor adaptation to prism is not simply a muscle potentiation effect, *Percept Psychophys* **18** (1975), 105–106.

[31] R. Cubelli, M. Pugliese and A.S. Gabellini, The effect of space location on neglect depends on the nature of the task, *J Neurol* **241** (1994), 611–614.

[32] S. Dehaene, S. Bossini and P. Giraux, The mental representation of parity and number magnitude, *J Exp Psychol Gen* **122** (1993), 371–396.

[33] H.C. Dijkerman, R.D. McIntosh, A.D. Milner, Y. Rossetti, C. Tilikete and R.C. Roberts, Ocular scanning and perceptual size distortion in hemispatial neglect: effects of prism adaptation and sequential stimulus presentation, *Exp Brain Res* **153** (2003), 220–230.

[34] F. Dolcos, H.J. Rice and R. Cabeza, Hemispheric asymmetry and aging: right hemisphere decline or asymmetry reduction, *Neurosci Biobehav Rev* **26** (2002), 819–825.

[35] S.M. Ebenholtz, The possible role of eye-muscle potentiation in several forms of prism adaptation, *Perception* **3** (1974), 477–485.

[36] A. Farne, Y. Rossetti, S. Toniolo and E. Ladavas, Ameliorating neglect with prism adaptation: visuo-manual and visuo-verbal measures, *Neuropsychologia* **40** (2002), 718–729.

[37] S. Ferber, J. Dankert, M. Joanisse, H.C. Goltz and M.A. Goodale, Eye movements tell only half the story, *Neurology* **60** (2003), 1826,1929.

[38] S. Ferber and L.J. Murray, Are perceptual judgments dissociated from motor processes? A prism adaptation study, *Cogn Brain Res* **23** (2005), 453–456.

[39] B. Fierro, F. Brighina, M. Oliveri, A. Piazza, V. La Bua, D. Buffa and E. Bisiach, Contralateral neglect induced by right posterior parietal rTMS in healthy subjects, *Neuroreport* **11** (2000), 1519–1521.

[40] B. Fierro, F. Brighina, A. Piazza, M. Oliveri and E. Bisiach, Timing of right parietal and frontal cortex activity in visuo-spatial perception: a TMS study in normal individuals, *Neuroreport* **12** (2001), 2605–2607.

[41] G.R. Fink, J.C. Marshall, P.H. Weiss and K. Zilles, The neural basis of vertical and horizontal line bisection judgments: an fMRI study of normal volunteers, *Neuroimage* **14** (2001), 59–67.

[42] J. Fleming and M. Behrmann, Visuospatial neglect in normal subjects: altered spatial representations induced by a perceptual illusion, *Neuropsychologia* **36** (1998), 469–475.

[43] T. Fujii, R. Fukatsu, A. Yamadori and I. Kimura, Effect of age on the line bisection test, *J Clin Exp Neuropsychol* **17** (1995), 941–944.

[44] R. Fukatsu, T. Fujii, I. Kimura, S. Saso and K. Kogure, Effects of hand and spatial conditions on visual line bisection, *Tohoku J Exp Med* **161** (1990), 329–333.

[45] G.M. Gauthier, J.M. Hofferer, W.F. Hoyt and L. Stark, Visual-motor adaptation. Quantitative demonstration in patients with posterior fossa involvement, *Arch Neurol* **36** (1979), 155–160.

[46] M. Girardi, R.D. McIntosh, C. Michel, G. Vallar and Y. Rossetti, Sensorimotor effects on central space representation: prism adaptation influences haptic and visual representations in normals subjects, *Neuropsychologia* **42** (2004), 1477–1487.

[47] P.W. Halligan and J.C. Marshall, Line bisection in visuo-spatial neglect: disproof of a conjecture, *Cortex* **25** (1989), 517–521.

[48] P.W. Halligan, L. Manning and J.C. Marshall, Hemispheric activation vs spatio-motor cueing in visual neglect: a case study, *Neuropsychologia* **29** (1991), 165–176.

[49] P.W. Halligan and J.C. Marshall, Spatial compression in visual neglect: a case study, *Cortex* **27** (1991), 623–629.

[50] M. Harvey and A.D. Milner, Residual perceptual distortion in recovered hemispatial neglect, *Neuropsychologia* **37** (1999), 745–750.

[51] M. Harvey, T.D. Pool, M.J. Roberson and B. Olk, Effects of visible and invisible cueing procedures on perceptual judgments in young and elderly subjects, *Neuropsychologia* **38** (2000), 22–31.

[52] M. Harvey, T. Kramer-McCaffery, L. Dow, P.J. Murphy and I.D. Gilchrist, Categorisation of perceptual and premotor neglect patients across different tasks: is there strong evidence for a dichotomy? *Neuropsychologia* **40** (2002), 1387–1395.

[53] K.M. Heilman and E. Valenstein, Mechanisms underlying hemispatial neglect, *Ann Neurol* **5** (1979), 166–170.

[54] K. Heilman, R.T. Watson and E. Valenstein, Neglect and related disorders, in: *Clinical Neuropsychology*, K.M. Heilman and E. Valenstein, eds, Oxford University Press, New York, 1993, pp. 279–336.

[55] R. Held, Exposure-History as a factor in maintaining stability of perception and coordination, *J Neuro Mental Disease* **132** (1961), 26–32.

[56] R. Held and S.J. Freedman, Plasticity in human sensori-motor control, *Science* **142** (1963), 455–462.

[57] R. Held and A. Hein, Movement produced stimulation in the development of visually guided behaviour, *J comp Physiol Psychol* **56** (1963), 872–876.

[58] K. Inoue, R. Kawashima, K. Satoh, S. Kinomura, R. Goto, M. Sugiura, M. Ito and H. Fukuda, Activity in the parietal area during visuomotor learning with optical rotation, *Neuroreport* **8** (1997), 3979–3983.

[59] M. Jeannerod and Y. Rossetti, Visuomotor coordination as a dissociable visual function: experimental and clinical evidence, in: *Visual perceptual defect*, C. Kennard, ed., I.P.R. Baillere Tindall Ltd, Baillere's Clinical Neurology, 1993, pp. 439–460.

[60] G. Jewell and M.E. McCourt, Pseudoneglect: a review and meta-analysis of performance factors in line bisection tasks, *Neuropsychologia* **38** (2000), 93–110.

[61] H.O. Karnath, D. Sievering and M. Fetter, The interactive contribution of neck muscle proprioception and vestibular stimulation to subjective "Straight ahead" orientation in man, *Exp Brain Res* **101** (1994), 140–146.

[62] H.O. Karnath, M. Fetter and J. Dichgans, Ocular exploration of space as a function of neck proprioceptive and vestibular input – observations in normal subjects and patients with neglect after parietal lesions, *Exp Brain Res* **109** (1996), 333–342.

[63] H.O. Karnath, M. Himmelbach and M.T. Perenin, Neglect-like behaviour in healthy subjects: dissociation of space exploration and goal-directed pointing after vestibular stimulation, *Exp Brain Res* **153** (2003), 231,238.

[64] A.S. Kornheiser, Adaptation to laterally displaced vision: a review, *Psychol Bull* **83** (1976), 783–816.

[65] K. Kurata and E. Hoshi, Reacquisition deficits in prism adaptation after muscimol microinjection into the ventral premotor cortex of monkeys, *J Neurophysiol* **81** (1999), 1927–1938.

[66] J.R. Lackner, Influence of abnormal postural and sensory conditions on human sensorimotor localization, *Environ Biol Med* **2** (1976), 137–177.

[67] B. Laeng and M. Peters, Cerebral lateralization for the processing of spatial coordinates and categories in left-and right-handers, *Neuropsychologia* **33** (1995), 421–439.

[68] D.J. Lewkowicz and G. Turkewitz, Intersensory interaction in newborns: modification of visual preferences following exposure to sound, *Child Dev* **52** (1981), 827–832.

[69] J. Luauté, C. Michel, G. Rode, D. Boisson, P.W. Halligan, N. Costes, F. Lavenne and Y. Rossetti, Cerebral plasticity induced by prismatic adaptation in neglect patients. A PET study, in: Proceeding of third world congress in neurological rehabilitation, Venice Italy, 2002.

[70] J. Luauté, C. Michel, G. Rode, L. Pisella, S. Jacquin-Courtois, N. Costes, F. Cotton, D. Le Bars, D. Boisson, P.W. Halligan and Y. Rossetti, Functional anatomy of the therapeutic effects of prism adaptation on unilateral neglect, submitted.

[71] K.E. Luh, Line bisection and perceptual asymmetries in normal individuals: What you see is not what you get, *Neuropsychology* **9** (1995), 435–448.

[72] M.S. MacLeod and O.H. Turnbull, Motor and perceptual factors in pseudoneglect, *Neuropsychologia* **37** (1999), 707–713.

[73] A. Maravita, J. McNeil, P. Malhotra, R. Greenwood, M. Husain and J. Driver, Prism adaptation can improve contralesional tactile perception in neglect, *Neurology* **60** (2003), 1829–1831.

[74] R.S. Marshall, R.M. Lazar, J.W. Krakauer and R. Sharma, Stimulus context in hemineglect, *Brain* **121** (1998), 2003–2210.

[75] T.A. Martin, J.G. Keating, H.P. Goodkin, A.J. Bastian and W.T. Thach, Throwing while looking through prisms. I. Focal olivocerebellar lesions impair adaptation, *Brain* **119** (1996), 1183–1198.

[76] J.B. Mattingley, J.L. Bradshaw and J.A. Bradshaw, Horizontal visual motion modulates focal attention in left unilateral spatial neglect, *J Neurol Neurosurg Psychiatry* **57** (1994), 1228–1235.

[77] J.B. Mattingley, J.L. Bradshaw and J.A. Bradshaw, The effects of unilateral visuospatial neglect on perception of Muller-Lyer illusory figures, *Perception* **24** (1995), 415–433.

[78] M.E. McCourt and G. Jewell, Visuospatial attention in line bisection: stimulus modulation of pseudoneglect, *Neuropsychologia* **37** (1999), 843–855.

[79] R.D. McIntosh, Y. Rossetti and A.D. Milner, Prism adaptation improves chronic visual and haptic neglect: a single case study, *Cortex* **38** (2002), 309–320.

[80] A.N. Meltzoff and R.W. Borton, Intermodal matching by human neonates, *Nature* **282** (1979), 403–404.

[81] P.R. Meudell and M. Greenhalgh, Age related differences in left and right hand skill and in visuo-spatial performance: their possible relationships to the hypothesis that the right hemisphere ages more rapidly than the left, *Cortex* **23** (1987), 431–445.

[82] C. Michel, L. Pisella, P.W. Halligan, J. Luaute, G. Rode, D. Boisson and Y. Rossetti, Simulating unilateral neglect in normals using prism adaptation: implications for theory, *Neuropsychologia* **41** (2003), 25–39.

[83] C. Michel, Y. Rossetti, G. Rode and C. Tilikete, After-effects of visuo-manual adaptation to prisms on body posture in normal subjects, *Exp Brain Res* **148** (2003), 219–226.

[84] C. Michel, L. Pisella, C. Prablanc, G. Rode and Y. Rossetti, Enhancing visuo-motor adaptation by reducing error signals: Single-step (aware) versus multiple-step (unaware) exposure to wedge prisms, submitted.

[85] C. Michel, P. Vernet, G. Courtine, Y. Ballay and T. Pozzo, Both cognitive and sensori-motor after-effects of prism adaptation during goal directed locomotion? Submitted.

[86] A.D. Milner, Animal models for the syndrome of spatial neglect, in: *Neurophysiological and neuropsychological aspects of spatial neglect*, M. Jeannerod, ed., Elsevier, Amsterdam, 1987, pp. 259–288.

[87] A.D. Milner, M. Brechmann and L. Pagliarini, To halve and to halve not: an analysis of line bisection judgements in normal subjects, *Neuropsychologia* **30** (1992), 515–526.

[88] A.D. Milner, M. Harvey and C.L. Pritchard, Visual size processing in spatial neglect, *Exp Brain Res* **123** (1998), 192–200.

[89] S. Miyauchi, H. Egusa, M. Amagase, K. Sekiyama, T. Imaruoka and T. Tashiro, Adaptation to left-right reversed vision rapidly activates ipsilateral visual cortex in humans, *J Physiol* **98** (2004), 207–219.

[90] A.P. Morris, A. Kritikos, N. Berberovic, L. Pisella, C.D. Chambers and J.B. Mattingley, Prism adaptation and spatial attention: a study of visual search in normals and patients with unilateral neglect, *Cortex* **40** (2004), 703–721.

[91] M. Oliveri, E. Bisiach, F. Brighina, A. Piazza, V. La Bua, D. Buffa and B. Fierro, rTMS on the unaffected hemisphere transiently reduces controlesional visuospatial hemineglect, *Neurology* **57** (2001), 1338–1340.

[92] J. Piaget, La naissance de l'intelligence chez l'enfant, Actualités pédagogiques et psychologiques, Delachaux and Niestlé, eds, Neuchâtel – Paris, 1977.

[93] L. Pisella, G. Rode, A. Farne, D. Boisson and Y. Rossetti, Dissociated long lasting improvements of straight-ahead pointing and line bisection tasks in two hemineglect patients, *Neuropsychologia* **40** (2002), 327–334.

[94] L. Pisella, C. Michel, H. Gréa, C. Tilikete, A. Vighetto and Y. Rossetti, Preserved prism adaptation following a bilateral lesion of the posterior parietal cortex: Cognitive versus adaptive reaction to prisms, *Exp Brain Res* **156** (2004), 399–408.

[95] L. Pisella, Y. Rossetti, C. Michel, G. Rode, D. Boisson, D. Pelisson and C. Tilikete, Ipsidirectional impairment of prism adaptation after unilateral lesion of anterior cerebellum, *Neurology* **65** (2005), 150–152.

[96] W. Prinzmetal and A. Wilson, The effect of attention on phenomenal length, *Perception* **26** (1997), 193–205.

[97] P.A. Reuter-Lorenz, M. Kinsbourne and M. Moscovitch, Hemispheric control of spatial attention, *Brain Cogn* **12** (1990), 240–266.

[98] P.A. Reuter-Lorenz and M.I. Posner, Components of neglect from right-hemisphere damage: an analysis of line bisection, *Neuropsychologia* **28** (1990), 327–333.

[99] P. Reuter-Lorenz, New visions of the aging mind and brain, *Trends Cogn Sci* **6** (2002), 394.

[100] H. Richter, S. Magnusson, K. Imamura, M. Fredrikson, M. Okura, Y. Watanabe and B. Langstrom, Long-term adaptation to prism-induced inversion of the retinal images, *Exp Brain Res* **144** (2002), 445–457.

[101] I.H., Robertson, R. Tegner, S.J. Goodrich and C. Wilson, Walking trajectory and hand movements in unilateral left neglect: a vestibular hypothesis, *Neuropsychologia* **32** (1994), 1495–1502.

[102] D.L. Robinson and C. Kertzman, Visuospatial attention: effects of age, gender and spatial reference, *Neuropsychologia* **28** (1990), 291–301.

[103] G. Rode, Y. Rossetti, L. Li and D. Boisson, Improvement of mental imagery after prism exposure in neglect: a case study, *Behav Neurol* **11** (1998), 251–258.

[104] G. Rode, Y. Rossetti and D. Boisson, Improvement of mental imagery after prism exposure in neglect: a case study, *Behavioural Neurology* **11** (1999), 251–258.

[105] G. Rode, L. Pisella, Y. Rossetti, A. Farne and D. Boisson, Bottom-up transfer of sensory-motor plasticity to recovery of spatial cognition: visuomotor adaptation and spatial neglect, *Prog Brain Res* **142** (2003), 273–287.

[106] Y. Rossetti, G. Rode, L. Pisella, A. Farne, L. Li, D. Boisson and M.T. Perenin, Prism adaptation to a rightward optical deviation rehabilitates left hemispatial neglect, *Nature* **395** (1998), 166–169.

[107] Y. Rossetti and G. Rode, Reducing spatial neglect by visual and other sensory manipulations: non-cognitive (physiological) routes to the rehabilitation of cognitive disorder, in: *The cognitive and neuronal bases of spatial neglect*, H.O. Karnath, A.D. Milner and G. Vallar, eds, Oxford University Press, New York, 2002, pp. 375–396.

[108] Y. Rossetti, S. Jacquin-Courtois, G. Rode, H. Ota, C. Michel and D. Boisson, Does action make the link between number and space representation? Visuo-manual adaptation improves number bisection in unilateral neglect, *Psychol Sci* **15** (2004), 426–430.

[109] D.J. Scarisbrick, J.R. Tweedy and G. Kuslansky, Hand preference and performance effects on line bisection, *Neuropsychologia* **25** (1987), 695–699.

[110] K. Sekiyama, S. Miyauchi, T. Imaruoka, H. Egusa and T. Tashiro, Body image as a visuomotor transformation device revealed in adaptation to reversed vision, *Nature* **407** (2000), 374–377.

[111] J.E. Shuren, D.H. Jacobs and K.M. Heilman, The influence of center of mass effect on the distribution of spatial attention in the vertical and horizontal dimensions, *Brain Cogn* **34** (1997), 293–300.

[112] Y. Sugita, Global plasticity in adult visual cortex following reversal of visual input, *Nature* **380** (1996), 523–526.

[113] W.T. Thach, H.P. Goodkin and J.G. Keating, The cerebellum and the adaptive coordination of movement, *Annu Rev Neurosci* **15** (1992), 403–442.

[114] G. Thut, A. Nietzel and A. Pascual-Leone, Dorsal posterior parietal rTMS affects voluntary orienting of visuospatial attention, *Cereb Cortex* **15** (2005), 628–638.

[115] C. Tilikete, G. Rode, Y. Rossetti, J. Pichon, L. Li and D. Boisson, Prism adaptation to a rightward optical deviation improves postural imbalance in left-hemiparetic patients, *Current Biology* **11** (2001), 1–5.

[116] A. Toraldo, A ruler for measuring representational space, *Visual Cognition* **10** (2003), 567–603.

[117] G. Vallar, M.L. Rusconi, L. Bignamini, G. Geminiani and D. Perani, Anatomical correlates of visual and tactile extinction in humans: a clinical CT scan study, *J Neurol Neurosurg Psychiatry* **57** (1994), 464–470.

[118] G. Vallar, C. Guariglia and M.L. Rusconi, Modulation of the neglect syndrome by sensory stimulation, in: *Parietal Lobe Contribution to Orientation in 3D Space*, P. Thier and H.O. Karnath, eds, Parietal Lobe Contribution to Orientation in 3D Space, Springer, Heidelberg, 1997, pp. 555–579.

[119] B. Wallace, L.E. Melamed and C. Kaplan, Movement and illumination factors in adaptation to viewing, *Percept Psychophys* **13** (1973), 164–168.

[120] R.T. Watson, B.D. Miller and K.M. Heilman, Nonsensory neglect, *Ann Neurol* **3** (1978), 505–508.

[121] M.J. Weiner, M. Hallet and H.H. Funkenstein, Adaptation to lateral displacement of vision in patients with lesions of the central nervous system, *Neurology* **33** (1983), 766–772.

[122] R.B. Welch, C.S. Cho and D.R. Heinrich, Evidence for a three-component model of prism adaptation, *J Exp Psychol* **103** (1974), 700–705.

[123] M. Zorzi, K. Priftis and C. Umilta, Brain damage: neglect disrupts the mental number line, *Nature* **417** (2002), 138–139.

Virtual reality applications for the remapping of space in neglect patients

Caterina Ansuini[a], Andrea Cristiano Pierno[a], Dean Lusher[b] and Umberto Castiello[a,c,*]
[a]*Dipartimento di Psicologia Generale, Università di Padova, Italy*
[b]*Department of Psychology, University of Melbourne, Australia*
[c]*Department of Psychology, Royal Holloway, University of London, UK*

Received 1 November 2005
Revised 13 April 2006
Accepted 22 June 2006

Abstract. *Purpose:* The aims of the present article were the following: (i) to provide some evidence of the potential of virtual reality (VR) for the assessment, training and recovery of hemispatial neglect; (ii) to present data from our laboratory which seem to confirm that the clinical manifestation of neglect can be improved by using VR techniques; and (iii) to ascertain the neural bases of this improvement.
Methods: We used a VR device (DataGlove) interfaced with a specially designed computer program which allowed neglect patients to reach and grasp a real object while simultaneously observing the grasping of a virtual object located within a virtual environment by a virtual hand. The virtual hand was commanded in real time by their real hand.
Results: After a period of training, hemispatial neglect patients coded the visual stimuli within the neglected space in an identical fashion as those presented within the preserved portions of space. However it was also found that only patients with lesions that spared the inferior parietal/superior temporal regions were able to benefit from the virtual reality training.
Conclusions: It was concluded that using VR it is possible to re-create links between the affected and the nonaffected space in neglect patients. Furthermore, that specific regions may play a crucial role in the recovery of space that underlies the improvement of neglect patients when trained with virtual reality. The implications of these results for determining the neural bases of a higher order attentional and/or spatial representation, and for the treatment of patients with unilateral neglect are discussed.

Keywords: Visual neglect, rehabilitation, virtual reality, reach-to-grasp, space remapping

1. Introduction

Unilateral neglect is a common consequence of damage to the right hemisphere in humans [1]. The syndrome of neglect is characterised by a failure to respond to stimuli in the contralesional half of space, with patients often behaving as if these stimuli do not exist. Although neglect is most commonly seen after damage involving the right inferior parietal lobe near the temporal-parietal junction, it may also occur after damage to the frontal lobes, temporal lobes, or subcortical structures [1]. The real life implications of neglect can be devastating, with patients failing to eat food off the left side of the plate, only dressing the right half of their bodies, and often being unaware of half of their world. Understanding the functional and neurological bases of unilateral neglect has been an imposing task and in recent years several promising advances have been made in its treatment as reviewed by various authors within this special issue. Further, although improvements in unilateral neglect have been reported with a number of patients with various lesions, it remains to be seen precisely what spared tissue could be responsible for the recovery of space.

---
*Corresponding author: Umberto Castiello, Dipartimento di Psicologia Generale, Università di Padova, Via Venezia, 8, 35131, Padova, Italy. E-mail: umberto.castiello@unipd.it.

Here we propose the use of virtual reality (VR) techniques as a mean for improving the visual representation of space deficits observed in hemispatial neglect patients and to ascertain possible neural loci for recovery. As explained below the impetus for using such techniques comes from recent VR applications which appear to be successful as to rehabilitate neglect.

1.1. Virtual reality applications and neglect

Virtual reality entails the use of advanced technologies, including computers and various multimedia peripherals, to produce a simulated (i.e., virtual) environment that users may perceive as comparable to real world objects and events. Users interact with displayed images, move and manipulate virtual objects, and perform other actions in a way that engenders a feeling of actual presence, and immerses their senses in the simulated environment. Virtual reality may be delivered to the user via a variety of different technologies (e.g., computer monitor, head-mounted display) that differ in their ability to determine a sense of immersion within the simulated environment. Until recently, the application of VR technology was limited by the lack of inexpensive, easy-to-maintain and easy-to-use VR systems, but recent technological developments have led to decreases in cost and increases in ease of use and in the availability of off-the-shelf programs.

An active area of research using VR is concerned with its use as an intervention tool in neurological rehabilitation [19,21]. In this respect, VR has the potential to assist current rehabilitation techniques in addressing the impairments associated with brain damage.

An essential part of the rehabilitation process is remediation of cognitive and motor deficits in order to improve the functional ability of the patient. The ultimate goal is to enable the patient to achieve greater independence in activities related to daily performance skills. In this respect, VR has the potential to be used as a novel modality in rehabilitation assessment and intervention due to a number of unique features. For one, the ability to objectively measure behaviour in challenging but safe and ecologically-valid environments, while maintaining strict experimental control over stimulus delivery. For another, the capacity to individualize treatment needs, while providing increased standardization of assessment and re-training protocols. Furthermore, virtual environments can provide repeated learning trials and offer the capacity to gradually increase the complexity of tasks while decreasing the support/feedback provided by the therapist.

Recently, a few attempts have been made to create VR environments which could be utilised for the rehabilitation of the neglect syndrome [13,26], but only a few experimental studies have been conducted. For example, Weiss and colleagues [27], see also [14] investigated the feasibility of using a PC-based, non-immersive VR system (i.e. a system in which the user has a reduced sense of actual presence in and control over the simulated environment) for training individuals with unilateral spatial neglect to cross streets in a safe and vigilant manner. A street crossing virtual environment was programmed as to run on a desktop computer, with successively graded levels of difficulty that provide users with an opportunity to decide when it is safe to cross a virtual street. The results indicated that the VR street crossing performance of neglect patients showed the effects of training. Specifically, there was improvement in the number of times participants looked to the left. More importantly, most patients made fewer accidents during the virtual street crossing. The results of this study clearly show that the VR intervention was effective both in terms of improving visual – spatial performance as measured in this study and for some improvement in the ability to cross a real street.

Kwanguk Kim and colleagues [11] deviced a virtual environment (VE) to assess and train unilateral neglect patients. This VE was composed by a branch road and a ball. A calibration and a main task were administered to patients. The patients' subjective visual middle line was measured during the calibration task whereas in the main task the participants had to detect the ball using their gaze (moving a small cross according to the subject's head motion). To measure the degree of visual neglect, the ball moved to a random direction with a specific velocity and distance. Visual and auditory cues helped the patients to detect the ball. The degree of difficulty was adjusted according to the result of the patient's achievement. The results suggest that in the VE patients could use a wider field of view. In particular, patients showed no difference in tracking the ball in both the right and left visual field.

All in all the above studies show that through VR programs it might be possibile to assess, train and rehabilitate hemispatial neglect. In the following sections we shall describe an experiment carried out with a VR methodology developed within our laboratory [3, 8] which might be used to rehabilitate neglect and to ascertain which brain areas might be implicated in such recovery. We created a real-time coincidence of the movement of the patients' real hand with the representation of a virtual hand moving within a virtual environment, so that the patient could be trained to use the virtual image of their hand to guide their real hand in the neglected space. The results indicate that after a period of training the patients coded in an identical fashion stimuli presented within the preserved and the neglected space.

2. Methods

2.1. Subjects

Subjects were six patients with left visual neglect following right hemisphere stroke (Table 1). Patients were classified on the basis of neurological assessment, behavioural observation, and standard clinical tests (Table 1). All patients were right-handed and had normal or corrected-to-normal vision with no signs of severe gaze palsy, dementia, or previous neurological illness. Lesions were confirmed by CT scan. Lesions were plotted (Fig. 1) using the template of Damasio and Damasio [4]. On the basis of lesion location we divided the patients into a dorsal fronto-parietal group (FP) and a ventral temporo-parietal group (TP). In addition three neurologically healthy control subjects were included. One-way analyses of variance (ANOVA) revealed that there was no significant difference ($F_{(2,2)} < 1$, ns) between the mean ages of the neglect patients for the FP group (69 years), the TP group (73 years) and the controls (73 years), or for the mean days after stroke for the FP and the TP neglect patients [FP: 59; TP: 58; $F_{(1,2)} < 1$, ns]. All subjects gave informed written consent before testing began.

The two groups of patients with neglect were well matched for degree of neglect (see Table 1). For example, on the star cancellation test the FP patients found a mean of only 17 targets (range, 12.2–21.2) out of 54, all on the right side of the sheet. Similarly, the TP patients found a mean of 13 out of 54 targets (range, 8–20), again all on the right side of the sheet.

2.2. Apparatus

The apparatus consisted of a monitor placed on top of a hollow box into which the subjects could reach (see Fig. 2). The computer screen was located approximately 50 cm from the subject's eyes. Vision of the reaching limb within the box was occluded by means of a black partition between the reaching limb and eyes. The targets for grasping consisted of either a) a real object (white polystyrene sphere 8 cm in diameter), resting on the table at a distance of 30 cm from a starting position located 20 cm in front of the subject, or b) a virtual object presented on the computer screen. The virtual object was an exact replica of the real object; its size was manipulated such that it had the same appearance as the target object for each given distance.

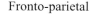
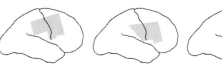
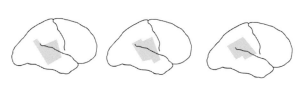

Fig. 1. Reconstruction of lesion location in the frontoparietal (FP) (top) and the temporo-parietal (TP) (bottom) patients who took part in this study.

2.3. Virtual reality devices and movement recordings

A data glove (Virtual Realities: Fifth Dimension Technologies, Irvine, CA) allowed the subjects to control the virtual hand that moved in real time within a computer-generated environment. The sampling rate was 200 Hz. All devices were operated via PC. We were able to resolve issues of real-virtual compatibility that can arise when the glove is worn by different subjects with different-sized hands. Reaching movements were recorded using a magnetic sensor placed on the wrist (Flock of Birds, Ascension Technology). Recordings of marker position were taken at 100 Hz, and stored in the computer for analysis offline. Following the testing, movement trajectories were computed from the stored data.

2.4. Procedure

Subjects sat at the table and reached to grasp either the real or the virtual object. As per Fig. 2, the real and virtual objects could be located either centrally (mid-sagittal plane), or 30° to the left or right of midline. The experiment was carried out in three sessions within the same day, one in the morning and two in the afternoon.

Table 1
Demographic and clinical data for the neglect patients who participated in the Experiment

Patient no.	Age	Sex	Lesion	Visual field	Post stroke (days)		Clinical tests		
							Line bisection test (mm)	Albert's line test (/36)	Star cancellation test (/54)
FP patients									
1	67	M	FP	Normal	56		12.2	15	13
2	69	M	FP	Normal	64		17.3	34	24
3	71	F	FP	Normal	58		21.2	26	14
						Mean	16.9	25	17
TP patients									
1	77	M	TP	Normal	59		10.8	22	8
2	70	M	TP	Normal	55		13.4	36	20
3	73	F	TP	Normal	61		18.7	32	13
						Mean	14.3	30	13

Notes. FP: fronto-parietal; TP: temporal-parietal.

2.4.1. Session 1: Baseline task

Subjects performed one of two types of task within either the real or virtual environment. An object (or its virtual counterpart) was presented in one of the three positions (midline or $+/-30°$ laterally), and in the 'sensory' task subjects were required to report the location in which the object appeared (left, right, or center). In the 'motor' task subjects had to reach out and grasp the object. Each participant performed four blocks, one of each combination of real/virtual and sensory/motor. The baseline task consisted of 10 trials at each location in each of four blocks. The total number of trials in the baseline task was thus 120. The experimental tasks were preceded by a block of randomly-determined 20 practice trials. Stimulus presentation was counterbalanced across participants.

2.4.2. Session 2: Training task

Subjects were required to reach for the real object located at one of the three locations within the real environment while simultaneously viewing the real-time virtual representation of the hand. While moving towards the real object, subjects observed the virtual hand moving toward the virtual object. This task consisted of two types of trial: a) congruent trials in which the real and virtual objects were spatially congruent (Fig. 3, top panels), or b) incongruent trials in which the real and virtual objects occupied different spatial locations (Fig. 3, lower panels). Crucial to the present study were the left incongruent trials (Fig. 3, panels f and g), in which the target was located to the left within the virtual environment whereas the real object appeared to the right or middle. We choose to give particular emphasis to this type of trials because we reasoned that the match between the 'good' proprioceptive input coming from the movement performed towards the object located in the preserved parts of the visual field (i.e., right and centre) and the visual input coming from the virtual hand moving towards the 'bad' portion of the visual field (i.e. left) would create a novel association. This novel association could be used later on to reach towards the 'bad' portion of space during the 'congruous left' trials and those incongruous trials in which a movement towards the real stimulus located on the left was required. Subjects performed 240 trials, 20 per each location/trial combination. Order of object presentation was counterbalanced. In order to avoid fatigue effects participants were given a 5 min. rest every 60 trials.

2.4.3. Session 3: Post-training sensory task

Subjects were required to perform the 'sensory' task in virtual and real conditions as in Session 1 to measure the effect of the training on performance of the sensory task.

2.4.4. Criteria for accuracy

Accuracy was analysed in the sensory and motor tasks (Sessions 1 and 3). Performance in the sensory task was considered correct when subjects successfully reported the location in which the object appeared within four seconds of its presentation. A correct movement was considered to be one in which the subject completed a successful reach and grasp, closing their hand around the target within four seconds of its appearance.

3. Results

3.1. Baseline tasks

For the baseline session (Session 1), the percentages of trials in which the object was successfully detected

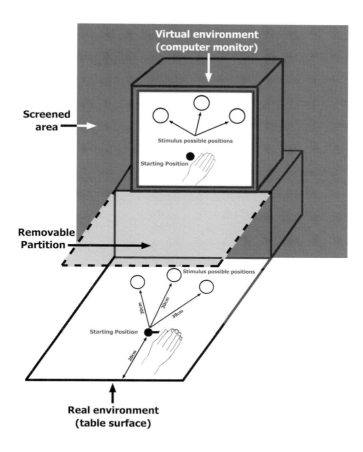

Fig. 2. Schematic of the experimental setup.

(sensory task) and in which the reaching movement was successfully carried out (motor tasks) were analyzed using ANOVA. The between-subjects factor was group (TP, FP, controls). The within-subjects factors were type of task (sensory, motor), environment (real, virtual), and location (left, middle, right). Post-hoc contrasts were performed using t-tests. Bonferroni corrections were applied (Alpha level, $p < 0.05$). For this analysis, the interaction group by location was significant ($F_{(1,2)} = 43.21$, $p < 0.0001$). Post-hoc contrasts revealed that both the FP and TP patients showed a clear inability to respond to leftward targets when compared to control subjects ($p_s < 0.01$). However, the performance for the neglect patients and the control subjects to targets presented to the right and to the centre in both the baseline sensory task and the baseline motor task was similar ($p_s > 0.5$). Similarly, for the right and the centre targets no differences in performance were found between the two neglect groups and the control groups ($p_s > 0.05$). These results confirmed the presence of similar severe unilateral neglect in both groups of patients prior to training with VR (see Fig. 4).

3.2. Training task

During the training task subjects were exposed to the spatially congruous and spatially incongruous trials (see Fig. 3). An ANOVA was carried out to test the effect of the left-incongruous trials (see Fig. 3f and 3g) on the performance for the left-congruous trials (see Fig. 3a) and the center-incongruous and right-incongruous trials (see Fig. 3d, 3e). In these latter two types of trials a movement towards the real stimulus located on the left was required. For this analysis the data for left-congruous trials and for center-incongruous and right-incongruous trials were divided based on occurrence (before or after) relative to the left-incongruous trials. Though the exact number varied,

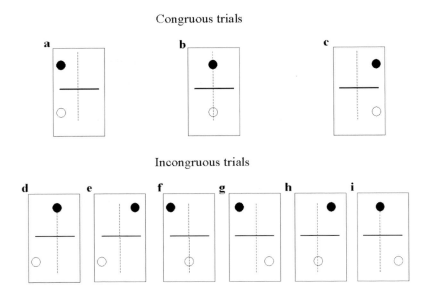

Fig. 3. Schematic of the various trial types in the training task. Virtual targets are shown as black circles, real targets as white circles. The top three panels represent congruent trials in which the location of real and virtual targets matched. The bottom six panels represent incongruent trials in which the locations of real and virtual targets did not match. The crucial left incongruent trials are represented in the third and fourth panels from the left – bottom row.

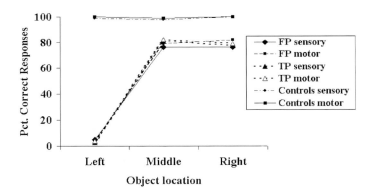

Fig. 4. Performance of patients and controls in baseline sensory and motor response tasks, real environment only. Percentage of correct responses is plotted as a function of group, location and task.

all subjects experienced at least 8 left-incongruous trials before the left-congruous, center-incongruous, and right-incongruous trials. Here, the between-subjects factor was group (FP, TP, controls) and the within-subjects factors were type of trial (congruous, incongruous), occurrence (before training vs. after training), and location (left, middle, right). Post-hoc contrasts were carried out using t-test. Bonferroni's corrections were applied (Alpha level $= p < 0.05$). The interaction between group, occurrence and location was significant ($F_{(1,2)} = 23.18$, $p < 0.0001$). Post-hoc contrasts revealed that there was a clear dissociation in performance for the training tasks for the FP and the TP patients (see Fig. 5). That is only the FP group show a significant improvement in their responses to leftward targets after training ($p_s < 0.01$). The lack of interaction between the main factor type of trial and the other measures signifies that the increase in percentage of correct responses for left trials was similar for both congruous and incongruous trials. In contrast, the TP group failed to show any signs of improvement after having experienced the left-incongruous trials ($p > 0.05$). Figure 5 shows that patients in the TP group hardly move at all towards the leftward target whenever it appeared on the left in virtual space, and failed to attain the leftward target even when it appeared in the central location in virtual space. The administration of right – and centre – incongruous trials did not bring to any sign of improvement on the performance for subsequent leftwards trials (congruous and incongruous; $p_s > 0.05$). Post – hoc analysis revealed also that there were no differences in the performance for the control group between congruous and incongruous trials, regardless of whether they experienced the incongruous left trials.

3.3. Post-training sensory task

In order to verify that an improvement also occurred for tests that did not require a motor response, in a third session FP and TP patients were asked to repeat the sensory task performed in the first session within the real space. This took place 1–2 hours after the training session. An ANOVA with group (FP, TP) as between subjects factor and session (first and third) and location (left, centre and right) as within-subjects factors was performed. The three way interaction group by session by location ($F_{(1,2)} = 24.12$, $p < 0.001$) revealed that the percentage of correct responses for the left trials was significantly greater for the third session than for the first session only for the FP group ($F_{(1,2)} = 24.12$, $p < 0.001$; 5% vs. 83%). No improvement was noticed for the TP group (4% vs. 5%; $p > 0.5$). This suggests that exposure to left-incongruous trials also had an effect on the perceptual component of neglect, but only for the FP group (Fig. 6).

4. Discussion

We examined the effect of VR manipulation in patients with left neglect. After being exposed to a certain number of trials in which the virtual object was located to the left within the virtual environment and the real object appeared to the right or in the middle in the real environment (i.e., left-incongruous trials), neglect patients were subsequently able to reach toward objects located to the portion of space of which they were previously unaware (i.e., the left hemifield). These results show an active process stimulated by VR resulting in the recalibration of visuomotor coordination and the ability to act on the organisation of high levels spatial representations such as those usually impaired in patients with visual neglect.

Further, the present study addressed the issue of the neurological bases of space recovery in unilateral neglect. We observed that patients with fronto-parietal lesions (the FP group), sparing the posterior inferior parietal and superior temporal regions, were able to acquire the ability to respond into the left visual field. However, this benefit did not accrue to patients with damage involving the posterior IPL and superior temporal lobe (the TP group). We now discuss these results in terms of the putative representational functions of areas of the posterior half of the brain.

To address this issue, it is worthwhile to consider what processes are required in the recovery of space and to examine what regions of the brain might subserve these processes. Bearing in mind that recovery of space can also occur after vestibular [2] and somatosensory stimulation, the most likely candidate would be a region that represents space in a multimodal fashion. At least two such areas are known to exist in the human brain, namely the prefrontal cortex and the posterior parietal cortex. Yet, only the latter area was affected in any of the patients studied here.

The inferior parietal lobes in humans acquire multimodal information from all of visual, somatosensory, and auditory senses and have been hypothesised to represent a region of higher order spatial representation [5, 12,17]. This region thus seems uniquely poised to perform a major role in the function of recovering space. Note also that in both the present and past studies, the recovery of space effected through a motor task has transferred rather easily to other, more sensory-based tasks (e.g., verbal response). This supports the contention that the recovery of space is at an attentional or representational level rather than a purely motor or purely perceptual level.

A second alternative explanation might be that damage to cells in the IPL region of the TP group remotely affected the functioning of cells in the SPL as a consequence of the intimate connectivity of these two regions [15,25]. This in turn may have impaired the SPL in what might be its normal function. Indeed, it is well known that naturally occurring brain damage can have effects on brain areas outside of the lesion [10]. However, if one accepts this contention then it becomes difficult to explain why damage to the premotor cortex in the FP group did not also lead to such a disruption, given that it also possesses strong connections with the SPL [16]. Further, both groups of patients showed intact on-line monitoring and control of their movements once initiated, a function ascribed to the SPL [7,9,18, 22], suggesting that at least one major function of the SPL remained intact. Thus, we are also confident in dismissing this argument.

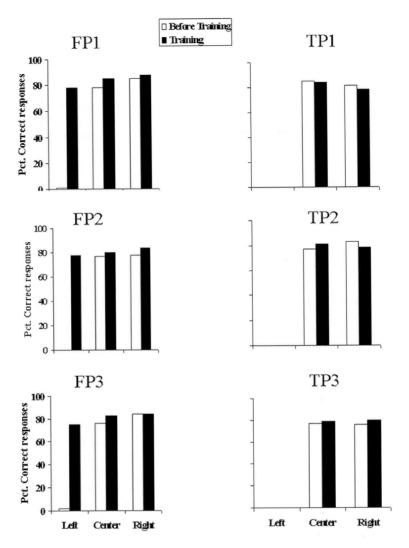

Fig. 5. Performance in the motor task prior to and after training. Correct responses to targets presented on the left, in the center, and on the right are plotted in the baseline (white bars) and post-training (black bars) sessions for individual patients in the FP (left column) and TP (right column) groups.

We suggest that the regions damaged in the TP group may play a crucial function in the specification of a target for an upcoming action in conjunction with attentional processes. In neglect, attention is typically diverted to the ipsilesional visual field and stimuli in the neglected field are ignored as targets for action. When these same stimuli are made to appear in central space, however, the attentional premotor requirement of target selection is enabled, allowing for the stimuli to be coded as the target of an upcoming action. However, when the inferior parietal/superior temporal regions are damaged, the result is an inability to recruit a motor plan for acting in the left side of space, despite the fact that the stimulus is now present in central vision.

The results of the present study suggest that attempts to treat unilateral neglect may be much more beneficial to those patients whose lesions spare the posterior IPL and possibly the superior aspects of the temporal lobe. A concern with this claim relates to the findings of previous studies involving attempts to improve unilateral neglect using prism adaptation [6,20,23]. In those studies, involving a similar shift in the perception of space as we engendered with our VR paradigm, some patients with temporo-parietal lesions did show improvements following training. Of those studies, precise localisa-

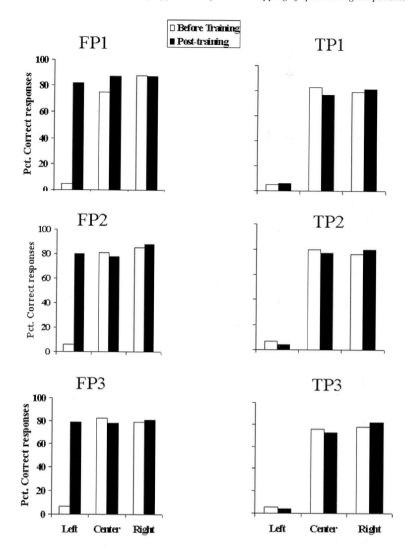

Fig. 6. Performance in the sensory task prior and after training. Conventions as in Fig. 5.

tion was only reported in Frassinetti et al. [6], however, in that case two of three patients whose lesions included the IPL did improve following training with prisms. One reason for the discrepancies across studies may have been the difficulty of the motor tasks involved (pointing in the prism studies versus reaching and grasping in the present study), or some more basic difference between the two techniques themselves. It would be beneficial to test our findings using larger samples of neglect patients, as well as to examine patients with varying lesion locations, and using different techniques, for the purpose of further clarifying these issues.

The question may also be raised as to why the VR training only led to improvement for leftward targets and not for targets presented in the center or right side of space. We suggest that the improvement in the former case resulted from the requirement to make movements into the previously neglected left side of space. Conversely, movements to the center or right side of space were not a novel occurrence, and so did not affect the ability to respond to these targets. Along these lines, it might be hypothesised that the VR training created a coincidence of the movement of the real hand and the hand's virtual image, allowing us to 'train' the patient to use the virtual image to guide their real hand in neglected space. This would presumably result in the formation of novel neural circuitry governing a novel mode of visuo-proprioceptive integration.

5. General conclusions

We here tested the ability of patients with unilateral neglect to recover space with the aid of virtual reality. The results of the present study suggest that space-recovery techniques such as virtual reality may lead to at least temporary relief for patients suffering from unilateral neglect. However, the usefulness of these techniques may depend, at least in part, on the integrity of structures in the inferior parietal/superior temporal lobe of the right hemisphere that may play a critical role in higher order attentional and/or spatial representation. Whereas FP patients showed a dramatic improvement in both motor and perceptual performance following training with virtual reality, TP patients did not benefit from the very same training. These results suggest that the recovery of space required for the recalibration of motor and perceptual responses into a neglected visual field may depend on the integrity of a multimodal attentional and/or spatial representation region in and around the right inferior parietal lobe. As the present study represents the first attempt to localise the areas responsible for the recovery of space, any conclusions reached must be cautious ones. Future studies using techniques such as virtual reality and prism adaptation will undoubtedly be needed to shed more light on both the treatment of neglect and the neural substrates responsible for its efficacy.

An important question is whether the improvement in the patients who took part in the current studies is transient or sustained. Various rehabilitation procedures using single applications of a variety of methods (caloric stimulation (e.g. [24]), neck vibration (e.g. [2]), optokinetic stimulation) have resulted in improvements lasting only a few minutes. Conversely, prism adaptation techniques can lead to improvements ranging from 2 hours to 5 weeks [6,23]. The patients of this study were given a pause ranging from 1 to 2 hours between the crucial second VR session and the final session in which the adaptation effects were still evident. Thus, we can be quite confident that the period of improvement produced by our VR manipulation lasted at least as long as the shortest period reported following prism adaptation and longer than the few minutes reported using other techniques. This suggests that VR techniques can potentially lead to long-lasting improvements in neglect patients, although the exact length of the amelioration will require further investigation.

Acknowledgements

The study was funded by the National Health and Medical Research Council (UC).

The presented data are part of a data set which has been published in full elsewhere (see [8]).

References

[1] E. Bisiach and G. Vallar, Hemineglect in humans, in: *Handbook of Neuropsychology*, (Vol. 1). F. Boller and J. Grafman, eds, Elsevier: Amsterdam, 1988, pp. 195–222.

[2] S. Cappa, R. Sterzi, G. Vallar and E. Bisiach, Remission of hemineglect and anosognosia during vestibular stimulation, *Neuropsychol* **25** (1987), 775–782.

[3] U. Castiello, D. Lusher, C. Burton, S. Glover and P. Disler, Improving left hemispatial neglect using virtual reality, *Neurology* **62** (2004), 1958–1962.

[4] H. Damasio and A.R. Damasio, *Lesion Analysis in Neuropsychology*, New York: Oxford University Press, 1989.

[5] J. Driver and P. Vuilleumier, Perceptual awareness and its loss in unilateral neglect and extinction, *Cognition* **79** (2001), 39–88.

[6] F. Frassinetti, V. Angeli, F. Meneghello, S. Avanzi and E. Ladavas, Long-lasting amelioration of visuospatial neglect by prism adaptation, *Brain* **125** (2002), 608–623.

[7] S. Glover, Separate visual representations in the planning and control of action, *Behav Brain Scie* **27** (2004), 3–28.

[8] S. Glover and U. Castiello, Recovering Space in Unilateral Neglect: A Neurological Dissociation Revealed by Virtual Reality, *Journal of Cognitive Neuroscience* **18** (2006), 833–843.

[9] H. Grea, L. Pisella, Y. Rossetti, M. Desmurget, C. Tilikete, S. Grafton, C. Prablanc and A. Vighetto, A lesion of the posterior parietal cortex disrupts on-line adjustments during aiming movements, *Neuropsychologia* **40** (2002), 2471–2480.

[10] B. Kolb and I.Q. Whishaw, *Fundamentals of human neuropsychology*, Freeman: New York, 2003.

[11] K. Kwanguk, K. Jaehun, K. Jeonghun, K. Deog Young, C. Won Hyek, S. Dong Ik, L. Jang Han, K. In Young and S. Kim, A virtual reality assessment and training system for unilateral neglect, *Cyberpsychol Behav* **7** (2004), 742–749.

[12] E. Ladavas, Functional and dynamic properties of visual peripersonal space, *Trends Cogn Sci* **6** (2002), 17–22.

[13] R.L. Myers and T.A. Bierig, Virtual reality and left hemineglect: A technology for assessment and therapy, *CyberPsychol Behav* **3** (2000), 465–468.

[14] Y. Naveh, N. Katz and P.L. Weiss, The effect of interactive virtual environment training on independent safe street crossing of right CVA patients with unilateral spatial neglect. Proceedings of the 3rd International Conference on Disability, Virtual Reality and Associated technologies, Alghero, Sardinia, September, 2000.

[15] D.N. Pandya and E. Yeterian, Architecture and connections of cortical association areas, in: *Cerebral Cortex Association and Auditory Cortices*, (Vol. 4), A. Peters and E. Jones, eds, 1985, pp. 3–62. New York: Plenum Press.

[16] R.E. Passingham, *The frontal lobes and voluntary action*, Oxford University Press: Oxford, UK, 1993.

[17] F. Pavani, E. Ladavas and J. Driver, Auditory and multisensory aspects of visuospatial neglect, *Trends Cogn Scie* **7** (2003), 407–414.

[18] L. Pisella, H. Grea, C. Tilikete, A. Vighetto, M. Desmurget, G. Rode, D. Boisson and Y. Rossetti, An automatic pilot for the hand in human posterior parietal cortex: Towards reinterpreting optic ataxia, *Nat Neurosci* **3** (2000), 729–736.

[19] A.A. Rizzo, M.T. Schultheis, K. Kerns and C. Mateer, Analysis of assets for virtual reality in neuropsychology, *Neuropsych rehab* **14** (2004), 207–239.

[20] G. Rode, Y. Rossetti and D. Boisson, Prism adaptation improves representational neglect, *Neuropsychologia* **39** (2001), 1250–1254.

[21] F.D. Rose, B.M. Brooks and A.A. Rizzo, Virtual reality in brain damage rehabilitation: review, *Cyberpsychol Behav* **8** (2005), 241–262.

[22] Y. Rossetti and L. Pisella, Several 'vision for action' systems: A guid to dissociating and integrating dorsal and ventral functions, in: *Attention and Performance XIX: Common mechanisms in perception and action*, W. Prinz and B. Hommel, eds, 2002, pp. 62–119. Oxford University Press: Oxford, UK.

[23] Y. Rossetti, G. Rode, L. Pisella, A. Farne, L. Li, D. Boisson and M.T. Perenni, Prism adaptation to a rightwards optical deviation rehabilitates left hemispatial neglect, *Nature* **395** (1998), 166–169.

[24] A.B. Rubens, Caloric stimulation and unilateral visual neglect, *Neurology* **35** (1985), 1019–1024.

[25] B. Seltzer and D.N. Pandya, Further observations on parieto-temporal connections in the rhesus monkey, *Exp Brain Res* **55** (1984), 301–312.

[26] P. Tripathi, K. Kahol, L.C. Baxter, T. McDaniel, A. Baker and S. Panchanathan, Rehabilitation of patients with hemispatial neglect using virtual – haptic feedback in virtual reality environment, accepted for publication at International Conference on Human – Computer Interfaces to be held in Las Vegas, 2005.

[27] P.L. Weiss, Y. Naveh and N. Katz, Design and testing of a virtual environment to train CVA patients with unilateral spatial neglect to cross a street safely, *Occup Ther Int* **10** (2003), 39–55.

Author Index Volume 24 (2006)

The issue number is given in front of the pagination

Ahn, S.H., see Jang, S.H. (2) 65–68
Ahn, Y.H., see Jang, S.H. (1) 25–29
Ahn, Y.H., see Jang, S.H. (2) 65–68
Almaguer-Melian, W., see Bergado, J.A. (2) 115–121
Ansuini, C., A.C. Pierno, D. Lusher and U. Castiello, Virtual reality applications for the remapping of space in neglect patients (4–6) 431–441
Antonucci, G., see Pizzamiglio, L. (4–6) 337–345
Azouvi, P., P. Bartolomeo, J.-M. Beis, D. Perennou, P. Pradat-Diehl and M. Rousseaux, A battery of tests for the quantitative assessment of unilateral neglect (4–6) 273–285

Bai, D., see Jang, S.H. (1) 25–29
Barth, T.M., see Byler, S.L. (3) 133–145
Bartolomeo, P., see Azouvi, P. (4–6) 273–285
Bazarian, J.J., C. Beck, B. Blyth, N. von Ahsen and M. Hasselblatt, Impact of creatine kinase correction on the predictive value of S-100B after mild traumatic brain injury (3) 163–172
Beck, C., see Bazarian, J.J. (3) 163–172
Beis, J.-M., see Azouvi, P. (4–6) 273–285
Bergado, J.A., Y. Rojas, V. Capdevila, O. González and W. Almaguer-Melian, Stimulation of the basolateral amygdala improves the acquisition of a motor skill (2) 115–121
Bittl, P., see Glocker, D. (4–6) 303–317
Blyth, B., see Bazarian, J.J. (3) 163–172
Boisson, D., see Luauté, J. (4–6) 409–418
Bowen, A., see Lincoln, N.B. (4–6) 401–408
Brelén, M.E., see Duret, F. (1) 31–40
Brenner, M.J., see Keune, J.D. (3) 181–190
Brozzoli, C., M.L. Dematté, F. Pavani, F. Frassinetti and A. Farnè, Neglect and extinction: Within and between sensory modalities (4–6) 217–232
Bublak, P., P. Redel and K. Finke, Spatial and non-spatial attention deficits in neurodegenerative diseases: Assessment based on Bundesen's theory of visual attention (TVA) (4–6) 287–301

Bunge, M.B., see Moon, L.D.F. (3) 147–161
Butler, B., see Eskes, G.A. (4–6) 385–398
Byler, S.L., M.C. Shaffer and T.M. Barth, Unilateral pallidotomy produces motor deficits and excesses in rats (3) 133–145
Byun, W.M., see Jang, S.H. (1) 25–29

Capdevila, V., see Bergado, J.A. (2) 115–121
Carey, J.R., F. Fregni and A. Pascual-Leone, rTMS combined with motor learning training in healthy subjects (3) 191–199
Carlson, B.M., see Dow, D.E. (1) 41–54
Castiello, U., see Ansuini, C. (4–6) 431–441
Cho, S.-H., see Chung, Y.-J. (3) 173–180
Chung, Y.-J., S.-H. Cho and Y.-H. Lee, Effect of the knee joint tracking training in closed kinetic chain condition for stroke patients (3) 173–180
Courtois-Jacquin, S., see Rode, G. (4–6) 347–356

de Groat, W.C., see Tai, C. (2) 69–78
Delbeke, J., see Duret, F. (1) 31–40
Dematté, M.L., see Brozzoli, C. (4–6) 217–232
Dennis, R.G., see Dow, D.E. (1) 41–54
Dow, D.E., B.M. Carlson, C.A. Hassett, R.G. Dennis and J.A. Faulkner, Electrical stimulation of denervated muscles of rats maintains mass and force, but not recovery following grafting (1) 41–54
Duret, F., M.E. Brelén, V. Lambert, B. Gérard, J. Delbeke and C. Veraart, Object localization, discrimination, and grasping with the optic nerve visual prosthesis (1) 31–40

Eskes, G.A. and B. Butler, Using limb movements to improve spatial neglect: The role of functional electrical stimulation (4–6) 385–398

Farnè, A., see Brozzoli, C. (4–6) 217–232
Faulkner, J.A., see Dow, D.E. (1) 41–54

Federico, F., M.G. Leggio, L. Mandolesi and L. Petrosini, The NMDA receptor antagonist CGS 19755 disrupts recovery following cerebellar lesions (1) 1–7

Fink, G.R., see Sturm, W. (4–6) 371–384

Finke, K., see Bublak, P. (4–6) 287–301

Fox, I.K., see Keune, J.D. (3) 181–190

Frassinetti, F., see Brozzoli, C. (4–6) 217–232

Fregni, F., see Carey, J.R. (3) 191–199

Gage, F.H., see Moon, L.D.F. (3) 147–161

Gérard, B., see Duret, F. (1) 31–40

Glocker, D., P. Bittl and G. Kerkhoff, Construction and psychometric properties of a novel test for body representational neglect (Vest Test) (4–6) 303–317

González, O., see Bergado, J.A. (2) 115–121

Guariglia, C., see Pizzamiglio, L. (4–6) 337–345

Ha, J.S., see Jang, S.H. (2) 65–68

Hämäläinen, H., see Julkunen, L. (2) 123–132

Hagner, A.P., see Thompson, H.J. (2) 109–114

Halligan, P., see Luauté, J. (4–6) 409–418

Han, B.S., see Jang, S.H. (1) 25–29

Hasselblatt, M., see Bazarian, J.J. (3) 163–172

Hassett, C.A., see Dow, D.E. (1) 41–54

Hillered, L., see Kunz, T. (1) 55–63

Hiltunen, J., see Julkunen, L. (2) 123–132

Hunter, D.A., see Keune, J.D. (3) 181–190

Isenmann, S., see Schmeer, C. (2) 79–95

Ishiai, S., What do eye-fixation patterns tell us about unilateral spatial neglect? (4–6) 261–271

Jääskeläinen, S.K., see Julkunen, L. (2) 123–132

Jacquin-Courtois, S., see Luauté, J. (4–6) 409–418

Jang, S.H., S.H. Ahn, J.S. Ha, S.J. Lee, J. Lee and Y.H. Ahn, Peri-infarct reorganization in a patient with corona radiata infarct: A combined study of functional MRI and diffusion tensor image tractography (2) 65–68

Jang, S.H., W.M. Byun, B.S. Han, H.-J. Park, D. Bai, Y.H. Ahn, Y.-H. Kwon and M.Y. Lee, Recovery of a partially damaged corticospinal tract in a patient with intracerebral hemorrhage: A diffusion tensor image study (1) 25–29

Jehkonen, M., M. Laihosalo and J.E. Kettunen, Impact of neglect on functional outcome after stroke – a review of methodological issues and recent research findings (4–6) 209–215

Jolkkonen, J., see Sonninen, R. (1) 17–23

Julkunen, L., O. Tenovuo, V. Vorobyev, J. Hiltunen, M. Teräs, S.K. Jääskeläinen and H. Hämäläinen, Functional brain imaging, clinical and neurophysiological outcome of visual rehabilitation in a chronic stroke patient (2) 123–132

Karbe, H., see Sturm, W. (4–6) 371–384

Keller, I., see Kerkhoff, G. (4–6) 357–369

Kerkhoff, G. and Y. Rossetti, Editorial (4–6) 201–206

Kerkhoff, G., I. Keller, V. Ritter and C. Marquardt, Repetitive optokinetic stimulation induces lasting recovery from visual neglect (4–6) 357–369

Kerkhoff, G., see Glocker, D. (4–6) 303–317

Kettunen, J.E., see Jehkonen, M. (4–6) 209–215

Keune, J.D., M.J. Brenner, K.E. Schwetye, J.W. Yu, I.K. Fox, D.A. Hunter and S.E. Mackinnon, Temporal factors in peripheral nerve reconstruction with suture scaffolds: An experimental study in rodents (3) 181–190

Klos, T., see Rode, G. (4–6) 347–356

Kretz, A., see Schmeer, C. (2) 79–95

Kunz, T., N. Marklund, L. Hillered and E.H. Oliw, Effects of the selective cyclooxygenase-2 inhibitor rofecoxib on cell death following traumatic brain injury in the rat (1) 55–63

Küst, J., see Sturm, W. (4–6) 371–384

Kwon, Y.-H., see Jang, S.H. (1) 25–29

Laihosalo, M., see Jehkonen, M. (4–6) 209–215

Lambert, V., see Duret, F. (1) 31–40

Laubis-Herrmann, U., see Lotze, M. (2) 97–107

Leasure, J.L., see Moon, L.D.F. (3) 147–161

LeBold, D.G., see Thompson, H.J. (2) 109–114

Lee, J., see Jang, S.H. (2) 65–68

Lee, M.Y., see Jang, S.H. (1) 25–29

Lee, S.J., see Jang, S.H. (2) 65–68

Lee, Y.-H., see Chung, Y.-J. (3) 173–180

Leggio, M.G., see Federico, F. (1) 1–7

Lincoln, N.B. and A. Bowen, The need for randomised treatment studies in neglect research (4–6) 401–408

Lotze, M., U. Laubis-Herrmann and H. Topka, Combination of TMS and fMRI reveals a specific pattern of reorganization in M1 in patients after complete spinal cord injury (2) 97–107

Luauté, J., P. Halligan, G. Rode, S. Jacquin-Courtois and D. Boisson, Prism adaptation first among equals in alleviating left neglect: A review (4–6) 409–418

Lusher, D., see Ansuini, C. (4–6) 431–441

Mackinnon, S.E., see Keune, J.D. (3) 181–190
Mandolesi, L., see Federico, F. (1) 1–7
Marklund, N., see Kunz, T. (1) 55–63
Marklund, N., see Thompson, H.J. (2) 109–114
Marquardt, C., see Kerkhoff, G. (4–6) 357–369
Mattingley, J.B., see Snow, J.C. (4–6) 233–245
McIntosh, T.K., see Thompson, H.J. (2) 109–114
Michel, C., Simulating unilateral neglect in normals: Myth or reality? (4–6) 419–430
Moon, L.D.F., J.L. Leasure, F.H. Gage and M.B. Bunge, Motor enrichment sustains hindlimb movement recovered after spinal cord injury and glial transplantation (3) 147–161
Morales, D.M., see Thompson, H.J. (2) 109–114

Oliw, E.H., see Kunz, T. (1) 55–63

Park, H.-J., see Jang, S.H. (1) 25–29
Pascual-Leone, A., see Carey, J.R. (3) 191–199
Pavani, F., see Brozzoli, C. (4–6) 217–232
Pérennou, D., Postural disorders and spatial neglect in stroke patients: A strong association (4–6) 319–334
Perennou, D., see Azouvi, P. (4–6) 273–285
Petrosini, L., see Federico, F. (1) 1–7
Pierno, A.C., see Ansuini, C. (4–6) 431–441
Pisella, L., see Rode, G. (4–6) 347–356
Pizzamiglio, L., C. Guariglia, G. Antonucci and P. Zoccolotti, Development of a rehabilitative program for unilateral neglect (4–6) 337–345
Pradat-Diehl, P., see Azouvi, P. (4–6) 273–285

Redel, P., see Bublak, P. (4–6) 287–301
Ritter, V., see Kerkhoff, G. (4–6) 357–369
Rode, G., see Luauté, J. (4–6) 409–418
Rode, G., T. Klos, S. Courtois-Jacquin, Y. Rossetti and L. Pisella, Neglect and prism adaptation: A new therapeutic tool for spatial cognition disorders (4–6) 347–356
Rojas, Y., see Bergado, J.A. (2) 115–121
Ronchi, R., see Vallar, G. (4–6) 247–257
Roppolo, J.R., see Tai, C. (2) 69–78
Rossetti, Y., see Kerkhoff, G. (4–6) 201–206
Rossetti, Y., see Rode, G. (4–6) 347–356
Rousseaux, M., see Azouvi, P. (4–6) 273–285

Schmeer, C., A. Kretz and S. Isenmann, Statin-mediated protective effects in the central nervous system: General mechanisms and putative role of stress proteins (2) 79–95
Schwetye, K.E., see Keune, J.D. (3) 181–190
Shaffer, M.C., see Byler, S.L. (3) 133–145
Sivenius, J., see Sonninen, R. (1) 17–23
Snow, J.C. and J.B. Mattingley, Stimulus- and goal-driven biases of selective attention following unilateral brain damage: Implications for rehabilitation of spatial neglect and extinction (4–6) 233–245
Sonninen, R., T. Virtanen, J. Sivenius and J. Jolkkonen, Gene expression profiling in the hippocampus of rats subjected to focal cerebral ischemia and enriched environment housing (1) 17–23
Sturm, W., M. Thimm, J. Küst, H. Karbe and G.R. Fink, Alertness-training in neglect: Behavioral and imaging results (4–6) 371–384

Tai, C., J.R. Roppolo and W.C. de Groat, Spinal reflex control of micturition after spinal cord injury (2) 69–78
Taupin, P., Adult neurogenesis and neuroplasticity (1) 9–15
Tenovuo, O., see Julkunen, L. (2) 123–132
Teräs, M., see Julkunen, L. (2) 123–132
Thimm, M., see Sturm, W. (4–6) 371–384
Thompson, H.J., D.G. LeBold, N. Marklund, D.M. Morales, A.P. Hagner and T.K. McIntosh, Cognitive evaluation of traumatically brain-injured rats using serial testing in the Morris water maze (2) 109–114
Topka, H., see Lotze, M. (2) 97–107

Vallar, G. and R. Ronchi, Anosognosia for motor and sensory deficits after unilateral brain damage: A review (4–6) 247–257
Veraart, C., see Duret, F. (1) 31–40
Virtanen, T., see Sonninen, R. (1) 17–23
von Ahsen, N., see Bazarian, J.J. (3) 163–172
Vorobyev, V., see Julkunen, L. (2) 123–132

Yu, J.W., see Keune, J.D. (3) 181–190

Zoccolotti, P., see Pizzamiglio, L. (4–6) 337–345

Alzheimer's Disease: A Century of Scientific and Clinical Research

New IOS Press Book

This landmark book commemorates the centennial of Alois Alzheimer's original description of the disease that would come to bear his name and offers a vantage point from which to revisit and reflect on the seminal discoveries in the field. It brings to life the classic studies that have essentially defined Alzheimer's disease research.

This milestone work has been guided by four of the most prominent voices in the field today. It traces how the true importance of AD as the major cause of late life dementia ultimately came to light and narrates the evolution of the concepts related to AD throughout the years and its recognition as a major public health problem, with an estimated 30-40 million people affected by AD today.

Attendees of the 10th International Conference on Alzheimer's Disease and Related Disorders, Madrid, July 15-20, 2006 receive a softcover copy of this book with the compliments of GlaxoSmithKline.

The book covers:
- Historical Perspective
- Neuropathology
- Synaptic Changes
- Amyloid
- Tau
- Disease Mechanisms
- Genetics
- Genetics
- Diagnosis and Treatment

Edited by:

George Perry
Dean of the University of Texas at San Antonio College of Sciences
Professor of Pathology and Neurosciences, Case Western Reserve University
Editor-in-Chief, Journal of Alzheimer's Disease

Jesús Avila
Center for Molecular Biology, University Autónoma of Madrid
Senior Editor, Journal of Alzheimer's Disease

June Kinoshita
Executive Editor, Alzheimer Research Forum

Mark A. Smith
Department of Pathology, Case Western Reserve University
Co-Editor-in-Chief, Journal of Alzheimer's Disease

These writings bring to the practitioner, student and interested lay person a perspective not only on the past, but also on where the Alzheimer's disease field is likely to go in the future. Only time will tell whether these milestones have charted the future accurately, but they are unquestionably the foundation upon which the future will be built.

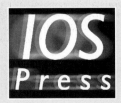

July 2006, 468 pp., hardcover
ISBN: 1-58603-619-x
Price: US$150 / €120 / £82

www.j-alz.com   www.iospress.nl